Applications of Nanomaterials in Biomedical Imaging and Cancer Therapy II

Applications of Nanomaterials in Biomedical Imaging and Cancer Therapy II

James C. L. Chow

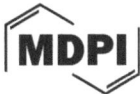

Basel • Beijing • Wuhan • Barcelona • Belgrade • Novi Sad • Cluj • Manchester

Editor
James C. L. Chow
Department of Radiation Oncology
University of Toronto
Toronto
Canada

Editorial Office
MDPI AG
Grosspeteranlage 5
4052 Basel, Switzerland

This is a reprint of articles from the Special Issue published online in the open access journal *Nanomaterials* (ISSN 2079-4991) (available at: www.mdpi.com/journal/nanomaterials/special_issues/Biomedical_Imaging_II).

For citation purposes, cite each article independently as indicated on the article page online and as indicated below:

Lastname, A.A.; Lastname, B.B. Article Title. *Journal Name* **Year**, *Volume Number*, Page Range.

ISBN 978-3-7258-2410-6 (Hbk)
ISBN 978-3-7258-2409-0 (PDF)
doi.org/10.3390/books978-3-7258-2409-0

© 2024 by the authors. Articles in this book are Open Access and distributed under the Creative Commons Attribution (CC BY) license. The book as a whole is distributed by MDPI under the terms and conditions of the Creative Commons Attribution-NonCommercial-NoDerivs (CC BY-NC-ND) license.

Contents

About the Editor vii

James C. L. Chow
Application of Nanomaterials in Biomedical Imaging and Cancer Therapy II
Reprinted from: *Nanomaterials* **2024**, *14*, 1627, doi:10.3390/nano14201627 1

Hayden Carlton, Nageshwar Arepally, Sean Healy, Anirudh Sharma, Sarah Ptashnik and Maureen Schickel et al.
Magnetic Particle Imaging-Guided Thermal Simulations for Magnetic Particle Hyperthermia
Reprinted from: *Nanomaterials* **2024**, *14*, 1059, doi:10.3390/nano14121059 4

Reju George Thomas, Subin Kim, Thi-Anh-Thuy Tran, Young Hee Kim, Raveena Nagareddy and Tae-Young Jung et al.
Magnet-Guided Temozolomide and Ferucarbotran Loaded Nanoparticles to Enhance Therapeutic Efficacy in Glioma Model
Reprinted from: *Nanomaterials* **2024**, *14*, 939, doi:10.3390/nano14110939 19

M. A. Ruiz-Robles, Francisco J. Solís-Pomar, Gabriela Travieso Aguilar, Maykel Márquez Mijares, Raine Garrido Arteaga and Olivia Martínez Armenteros et al.
Physico-Chemical Properties of CdTe/Glutathione Quantum Dots Obtained by Microwave Irradiation for Use in Monoclonal Antibody and Biomarker Testing
Reprinted from: *Nanomaterials* **2024**, *14*, 684, doi:10.3390/nano14080684 34

Melani Fuentealba, Alejandro Ferreira, Apolo Salgado, Christopher Vergara, Sergio Díez and Mauricio Santibáñez
An Optimized Method for Evaluating the Potential Gd-Nanoparticle Dose Enhancement Produced by Electronic Brachytherapy
Reprinted from: *Nanomaterials* **2024**, *14*, 430, doi:10.3390/nano14050430 52

Michael S. Petronek, Nahom Teferi, Chu-Yu Lee, Vincent A. Magnotta and Bryan G. Allen
MRI Detection and Therapeutic Enhancement of Ferumoxytol Internalization in Glioblastoma Cells
Reprinted from: *Nanomaterials* **2024**, *14*, 189, doi:10.3390/nano14020189 66

Barbara Wenzel, Maximilian Schmid, Rodrigo Teodoro, Rareş-Petru Moldovan, Thu Hang Lai and Franziska Mitrach et al.
Radiofluorination of an Anionic, Azide-Functionalized Teroligomer by Copper-Catalyzed Azide-Alkyne Cycloaddition
Reprinted from: *Nanomaterials* **2023**, *13*, 2095, doi:10.3390/nano13142095 76

Vincenzo Patamia, Chiara Zagni, Roberto Fiorenza, Virginia Fuochi, Sandro Dattilo and Paolo Maria Riccobene et al.
Total Bio-Based Material for Drug Delivery and Iron Chelation to Fight Cancer through Antimicrobial Activity
Reprinted from: *Nanomaterials* **2023**, *13*, 2036, doi:10.3390/nano13142036 91

Tainah Dorina Marforio, Edoardo Jun Mattioli, Francesco Zerbetto and Matteo Calvaresi
Exploiting Blood Transport Proteins as Carborane Supramolecular Vehicles for Boron Neutron Capture Therapy
Reprinted from: *Nanomaterials* **2023**, *13*, 1770, doi:10.3390/nano13111770 103

Radek Ostruszka, Denisa Půlpánová, Tomáš Pluháček, Ondřej Tomanec, Petr Novák and Daniel Jirák et al.
Facile One-Pot Green Synthesis of Magneto-Luminescent Bimetallic Nanocomposites with Potential as Dual Imaging Agent
Reprinted from: *Nanomaterials* **2023**, *13*, 1027, doi:10.3390/nano13061027 123

André Q. Figueiredo, Carolina F. Rodrigues, Natanael Fernandes, Duarte de Melo-Diogo, Ilídio J. Correia and André F. Moreira
Metal-Polymer Nanoconjugates Application in Cancer Imaging and Therapy
Reprinted from: *Nanomaterials* **2022**, *12*, 3166, doi:10.3390/nano12183166 138

Afia Sadiq and James C. L. Chow
Evaluation of Dosimetric Effect of Bone Scatter on Nanoparticle-Enhanced Orthovoltage Radiotherapy: A Monte Carlo Phantom Study
Reprinted from: *Nanomaterials* **2022**, *12*, 2991, doi:10.3390/nano12172991 161

Sarkar Siddique and James C. L. Chow
Recent Advances in Functionalized Nanoparticles in Cancer Theranostics
Reprinted from: *Nanomaterials* **2022**, *12*, 2826, doi:10.3390/nano12162826 173

Yuanfei Lu, Na Feng, Yongzhong Du and Risheng Yu
Nanoparticle-Based Therapeutics to Overcome Obstacles in the Tumor Microenvironment of Hepatocellular Carcinoma
Reprinted from: *Nanomaterials* **2022**, *12*, 2832, doi:10.3390/nano12162832 189

About the Editor

James C. L. Chow

James Chow is a Medical Physicist at the Princess Margaret Cancer Centre and an Associate Professor at the Department of Radiation Oncology at the University of Toronto. He is also a Clinician Investigator at the Princess Margaret Cancer Research Institute, an Associate Member of the Temerty Centre for AI Research and Education in Medicine, and an Affiliate Member of the Acceleration Consortium at the University of Toronto. In addition to being a Fellow of the Canadian College of Physicists in Medicine in Canada (FCCPM), a Fellow at the Institution of Engineering and Technology (FIET), and a Fellow in the Institute of Physics (FInstP) in the UK, James is also a Senior Member of the Institute of Electrical and Electronics Engineers (SMIEEE) in the USA. James is a Certified Medical Physicist in Canada, a Professional Physicist in Canada (PPhys), a Chartered Physicist in the UK (CPhys), and a Chartered Scientist (CSci) in the UK. His research interests span a diverse array of areas, including medical physics, radiotherapy, nanotechnology, computer simulation, machine learning/large language models, radiation dosimetry, and quantum computing.

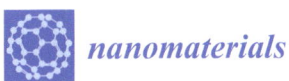

Editorial

Application of Nanomaterials in Biomedical Imaging and Cancer Therapy II

James C. L. Chow [1,2]

1. Radiation Medicine Program, Princess Margaret Cancer Centre, University Health Network, Toronto, ON M5G 1X6, Canada; james.chow@uhn.ca
2. Department of Radiation Oncology, University of Toronto, Toronto, ON M5T 1P5, Canada

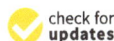

Citation: Chow, J.C.L. Application of Nanomaterials in Biomedical Imaging and Cancer Therapy II. *Nanomaterials* **2024**, *14*, 1627. https://doi.org/10.3390/nano14201627

Received: 12 September 2024
Accepted: 22 September 2024
Published: 11 October 2024

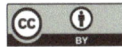

Copyright: © 2024 by the author. Licensee MDPI, Basel, Switzerland. This article is an open access article distributed under the terms and conditions of the Creative Commons Attribution (CC BY) license (https://creativecommons.org/licenses/by/4.0/).

Following the successful publication of the first edition of our Special Issue entitled "Application of Nanomaterials in Biomedical Imaging and Cancer Therapy" [1], we are pleased to present this second edition, which continues to explore cutting-edge advances in the application of nanomaterials for cancer imaging and therapy. Nanotechnology has emerged as a transformative tool in oncology, offering novel solutions for diagnosis, treatment, and theranostics [2]. In this edition, we focus on the integration of nanoparticles in cancer research, addressing key challenges such as treatment specificity, overcoming biological barriers, and enhancing the effectiveness of traditional therapies. The selected studies provide valuable insights into the development of multifunctional nanocomposites, the design of nanoparticle-based drug delivery systems, and innovations in imaging modalities and radiotherapy dose enhancement. This Special Issue aims to advance our understanding of how nanomaterials can be harnessed to improve cancer treatment outcomes and pave the way for clinical translation, while addressing challenges such as biocompatibility, stability, and safety. We hope this collection serves as a valuable resource for researchers and clinicians alike, pushing the frontiers of nanotechnology in cancer care.

Studies on nanoparticle-based imaging and therapeutic applications present a wide range of innovative approaches. Carlton et al. [3] introduce a clinically translatable protocol using Magnetic Particle Imaging (MPI) to guide thermal simulations for Magnetic Particle Hyperthermia (MPH), enhancing treatment planning accuracy. Thomas et al. [4] demonstrate the efficacy of magnet-guided liposomal nanoparticles loaded with temozolomide and ferucarbotran in glioma treatment, overcoming blood–brain barrier challenges while improving imaging and therapy. Petronek et al. [5] further explore MR-based nanotheranostics by using ferumoxytol and pharmacological ascorbate (AscH−) for glioblastoma treatment, highlighting increased toxicity when ferumoxytol is internalized in cancer cells.

Nanoparticles are also employed to enhance imaging techniques. Ostruszka et al. [6] develop a green synthesis method for magneto-luminescent bimetallic nanocomposites (AuNCs-BSA-SPIONs) as dual imaging agents, combining luminescence and MRI contrast for potential clinical use. Wenzel et al. [7] describe the radiofluorination of an amphiphilic teroligomer for stabilizing siRNA-loaded calcium phosphate nanoparticles, enabling PET imaging of brain tumors and providing a tool for tracking nanoparticle distribution.

Theranostic applications in cancer therapy are highlighted by Ruiz-Robles et al. [8], who report the synthesis and characterization of CdTe quantum dots for precise monoclonal antibody and biomarker testing in cellular labeling. Fuentealba et al. [9] present an optimized method for evaluating Gd-nanoparticle dose enhancement in electronic brachytherapy, emphasizing the importance of K-edge interactions in enhancing radiation dose.

Sadiq et al. [10] take a dosimetric approach, using Monte Carlo simulations to study the impact of bone scatter on dose enhancement in nanoparticle-enhanced orthovoltage radiotherapy. Their findings indicate significant underestimation of dose enhancement when bone presence is neglected, particularly at higher nanoparticle concentrations.

From a materials science perspective, Patamia et al. [11] combine halloysite nanotubes with kojic acid to create an antibacterial nanomaterial capable of drug delivery, demonstrating a bio-based approach to antimicrobial cancer therapy. Marforio et al. [12] focus on overcoming the hydrophobicity of carboranes for Boron Neutron Capture Therapy (BNCT) by utilizing blood transport proteins as carriers.

In the realm of reviews, Figueiredo et al. [13] examine metal–polymer nanoconjugates in cancer imaging and therapy, noting that while metallic nanoparticles have unique properties, combining them with polymers enhances biocompatibility, stability, and tumor specificity. Lu et al. [14] review nanoparticle-based therapies targeting the tumor microenvironment (TME) in hepatocellular carcinoma (HCC), addressing the challenges of short drug retention and providing insights into the future of TME-targeting nanomedicine. Siddique et al. [15] highlight advances in functionalized nanoparticles for cancer theranostics, focusing on MRI-guided therapies and photothermal treatments, and discussing their potential to revolutionize personalized cancer care.

The studies presented in this Special Issue underscore significant advancements in the use of nanomaterials for cancer imaging, therapy, and theranostics, offering innovative solutions for more personalized and targeted treatments. These contributions highlight the development of dual-functional nanocomposites for improved imaging and treatment precision, the integration of nanoparticles to overcome challenges like drug retention and the blood–brain barrier, and the critical role of accurate dosimetric planning in radiotherapy. Moreover, the reviews on metal–polymer nanoconjugates, tumor-microenvironment-targeting nanoparticles, and functionalized nanoparticles for theranostics emphasize the potential of these nanomaterials to enhance therapeutic specificity, biocompatibility, and multifunctionality. Together, these findings pave the way for future clinical applications of nanotechnology in cancer care, while addressing ongoing challenges like toxicity, stability, and effective translation to clinical settings.

Funding: This research received no external funding.

Data Availability Statement: Not applicable.

Acknowledgments: The author extends sincere gratitude to all of the contributors and editors of this Special Issue for their invaluable efforts and dedication.

Conflicts of Interest: The author declares no conflicts of interest.

References

1. Chow, J.C. Application of nanomaterials in biomedical imaging and cancer therapy. *Nanomaterials* **2022**, *12*, 726. [CrossRef] [PubMed]
2. Siddique, S.; Chow, J.C. Application of nanomaterials in biomedical imaging and cancer therapy. *Nanomaterials* **2020**, *10*, 1700. [CrossRef] [PubMed]
3. Carlton, H.; Arepally, N.; Healy, S.; Sharma, A.; Ptashnik, S.; Schickel, M.; Newgren, M.; Goodwill, P.; Attaluri, A.; Ivkov, R. Magnetic Particle Imaging-Guided Thermal Simulations for Magnetic Particle Hyperthermia. *Nanomaterials* **2024**, *14*, 1059. [CrossRef] [PubMed]
4. Thomas, R.G.; Kim, S.; Tran, T.A.; Kim, Y.H.; Nagareddy, R.; Jung, T.Y.; Kim, S.K.; Jeong, Y.Y. Magnet-Guided Temozolomide and Ferucarbotran Loaded Nanoparticles to Enhance Therapeutic Efficacy in Glioma Model. *Nanomaterials* **2024**, *14*, 939. [CrossRef] [PubMed]
5. Petronek, M.S.; Teferi, N.; Lee, C.Y.; Magnotta, V.A.; Allen, B.G. MRI Detection and Therapeutic Enhancement of Ferumoxytol Internalization in Glioblastoma Cells. *Nanomaterials* **2024**, *14*, 189. [CrossRef] [PubMed]
6. Ostruszka, R.; Půlpánová, D.; Pluháček, T.; Tomanec, O.; Novák, P.; Jirák, D.; Šišková, K. Facile One-Pot Green Synthesis of Magneto-Luminescent Bimetallic Nanocomposites with Potential as Dual Imaging Agent. *Nanomaterials* **2023**, *13*, 1027. [CrossRef] [PubMed]
7. Wenzel, B.; Schmid, M.; Teodoro, R.; Moldovan, R.P.; Lai, T.H.; Mitrach, F.; Kopka, K.; Fischer, B.; Schulz-Siegmund, M.; Brust, P.; et al. Radiofluorination of an Anionic, Azide-Functionalized Teroligomer by Copper-Catalyzed Azide-Alkyne Cycloaddition. *Nanomaterials* **2023**, *13*, 2095. [CrossRef] [PubMed]

8. Ruiz-Robles, M.A.; Solís-Pomar, F.J.; Travieso Aguilar, G.; Márquez Mijares, M.; Garrido Arteaga, R.; Martínez Armenteros, O.; Gutiérrez-Lazos, C.D.; Pérez-Tijerina, E.G.; Fundora Cruz, A. Physico-Chemical Properties of CdTe/Glutathione Quantum Dots Obtained by Microwave Irradiation for Use in Monoclonal Antibody and Biomarker Testing. *Nanomaterials* **2024**, *14*, 684. [CrossRef] [PubMed]
9. Fuentealba, M.; Ferreira, A.; Salgado, A.; Vergara, C.; Díez, S.; Santibáñez, M. An Optimized Method for Evaluating the Potential Gd-Nanoparticle Dose Enhancement Produced by Electronic Brachytherapy. *Nanomaterials* **2024**, *14*, 430. [CrossRef] [PubMed]
10. Sadiq, A.; Chow, J.C. Evaluation of dosimetric effect of bone scatter on nanoparticle-enhanced orthovoltage radiotherapy: A Monte Carlo phantom study. *Nanomaterials* **2022**, *12*, 2991. [CrossRef] [PubMed]
11. Patamia, V.; Zagni, C.; Fiorenza, R.; Fuochi, V.; Dattilo, S.; Riccobene, P.M.; Furneri, P.M.; Floresta, G.; Rescifina, A. Total Bio-Based Material for Drug Delivery and Iron Chelation to Fight Cancer through Antimicrobial Activity. *Nanomaterials* **2023**, *13*, 2036. [CrossRef] [PubMed]
12. Marforio, T.D.; Mattioli, E.J.; Zerbetto, F.; Calvaresi, M. Exploiting blood transport proteins as carborane supramolecular vehicles for boron neutron capture therapy. *Nanomaterials* **2023**, *13*, 1770. [CrossRef] [PubMed]
13. Figueiredo, A.Q.; Rodrigues, C.F.; Fernandes, N.; de Melo-Diogo, D.; Correia, I.J.; Moreira, A.F. Metal-polymer nanoconjugates application in cancer imaging and therapy. *Nanomaterials* **2022**, *12*, 3166. [CrossRef] [PubMed]
14. Lu, Y.; Feng, N.; Du, Y.; Yu, R. Nanoparticle-based therapeutics to overcome obstacles in the tumor microenvironment of hepatocellular carcinoma. *Nanomaterials* **2022**, *12*, 2832. [CrossRef] [PubMed]
15. Siddique, S.; Chow, J.C. Recent advances in functionalized nanoparticles in cancer theranostics. *Nanomaterials* **2022**, *12*, 2826. [CrossRef] [PubMed]

Disclaimer/Publisher's Note: The statements, opinions and data contained in all publications are solely those of the individual author(s) and contributor(s) and not of MDPI and/or the editor(s). MDPI and/or the editor(s) disclaim responsibility for any injury to people or property resulting from any ideas, methods, instructions or products referred to in the content.

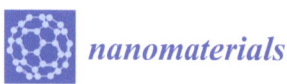

Article

Magnetic Particle Imaging-Guided Thermal Simulations for Magnetic Particle Hyperthermia

Hayden Carlton [1], Nageshwar Arepally [2], Sean Healy [1], Anirudh Sharma [1], Sarah Ptashnik [3], Maureen Schickel [3], Matt Newgren [4], Patrick Goodwill [4], Anilchandra Attaluri [2] and Robert Ivkov [1,5,6,7,*]

1. Department of Radiation Oncology and Molecular Radiation Sciences, The Johns Hopkins University School of Medicine, Baltimore, MD 21205, USA; hcarlto1@jhmi.edu (H.C.); shealy7@gatech.edu (S.H.); asharm55@jhmi.edu (A.S.)
2. Department of Mechanical Engineering, School of Science, Engineering, and Technology, The Pennsylvania State University—Harrisburg, Middletown, PA 17057, USA; nageshwar25150@gmail.com (N.A.); aua473@psu.edu (A.A.)
3. Materialise NV, 3001 Leuven, Belgium; sarah.ptashnik@materialise.com (S.P.); schickel.1@outlook.com (M.S.)
4. Magnetic Insight Inc., Alameda, CA 94502, USA; mnewgren@magneticinsight.com (M.N.); goodwill@magneticinsight.com (P.G.)
5. Department of Oncology, Sydney Kimmel Comprehensive Cancer Center, School of Medicine, Johns Hopkins University, Baltimore, MD 21205, USA
6. Department of Mechanical Engineering, Whiting School of Engineering, Johns Hopkins University, Baltimore, MD 21218, USA
7. Department of Materials Science and Engineering, Whiting School of Engineering, Johns Hopkins University, Baltimore, MD 21218, USA
* Correspondence: rivkov1@jhmi.edu

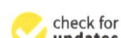

Citation: Carlton, H.; Arepally, N.; Healy, S.; Sharma, A.; Ptashnik, S.; Schickel, M.; Newgren, M.; Goodwill, P.; Attaluri, A.; Ivkov, R. Magnetic Particle Imaging-Guided Thermal Simulations for Magnetic Particle Hyperthermia. *Nanomaterials* 2024, *14*, 1059. https://doi.org/10.3390/nano14121059

Academic Editor: James Chow

Received: 20 April 2024
Revised: 13 June 2024
Accepted: 17 June 2024
Published: 20 June 2024

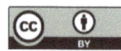

Copyright: © 2024 by the authors. Licensee MDPI, Basel, Switzerland. This article is an open access article distributed under the terms and conditions of the Creative Commons Attribution (CC BY) license (https://creativecommons.org/licenses/by/4.0/).

Abstract: Magnetic particle hyperthermia (MPH) enables the direct heating of solid tumors with alternating magnetic fields (AMFs). One challenge with MPH is the unknown particle distribution in tissue after injection. Magnetic particle imaging (MPI) can measure the nanoparticle content and distribution in tissue after delivery. The objective of this study was to develop a clinically translatable protocol that incorporates MPI data into finite element calculations for simulating tissue temperatures during MPH. To verify the protocol, we conducted MPH experiments in tumor-bearing mouse cadavers. Five 8–10-week-old female BALB/c mice bearing subcutaneous 4T1 tumors were anesthetized and received intratumor injections of Synomag®-S90 nanoparticles. Immediately following injection, the mice were euthanized and imaged, and the tumors were heated with an AMF. We used the Mimics Innovation Suite to create a 3D mesh of the tumor from micro-computerized tomography data and spatial index MPI to generate a scaled heating function for the heat transfer calculations. The processed imaging data were incorporated into a finite element solver, COMSOL Multiphysics®. The upper and lower bounds of the simulated tumor temperatures for all five cadavers demonstrated agreement with the experimental temperature measurements, thus verifying the protocol. These results demonstrate the utility of MPI to guide predictive thermal calculations for MPH treatment planning.

Keywords: magnetic nanoparticles; magnetic particle imaging; magnetic hyperthermia; image guidance; finite element analysis

1. Introduction

Magnetic particle hyperthermia (MPH) is an interstitial thermal therapy approved for treating recurrent glioblastoma with external beam radiation therapy [1]. First proposed in the mid-20th century, clinical MPH involves the intratumor delivery of magnetic nanoparticles (MNPs), which are heated via magnetic hysteresis loss by exposing the region to an alternating magnetic field (AMF) [2]. The magnetocaloric effect has garnered interest for applications in hyperthermia; however, it is prominent in doped manganite magnetic materials and not magnetite/maghemite [3]. For hyperthermia, treatment effectiveness requires the control of thermal energy to heat the tumor to a mild temperature (41–45 °C) for a prescribed time while minimizing the temperature rise in normal tissue. The duration of exposure at an elevated temperature (or "time-at-temperature") defines the thermal dose [4], which is often expressed by the isoeffect dose metric cumulative equivalent minutes of exposure referenced against 43 °C (CEM43), close to the thermal breakpoint temperature (42.5 °C) of human cells [5,6]. Depending on the thermal dose (typically >15 min), hyperthermia can sensitize cells to radiation [7–9] or chemotherapy [10,11], increase blood perfusion to reduce tumor hypoxia [12–14], stimulate anti-tumor immune signaling [15–17], or it can be directly cytotoxic [18].

While MPH offers substantial advantages for intervention, technical challenges continue to inhibit wider clinical acceptance. Among these, an inability to accurately measure the MNP concentration and its distribution in tissues presents barriers to developing reliable MPH clinical workflows that provide adequate quality assurance measures to compare the delivered thermal doses with the initial prescriptive treatment plan [19]. As sources of heat, the nanoparticle content and distribution determine the thermal dose for MPH; therefore, knowing these in both tumor and surrounding tissues becomes essential when addressing the clinical requirements for reliability and quality in patient care. Previous efforts to quantify the nanoparticles' distribution have relied on the analyses of computerized tomography (CT) scans [1,20], but there are some limitations. Foremost, the CT signal from the MNPs must be differentiated from the tissue signal; this can prove difficult for intratumor concentrations of less than ~10 g/L [1,19,21].

Magnetic particle imaging (MPI) [22] is a tracer imaging modality that measures time-varying responses of the magnetization vector of a sample and offers advantages for MPH over anatomical imaging. Early efforts demonstrated that the MPI signal correlated with the intratumor nanoparticle content, which can be used to predict a temperature rise when a region is exposed to AMFs [23]. These initial studies were extended to demonstrate how MPI can be used to monitor changes in MNP distribution after MPH [24]. Further advances integrated MPI with an AMF heater and used the MPI gradient field to restrict heating to a particular area within the AMF coil [25,26]. One group developed a computational model for predicting the spatio-thermal resolution of combined MPI/MPH systems [27]. A fully automated prototype AMF heating platform that enables spatially confined heating in a user-selected region of interest has also been described [28]. Buchholz et al. integrated MPI/MPH functionality into a platform that included MPI-based thermometry to monitor safety [29]; the same group also discussed proposed hyperthermia platforms that can integrate with commercial MPI scanners [30].

The technology exists to implement MPI-guided MPH; however, we must be able to incorporate MPI data into predictive thermal simulations to accurately estimate the intratumor temperature. Finite element (FEM) and finite difference methods (FDM) applications are available for other hyperthermia modalities. In those cases, the software enables the user to estimate the thermal dose within specified volumes to create thermal dose contours of the tumor and margins [31,32]. Treatment planning applications for hyperthermia include HyperPlan [33–35], SEMCAD X [36,37], and Plan2Heat [38,39]. In some cases, commercial finite element analysis (FEA) applications have been validated for hyperthermia [40]. We have previously validated COMSOL Multiphysics® for preclinical MPH [41]. Lacking in those previous efforts was a direct knowledge of the MNP distribution in tissue or a tissue-mimicking phantom [42]. MNP distribution in tumors and surrounding tissue is subject to considerable individual variability, irrespective of the method used to deliver MNPs [9]. This fact is understudied and often underappreciated, yet it can be a singular source of uncertainty and unreliability in predictive computations of tissue temperature with MPH. It thus becomes essential to develop robust methods to ascertain the MNP tissue content and distribution in each tumor after delivery. Previous work demonstrated integrating MPI data into heat transfer simulations; however, approaches and experimental verification were limited [43,44]. Here, we describe the results of an effort to develop and verify a clinically translatable thermal simulation workflow that uses 3D MPI data as input for finite element computations to predict tumor temperature during a simulated MPH (Figure 1). To process the MPI and micro CT data, we used an imaging-data processing suite that has clinical utility. Verification was achieved by comparing temperatures measured from tumors in mouse cadavers that were heated by AMF-activated MNPs with predicted temperatures of simulated MPHs, where we used experimental temperature data as the initial and boundary conditions for the simulations.

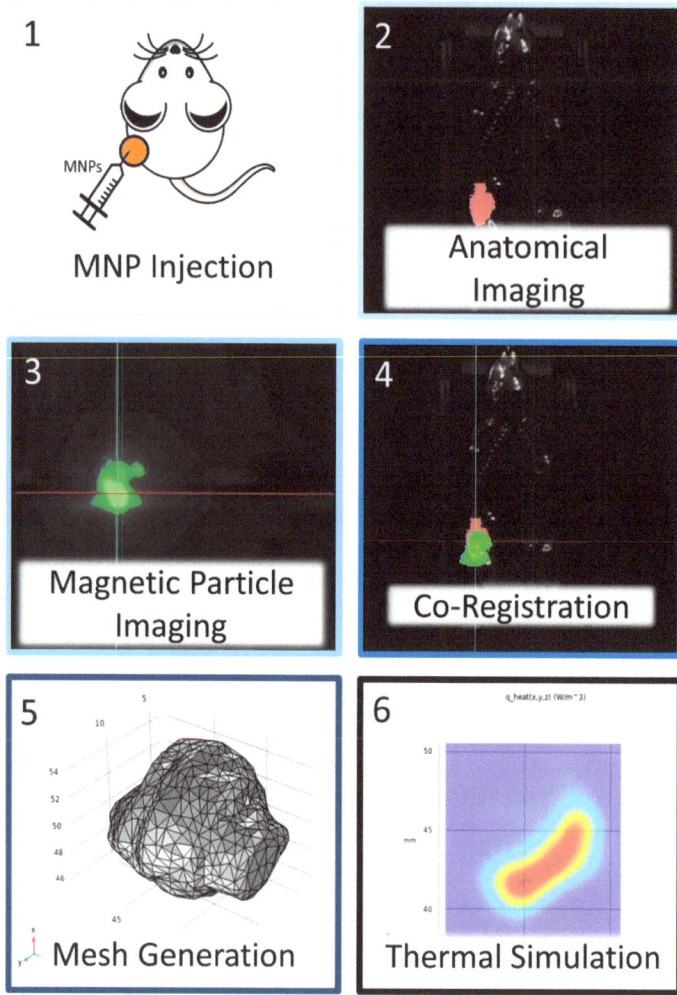

Figure 1. Schematic representation of workflow for magnetic particle imaging (MPI)-guided thermal simulations. Magnetic nanoparticles (MNPs) at a pre-determined dose were injected intratumorally. After MNP injection, the tumor was imaged with both MPI and microCT for anatomical reference. Using fiducial markers, the MPI data were co-registered with anatomical images to establish a common datum. The tumor geometry was segmented, converted to a 3D part, and volume-meshed and imported into FEA software (COMSOL Multiphysics 6.2); additionally, voxel intensities obtained from the MPI scan were converted into volumetric thermal output values from a calibration curve developed using measured MNP heating data. With the MPI values spatially registered and calibrated for heat output, the FEA simulation was performed.

2. Materials and Methods

2.1. Postmortem Animal Studies

2.1.1. Mouse Models

All animal study procedures were conducted according to the protocol approved by the Johns Hopkins University Animal Care and Use Committee (JHU ACUC). The project/protocol identification number is not publicly available due to the JHU institutional policy and can be provided on request from the corresponding author. Five 8–10-week-old female BALB/c mice (Jackson Laboratory, Bar Harbor, ME, USA) were used. All mice were fed a normal diet and water ad libitum, maintained at a 12 h light/12 h dark cycle, and monitored daily for signs of distress or pain.

2.1.2. Cell Line and Tumor Implantation

A vial of the 4T1 murine mammary carcinoma cell line [ER/PR/HER2 negative] was purchased from the American Type Culture Collection (ATCC, Manassas, VA, USA) and maintained according to the supplier's recommendations. Roswell Park Memorial Institute (RPMI) 1640 media with 10% heat-inactivated fetal bovine serum (FBS) was used to grow the cells. For each mouse, approximately 50,000 cells were suspended in 100 µL of PBS and injected subcutaneously into the right thigh. Once the tumors were palpable, we measured them daily using calipers until they reached a volume between 100–500 mm^3.

2.1.3. MNPs

Hydroxyethyl starch-coated Synomag®-S90 iron oxide (mixture of magnetite and maghemite) nanoparticles (Lot #: 14422105–01; micromod Partikeltechnologie GmbH, Rostock, Germany) suspended in water and 50 mg of Fe/mL were used as received [45]. Photon correlation spectroscopy data from the manufacturer indicated a z-average diameter of 109.8 nm with a polydispersity index of 0.092. The particle concentration was verified using a Ferene-s assay [46]. In brief, we first digested the nanoparticles in an acetate buffer with ascorbic acid for at least 20 h. The iron concentration was determined by comparison with reference standards using UV/vis spectrophotometry. The heating rate of the MNPs was estimated using our previously published transient pulse analysis and was reported as specific loss power (SLP) [47]. A sample of nanoparticles at a concentration of 1 mg of Fe/mL H$_2$O was heated at a peak AMF amplitude of 15 mT and at 50% duty (60 s ON/60 s OFF). Each pulse was analyzed and fitted to a non-adiabatic lumped mass heat transfer model, from which the SLP was calculated.

2.1.4. Intratumor MNP Injections

For the MNP dose (i.e., MNP mass) calculation, we used a heat transfer approach to model the MNPs as a spherical uniform heat source [48–50] to identify the minimum concentration (c) needed to increase the temperature, ΔT, of a tumor having radius R (Equation (1)):

$$c = \frac{3 \Delta T k}{SLP \times R^2}. \tag{1}$$

Here, k is the isotropic coefficient of the thermal conductivity of the tumor. Using the measured SLP (496 ± 28 W/g) for the nanoparticle lot used (Figure S4) and assuming idealized conditions, we estimated the minimum MNP concentration required to raise the temperature of a tumor having radius $R = 0.5$ cm and $k = 0.6$ W/(m°C) from 37 °C to 43 °C (Equation (2)):

$$c = \frac{3 \times 6°C \times 0.6 \frac{W}{m°C}}{496 \frac{W}{g} \times (0.005 m)^2} = 0.870 \frac{mgFe}{mLTumor}. \tag{2}$$

Then, we adjusted the injection volume and concentration to achieve a target intratumor concentration of ~2 mg Fe/mL tumor to compensate for particle loss and heterogeneous intratumor distribution. Tumor size, for dose determination, was measured with calipers, and the MNP injected volume was adjusted to achieve 2 mg of Fe/mL tumor concentration (Table 1).

Table 1. Tumor sizes were measured with calipers and associated MNP injection volume.

Sample	Caliper Measured Tumor Volume (mm^3)	MNP Injection Volume (μL) @ 50 mg Fe/mL
Tumor 1	144	5.6
Tumor 2	193	7.7
Tumor 3	280	11.2
Tumor 4	355	14.2
Tumor 5	455	18.2

Mice were anesthetized via inhalation of 1–2% isoflurane mixed with O$_2$ delivered through a nose cone. The nose cone remained in place for the duration of the MNP injection. MNPs were injected into each tumor at a rate of 2.5 μL/min using a syringe pump (Pump 11 Elite, Harvard Apparatus, Holliston, MA, USA), followed immediately by euthanasia. We decided to perform the experiments with mouse cadavers in order to remove the effects of temperature-dependent perfusion and tissue damage accumulation to better isolate the temperature change induced by the MNPs.

2.1.5. MPI Scanner and Imaging

We used a Momentum® MPI scanner (Magnetic Insight, Inc., Alameda, CA, USA) to generate 3D images of the MNPs within each tumor. The scanner was equipped with a custom mouse holder to limit lateral movement. We used three ~1 μL aliquots of Synomag®-S90 MNPs in microcentrifuge tubes secured to the sample holder within the scanning region as fiducial markers. Each isotropic scan was measured using the 'Standard mode' scanner configuration and an excitation field amplitude of 5 mT, with a gradient field of 5.7 T/m and a drive frequency of 45 kHz. Each 3D image consisted of 21 radial scans.

2.1.6. The microCT

We used an IVIS SpectrumCT In Vivo Imaging System (Perkin-Elmer, Shelton, CT, USA) for the anatomical imaging, which was co-registered with the MPI scans. The scans (50 kV at 1 mA) consisted of 720 projections, each with an exposure time of 20 ms. We performed microCT immediately after MPI using the MPI sample holder. A 3D-printed adapter enabled the integration of the MPI holder into the IVIS scanner. We adjusted the scan area to include the mouse cadaver as well as the fiducials within the area of interest.

2.1.7. AMF Heating

All tissue heating was performed on the HYPER device previously described [28]. The selected AMF amplitude for MNP heating by the solenoid was 15 mT ± 10% (12 kA/m) at a set frequency of 341.25 kHz, which is within the Hergt–Dutz biological limit of 5×10^9 A/(m-s) [51]. We verified the amplitude with a 1D magnetic field probe (AMF LifeSystems, LLC, Auburn Hills, MI, USA). The temperature in the sample area encompassed by the solenoid was maintained at 37 ± 0.1 °C by a closed-loop water circulating system.

Before heating the tumors, mouse cadavers were individually placed into plastic bags, which were sealed and immersed into a circulating water bath (Polyscience, Niles, IL, USA) set at 37 °C for 15 min. Mouse cadavers were then removed from the water bath and plastic bags and then placed into a custom 3D-printed sample holder, also maintained at 37.0 ± 0.1 °C by circulated heated water. After securing the cadaver to the sample holder, a single probe was inserted into the tumor to the approximate geometric center. Temperatures were recorded at 1 s intervals. An additional probe was inserted into the rectum to monitor the core body temperature at similar intervals. Each tumor underwent two separate, consecutive heating trials. The first trial consisted of continuous heating at

15 mT for 30 min, or until the tumor exceeded 51 °C. After the trial, the tumor was allowed to cool until 37 °C. When the tumor temperature returned to 37 °C, it was heated at 15 mT at a 67% duty cycle (60 s ON/30 s OFF) for 20 cycles. We performed pulsed heating in addition to continuous heating to mimic the power modulation that may occur during MPH therapy.

2.2. Image Analysis and Computational Modeling

2.2.1. Co-Registration

We used the Mimics Innovation Suite (MIS) Research v.25 (Materialise NV, Leuven, Belgium) with the FEA module for all image analyses, including segmentation, co-registration, conversion to 3D parts, and meshing. While we used the Research version of the software, MIS Medical has FDA 501k medical clearance. The suite consists of two main software: (1) Mimics v26.0®, which we used to create masks and 3D parts from the data, and (2) 3-matic® v18.0 for smoothing and re-meshing. For the MPI-guided simulations, MPI and anatomical imaging data were co-registered to ensure alignment of the shared scale and coordinate system. Mathematically, co-registration transforms each voxel, or 3D pixel, at point x (x, y, z) to point y (x', y', z'), as shown in Equation (3):

$$\begin{bmatrix} a_{11} & a_{12} & a_{13} & a_{14} \\ a_{21} & a_{22} & a_{23} & a_{24} \\ a_{31} & a_{32} & a_{33} & a_{34} \\ 0 & 0 & 0 & 1 \end{bmatrix}_A \times \begin{bmatrix} x \\ y \\ z \\ 1 \end{bmatrix}_x = \begin{bmatrix} x' \\ y' \\ z' \\ 1 \end{bmatrix}_y. \qquad (3)$$

Within matrix A, the top left 3×3 values scale or rotate the image, while the top right 3×1 values translate the image. Without this co-registration, the positions of the MNPs (heat generators) within the tumor would be unknown. Practically, we performed the co-registration using the Landmark Registration tool in Mimics®, where the locations of the fiducial markers in 3D space were matched in both the MPI and microCT image stacks (Figure 2). The application automatically generated a transformation matrix (matrix A), which we applied to the MPI data to spatially match the MNP locations within the tumor. The co-registered images for all 5 mice can be found in Figure S1 in the Supplementary Materials.

2.2.2. Imaging Data Calibration

To correlate the MPI signal within a single voxel to MNP thermal output, we prepared serial dilutions of the MNP suspension in 20 µL aliquots in plastic centrifuge tubes having concentrations 0, 0.25, 0.5, 2.5, 5.0, 25, and 50 mg of Fe/mL H_2O. The tubes were placed onto the MPI sample holder to ensure separate and distinguishable samples. The calibration samples were then measured with the MPI using the same scanning parameters used to image the tumors. We then used Mimics® to extract the maximum voxel intensity from each calibration sample. The MPI signal intensity of each voxel was mapped to an arbitrary grayscale by the Mimics® software; we will refer to the units simply as a grayscale value (GV). Afterward, we plotted the maximum GV against the estimated volumetric thermal output from each sample (SLP × concentration) and used linear least squares regression to fit the data points (Figure 3). We assumed the SLP did not vary with the concentration or aggregation effects. A representative MPI scan and segmentations of the calibration samples can be found in Figure S2 in the Supplementary Materials. The tabulated calibration curve can also be found in Table S1.

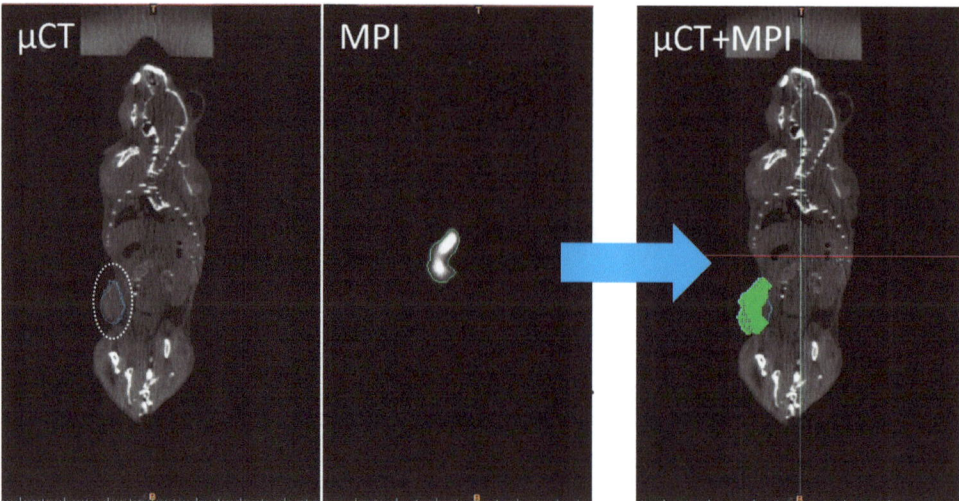

Figure 2. Co-registration is necessary to correlate MPI voxel intensity values with 3D coordinates within the segmented tumor (Mouse 1 is shown as an example). The micro(μ)CT and MPI of tumored mice after injection are shown, where the tumor is circled in white. The micro(μ)CT and MPI scans were co-registered within Mimics, and a transformation matrix was created. The transformation matrix obtained for each tumor was applied to the MPI scan and overlaid onto the micro(μ)CT scan.

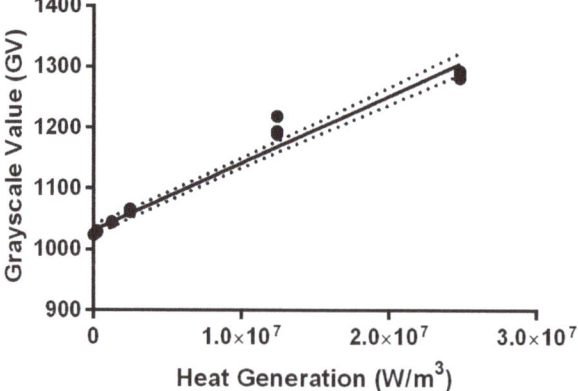

Figure 3. MNP calibration is essential to generate accurate MPI-guided simulations. The max grayscale and thermal generation values (calculated from SLP) were fitted to a linear equation using least squares regression to yield y-intercept of 1031 ± 4 GV and slope = (1.10 ± 0.04) × 10^{-5} W·m^{-3}·GV^{-1} with R^2 = 0.9746. Uncertainty is represented by 95% confidence bounds, which are shown as dashed lines in the figure.

2.2.3. Mesh Generation

We created masks for both the tumor and MNP distribution using the built-in functions within Mimics®. The tumor boundary was segmented, and the created mask was then converted to a .STL file (3D part). We then imported the tumor-part file into 3-matic® (Figure 4a), where the geometry surface was smoothed and re-meshed; a volume mesh was calculated (Figure 4b), and the final mesh was exported as a COMSOL® mesh-part file (Figure 4c), using the built-in functions within 3-matic®. Similarly, the MNP distribution was segmented (Figure 4d), except that the distribution was converted directly to a voxel mesh in Mimics from the image data rather than being converted to a 3D part before meshing (Figure 4e). The MPI mask was created using a threshold segmentation, where the upper bound was the highest GV, and the lower bound was selected manually for each tumor, such that the majority of the signal within the tumor bounds was encompassed. Then, under material assignment, we used the calibration curve to convert the GV of each voxel to units of volumetric thermal output (W/m^3), using the samples with the highest and lowest concentrations as references. A material property table was created, which contained the spatial coordinates of each voxel and the corresponding volumetric thermal energy generation (Figure 4f). A more detailed experimental procedure is described in the Supplementary Materials.

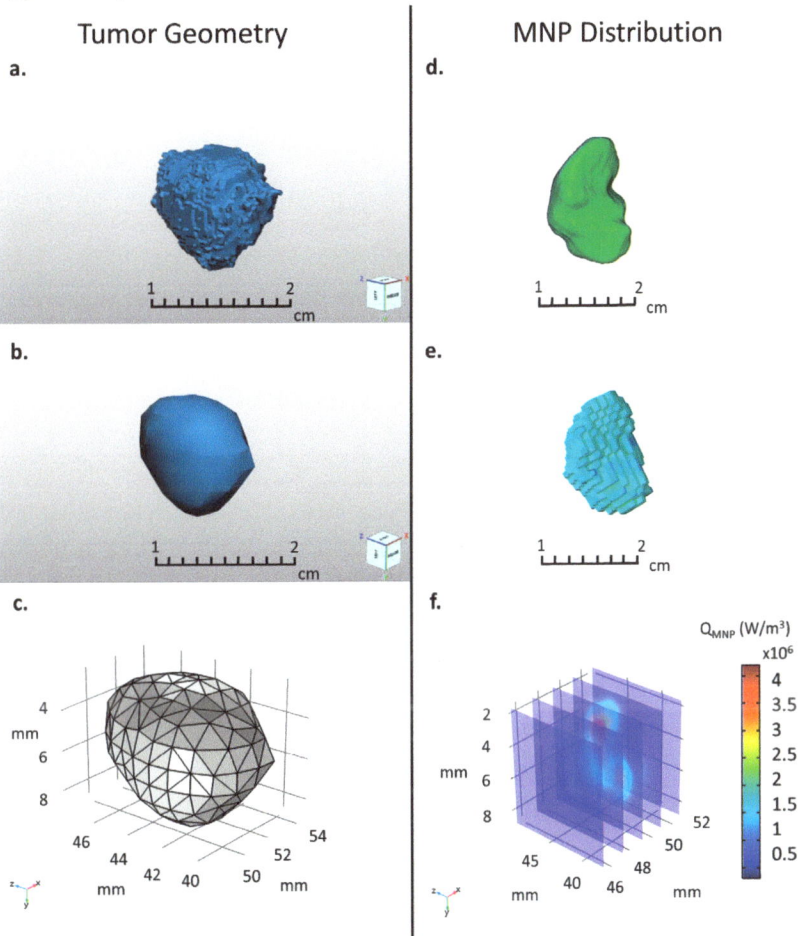

Figure 4. After co-registration and segmentation, the represented MNP distribution and tumor geometry (Mouse 3 shown as an example) were prepared for COMSOL. (**a**) After converting the tumor mask to a .stl file, it was imported into 3-matic, where it was (**b**) smoothed, re-meshed, and (**c**) converted to a COMSOL mesh file. (**d**) The MPI scan was segmented, and the resulting mask was used to represent the MNP distribution in the computational tumor phantom. (**e**) The voxel intensities were mapped onto the values of the MPI calibration curve using the Mimics® material assignment tab. (**f**) The calibrated voxel values were then imported into COMSOL as a 3-argument interpolation function.

2.2.4. FEA Software and Mathematical Models

We used the COMSOL Multiphysics® 6.2 (COMSOL, Burlington, MA, USA) advanced numerical methods software for all heat transfer calculations. The geometry of the computational model is illustrated schematically in Figure 5. The tumor mesh was modeled as a subcutaneous mass, where approximately 1/3 of the tumor volume was embedded within a cuboid geometry representing muscle. The computational phantom tumor and muscle resided within a cylindrical AMF coil, having dimensions similar to that of the experimental coil on the HYPER device.

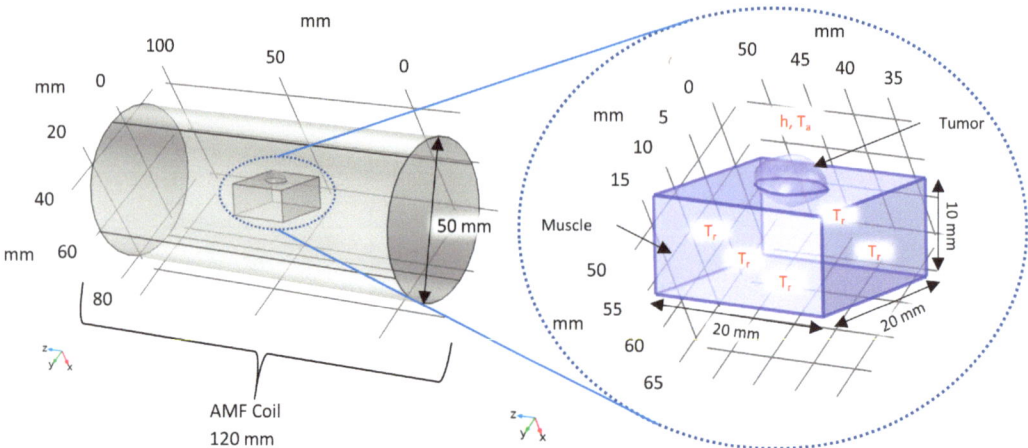

Figure 5. Schematic diagram of computational tumor and muscle phantom used to simulate MPH with COMSOL. The imported tumor geometry was embedded in a phantom body represented by a cuboid having properties of muscle, suspended in a phantom AMF coil with a diameter similar to that of the coil in the HYPER device. Constant temperature boundary conditions were assumed, having values obtained from experimental rectal temperatures, on the bottom and sides of the phantom body. We imposed a convective boundary condition on the top of the phantom tumor and muscle, with an assumed heat transfer coefficient and ambient temperature.

We used two physics modules available in COMSOL, Heat Transfer in Solids and Magnetic Fields, as well as the Electromagnetic Heating multiphysics module to simulate eddy current heating. The material properties used for the simulation are summarized in Table 2. The Heat Transfer in Solids module implemented the Fourier conduction equation (Equation (4)),

$$\rho c_p \frac{\partial T}{\partial t} = k \nabla^2 T + Q_{MNP} + Q_{eddy} \qquad (4)$$

where ρ is the density, c_p is the specific heat at constant pressure, k is the coefficient of thermal conductivity, T is the temperature, t is the time, and Q_{MNP} and Q_{eddy} are the volumetric thermal power outputs from the hysteresis heating of the MNPs and Joule heating from induced eddy currents, respectively. For Q_{MNP}, we imported the material properties table created in Mimics® from the MPI data as a 3D interpolation function, which was used as a spatially variant heat source.

Q_{eddy} was calculated by coupling the frequency domain of Maxwell's equations (Equations (4)–(7)) with the conduction equation (Equation (4)),

$$\nabla \times H = J, \qquad (5)$$

$$B = \nabla \times A, \qquad (6)$$

$$J = \sigma E + j\omega D, \qquad (7)$$

$$E = -j\omega A, \tag{8}$$

where J is the current density, H is the magnetic field amplitude, B is the magnetic flux density, A is the magnetic vector potential, σ is the electrical conductivity, E is the electric field amplitude, ω is the angular frequency, and D is the electric flux density. As an initial condition, A was assumed zero in all dimensions, and Ampere's law was applied to the phantom muscle and tumor geometries. The AMF coil was modeled as free space with a magnetic field of amplitude 12 kA/m, applied along the z-axis (along the coil length). Using the equation for Q_{eddy} (Equation (9)), COMSOL solved the Joule heating contribution as follows:

$$Q_{eddy} = 0.5 Re(J \cdot E) + 0.5 Re(i\omega B \cdot H). \tag{9}$$

On the top surface of the tumor and muscle, a convective boundary condition (Equation (10)) was implemented using Newton's law of cooling, with a constant ambient temperature (T_∞) of 37 °C and a heat transfer coefficient (h) of 20 W/(m²·K).

$$q = h(T - T_\infty), \tag{10}$$

where q is the convective heat flux.

Table 2. Material properties used for COMSOL electromagnetic heating simulations.

Property	Muscle	Tumor	Ref.
Specific Heat at Constant Pressure (cp)	3421 J/(kg-K)	3760 J/(kg-K)	[43]
Density (ρ)	1090 kg/m³	1045 kg/m³	[43]
Thermal Conductivity (k)	0.49 W/(m-K)	0.51 W/(m-K)	[43]
Relative Permeability (μ_r)	1	1	
Relative Permittivity (ε_r)	2000	2000	[52]
Electrical Conductivity (σ)	0.23 S/m	0.23 S/m	[52]

A uniform temperature boundary condition was used on the remaining five rectangular faces of the phantom muscle, where the temperature value was interpolated from the experimental cadaver rectal temperature at a given time point. The rectal temperature data can be seen in Figure S3 of the Supplementary Materials. Additionally, we used experimental data for our initial conditions, where the initial temperature of the phantom tumor(s) and muscle geometries corresponded with the respective initial experimental temperatures measured, i.e., at $t = 0$. A default physics-based "fine" mesh was selected in COMSOL. We performed a frequency-transient study at 341.25 kHz for each phantom tumor to mirror the experimental heating. Specifically, simulated heating was conducted as one continuous heating trial and one pulsed heating trial (60 s ON/30 s OFF). Predicted temperatures from tumor phantoms were reported as a volumetric maximum, minimum, and average of the entire tumor geometry.

2.3. Uncertainty Quantitation

We used the Type A uncertainty evaluation, where valid statistical methods were used to treat our data, as defined by the National Institutes of Standards and Technology [53]. The MPI calibration was performed in triplicate, where the values used to convert the MPI GV to a volumetric thermal output consisted of the average calculated from the 3 replicate measurements. All statistical testing, linear regression, and analyses were performed using Prism 6 software (GraphPad, Boston, MA, USA).

3. Results

All simulated tumor temperature values showed general agreement with the measured intratumor temperatures (Figure 6). For tumors 1, 3, and 4, the calculated average tumor phantom temperatures were ±3 °C of the experimental temperatures measured at the tumor center. Deviations between the simulated and experimental temperatures were observed with tumors 2 and 5, with the latter showing the largest discrepancy. In this case, most of the injected MNPs were concentrated on the left tumor boundary, while the remainder of the tumor (notably the tumor center and location of the probe) was virtually MNP-free. However, the experimental temperature plot for tumor 5 matches the minimum simulated temperature reasonably well, supporting the accuracy of the simulation. We observed significant variances of intratumor MNP and temperature distributions among the tumors after single-point injection, consistent with the previous observations from other tumor models (Figure 6) [9].

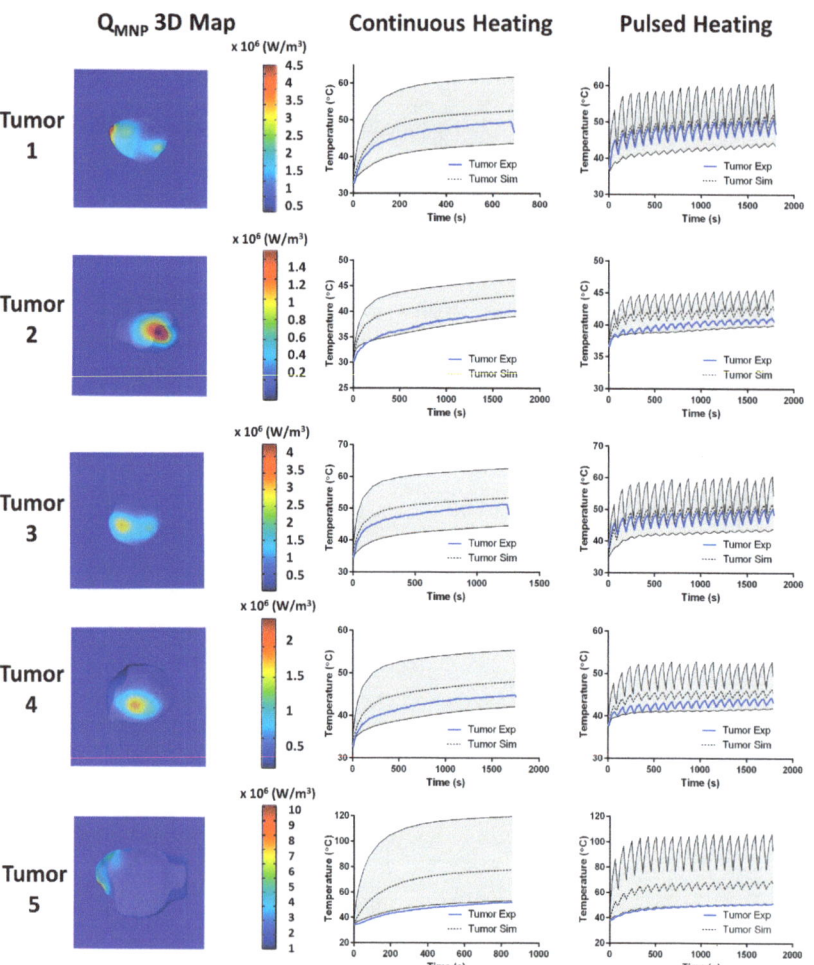

Figure 6. MPI-guided simulations of magnetic hyperthermia accurately predict intratumor temperatures measured experimentally in the center of murine 4T1 tumors. The left column shows the distribution of MNPs within the tumor from the MPI data that were used as inputs for simulated MPH in computational phantoms. The second column shows the results of the continuous heating trials, where the gray region encompasses the maximum and minimum predicted temperature values obtained from the computational phantoms, the dashed lines show the average simulation temperature, and the solid blue lines are the experimentally measured temperatures from the 4T1 tumor heating trials in mouse cadavers. The third column shows similar results, which were obtained from the pulsed heating trials.

4. Discussion

4.1. MNP Distribution and Thermal Probe Placement

The results demonstrate the challenges to achieving a uniform distribution of MNPs within any tumor (constant concentration of MNPs throughout), even with percutaneous delivery, thus highlighting the importance of accounting for the MNP content and distribution in tissues prior to activating them with an AMF. One strategy used to mitigate the effects of unknown and heterogeneous MNP distributions was by manual or automated temperature control mechanisms [42]; however, their success relies on the appropriate placement of the thermal probe within the tumor. Consider tumor 5 (Figure 6). Based solely on the experimental data, we observed temperatures in the range of 40–50 °C for the duration of testing, which is ideal for MPH. Yet, based on the MPI data, the largest concentration of MNPs was along the tumor periphery, away from the position of the probe at the tumor center, resulting in the predicted temperatures being >twofold what was measured experimentally. The MPI data imply that such conditions in a live subject could have produced significant ablative tissue damage at the tumor boundary, assuming a single thermal probe placed in the tumor center as a reference. During treatment, such a disparate probe placement from the concentration of MNPs provides little useful information for accurate thermal dosimetry in the tumor and, worse, fails to anticipate the damage to surrounding normal tissues. MPI, with its enhanced sensitivity to changes in MNP concentration, provides the necessary critical information to locate such potential "hot spot" regions and avoid damaging healthy tissue when compared to works that use anatomical imaging alone.

4.2. Implications for Treatment Planning

Our aim in this work was to develop and verify the capability of MPI to guide thermal simulations using clinically relevant software. To achieve this, we conducted the computational analysis after experimental heating trials, where experimental temperature data was used to provide both boundary and initial conditions for simulations. If simulations are to be used for MPH treatment planning, initial and boundary conditions would be required as initial inputs prior to treatments commencing. Our results here show that reasonable approximations, e.g., subject temperature, could suffice, provided the simulations are used to estimate average, maximum, and minimum temperatures in the target volume (tumor). In the context of treatment planning, these values could be used to generate thermal dose contours to guide AMF power management to ensure treatments achieve an outcome within a prescribed thermal dose range. Certainly, the accuracy of correspondence between planned and achieved treatments would improve if temperature probe placement is performed with imaging guidance. MPI-guided simulations thus can provide the basis of MPH quality control to the researcher or clinician who is able to follow a pre-determined, in silico treatment plan. Additional investigation is needed to ascertain the limits of MPI-guided simulations for treatment planning.

4.3. Limitations

For combined MPI/MPH treatment, the MNPs are both therapeutic and tracer imaging agents; therefore, the selected nanoparticles must generate adequate heat with acceptable MPI tracer quality. For this study, we use commercially available magnetic nanoflowers, Synomag®, that exhibit suitable properties for both MPI and MPH [54]; however, the effect of the MNP dose on MPI image quality bears consideration. The MPI signal varies linearly with the MNP spatial density, i.e., concentration. A high-intensity signal generally produces quality images, but if the concentration is too high, the signal saturates the MPI detector, resulting in image aberrations. Corrective actions can be implemented, such as lowering the excitation field amplitude and increasing the gradient field magnitude, but relatively high MNP concentrations (>1 mg Fe/mL) associated with MPH therapies will likely produce image artifacts when compared to tumor models injected with MNPs at tracer concentrations (~µg Fe/mL).

MPH requires accurate active thermometry to ensure that the prescribed thermal dose is achieved. Further, in vivo thermometry with MPH typically uses invasive probes (usually one) implanted directly within the tumor to measure the intratumor temperature. From a heat transfer perspective, single-point thermometry introduces severe limitations, especially for larger tumors, as seen with tumor 5 (Figure 6). To draw useful conclusions from a single temperature probe, one must assume the tumor is a lumped mass with a uniform spatial temperature distribution, which is only true for sufficiently small tumors that are uniformly loaded with MNPs. Future development of multi-point or volumetric thermometry would enhance the accuracy of MPI-guided simulations of MPH and reduce the associated uncertainties.

5. Conclusions

We developed and verified an MPI-guided thermal simulation workflow for use in MPH preclinical experiments. We conclude that our methodology successfully integrated MPI data into FEA software for thermal simulations. Verification of the proposed methodology was achieved by comparing the simulation results with corresponding experimentally heated tumor-bearing mouse cadavers that had been previously injected with MNPs. The general agreement between the experimental and simulated results raises confidence that this approach can overcome many of the technological limitations encountered with clinical MPH. Achieving further in vivo preclinical validation of this methodology will establish its potential for use in human patients.

Supplementary Materials: The following supporting information can be downloaded at: https://www.mdpi.com/article/10.3390/nano14121059/s1.

Author Contributions: Conceptualization: H.C., N.A., S.H. and R.I.; Resources: H.C., S.P., M.S., M.N., P.G. and R.I.; Funding acquisition: R.I.; Methodology: H.C., N.A., S.H., A.S., S.P., M.S., M.N., P.G. and A.A.; Investigation: H.C.; Data curation: H.C.; Formal analysis: H.C.; Validation: H.C., N.A., S.H., A.A. and R.I.; Visualization: H.C.; Project administration: A.A. and R.I.; Supervision: R.I.; Writing—original draft: H.C. and R.I.; Writing—review and editing: H.C., N.A., S.H., A.S., S.P., M.S., M.N., P.G., A.A. and R.I. All authors have read and agreed to the published version of the manuscript.

Funding: Funding for the experimental portion of this project was provided by the National Cancer Institute of the National Institutes of Health under Award Numbers 1R01 CA257557, 1R01 CA247290, 1S10 OD026740, 5P30 CA006973, 1R44CA285064 and R37 CA229417. The content is solely the responsibility of the authors and does not necessarily represent the official views of Johns Hopkins University, Pennsylvania State University, or the National Institutes of Health.

Institutional Review Board Statement: No human subjects were used. The animal study procedures were conducted according to the Johns Hopkins Institutional Animal Care and Use Committee (IACUC) approved protocol. The protocol/project identification number is not publicly available due to the JHU institutional policy and can be provided on request from the corresponding author.

Data Availability Statement: Data are publicly available on the Johns Hopkins Data Repository.

Conflicts of Interest: M.N. and P.G. are employees of Magnetic Insight, Inc., a company that manufactures and sells MPI scanners and technology used in this study. S.P. and M.S. are employees of Materialise, the company that manufactures and sells the imaging data processing software used in this study. R.I. is an inventor listed on several nanoparticle patents. All patents are assigned to either The Johns Hopkins University or Aduro Biosciences, Inc. All other authors report no other conflicts of interest.

References

1. Maier-Hauff, K.; Ulrich, F.; Nestler, D.; Niehoff, H.; Wust, P.; Thiesen, B.; Orawa, H.; Budach, V.; Jordan, A. Efficacy and safety of intratumoral thermotherapy using magnetic iron-oxide nanoparticles combined with external beam radiotherapy on patients with recurrent glioblastoma multiforme. *J. Neuro-Oncol.* **2011**, *103*, 317–324. [CrossRef]
2. Gilchrist, R.K.; Medal, R.; Shorey, W.D.; Hanselman, R.C.; Parrott, J.C.; Taylor, C.B. Selective inductive heating of lymph nodes. *Ann. Surg.* **1957**, *146*, 596–606. [CrossRef] [PubMed]
3. Rmili, N.; Riahi, K.; M'Nassri, R.; Ouertani, B.; Cheikhrouhou-Koubaa, W.; Hlil, E.K. Magnetocaloric and induction heating characteristics of $La_{0.71}Sr_{0.29}Mn_{0.95}Fe_{0.05}O_3$ nanoparticles. *J. Sol-Gel Sci. Technol.* **2024**. ahead of print. [CrossRef]

4. Dewhirst, M.W.; Viglianti, B.L.; Lora-Michiels, M.; Hanson, M.; Hoopes, P.J. Basic principles of thermal dosimetry and thermal thresholds for tissue damage from hyperthermia. *Int. J. Hyperth.* **2003**, *19*, 267–294. [CrossRef] [PubMed]
5. Sapareto, S.A.; Dewey, W.C. Thermal dose determination in cancer-therapy. *Int. J. Radiat. Oncol. Biol. Phys.* **1984**, *10*, 787–800. [CrossRef] [PubMed]
6. Oleson, J.R.; Samulski, T.V.; Leopold, K.A.; Clegg, S.T.; Dewhirst, M.W.; Dodge, R.K.; George, S.L. Sensitivity of hyperthermia trial outcomes to temperature and time—Implications for thermal goals of treatment. *Int. J. Radiat. Oncol. Biol. Phys.* **1993**, *25*, 289–297. [CrossRef] [PubMed]
7. Wust, P.; Hildebrandt, B.; Sreenivasa, G.; Rau, B.; Gellermann, J.; Riess, H.; Felix, R.; Schlag, P.M. Hyperthermia in combined treatment of cancer. *Lancet Oncol.* **2002**, *3*, 487–497. [CrossRef] [PubMed]
8. van der Zee, J.; van Rhoon, G.C. Hyperthermia is effective in improving clinical radiotherapy results. *Int. J. Radiat. Oncol. Biol. Phys.* **2006**, *66*, 633–634. [CrossRef]
9. Attaluri, A.; Kandala, S.K.; Wabler, M.; Zhou, H.; Cornejo, C.; Armour, M.; Hedayati, M.; Zhang, Y.; DeWeese, T.L.; Herman, C.; et al. Magnetic nanoparticle hyperthermia enhances radiation therapy: A study in mouse models of human prostate cancer. *Int. J. Hyperth.* **2015**, *31*, 359–374. [CrossRef]
10. Tohnai, I.; Goto, Y.; Hayashi, Y.; Ueda, M.; Kobayashi, T.; Matsui, M. Preoperative thermochemotherapy of oral cancer using magnetic induction hyperthermia (implant heating system: IHS). *Int. J. Hyperth.* **1996**, *12*, 37–47. [CrossRef]
11. Otsuka, T.; Yonezawa, M.; Kamiyama, F.; Matsushita, Y.; Matsui, N. Results of surgery and radio-hyperthermo-chemotherapy for patients with soft-tissue sarcoma. *Int. J. Clin. Oncol.* **2001**, *6*, 253–258. [CrossRef] [PubMed]
12. Iwata, K.; Shakil, A.; Hur, W.J.; Makepeace, C.M.; Griffin, R.J.; Song, C.W. Tumour pO(2) can be increased markedly by mild hyperthermia. *Br. J. Cancer* **1996**, *74*, S217–S221.
13. Brizel, D.M.; Scully, S.P.; Harrelson, J.M.; Layfield, L.J.; Dodge, R.K.; Charles, H.C.; Samulski, T.V.; Prosnitz, L.R.; Dewhirst, M.W. Radiation therapy and hyperthermia improve the oxygenation of human soft tissue sarcomas. *Cancer Res.* **1996**, *56*, 5347–5350. [PubMed]
14. Elming, P.B.; Sorensen, B.S.; Oei, A.L.; Franken, N.A.P.; Crezee, J.; Overgaard, J.; Horsman, M.R. Hyperthermia: The Optimal Treatment to Overcome Radiation Resistant Hypoxia. *Cancers* **2019**, *11*, 60. [CrossRef] [PubMed]
15. Zanker, K.S.; Lange, J. Whole-body hyperthermia and natural-killer cell-activity. *Lancet* **1982**, *1*, 1079–1080. [CrossRef] [PubMed]
16. Yan, X.Y.; Xiu, F.M.; An, H.Z.; Wang, X.J.; Wang, J.L.; Cao, X.T. Fever range temperature promotes TLR4 expression and signaling in dendritic cells. *Life Sci.* **2007**, *80*, 307–313. [CrossRef] [PubMed]
17. Dayanc, B.E.; Beachy, S.H.; Ostberg, J.R.; Repasky, E.A. Dissecting the role of hyperthermia in natural killer cell mediated anti-tumor responses. *Int. J. Hyperth.* **2008**, *24*, 41–56. [CrossRef] [PubMed]
18. Roizintowle, L.; Pirro, J.P. The response of human and rodent cells to hyperthermia. *Int. J. Radiat. Oncol. Biol. Phys.* **1991**, *20*, 751–756. [CrossRef] [PubMed]
19. Johannsen, M.; Gneveckow, U.; Eckelt, L.; Feussner, A.; Waldöfner, N.; Scholz, R.; Deger, S.; Wust, P.; Loening, S.A.; Jordan, A. Clinical hyperthermia of prostate cancer using magnetic nanoparticles:: Presentation of a new interstitial technique. *Int. J. Hyperth.* **2005**, *21*, 637–647. [CrossRef]
20. LeBrun, A.; Manuchehrabadi, N.; Attaluri, A.; Wang, F.; Ma, R.H.; Zhu, L. MicroCT image-generated tumour geometry and SAR distribution for tumour temperature elevation simulations in magnetic nanoparticle hyperthermia. *Int. J. Hyperth.* **2013**, *29*, 730–738. [CrossRef]
21. Gneveckow, U.; Jordan, A.; Scholz, R.; Brüss, V.; Waldöfner, N.; Ricke, J.; Feussner, A.; Hildebrandt, B.; Rau, B.; Wust, P. Description and characterization of the novel hyperthermia- and thermoablation-system MFH®300F for clinical magnetic fluid hyperthermia. *Med. Phys.* **2004**, *31*, 1444–1451. [CrossRef]
22. Gleich, B.; Weizenecker, R. Tomographic imaging using the nonlinear response of magnetic particles. *Nature* **2005**, *435*, 1214–1217. [CrossRef]
23. Murase, K.; Aoki, M.; Banura, N.; Nishimoto, K.; Mimura, A.; Kuboyabu, T.; Yabata, I. Usefulness of Magnetic Particle Imaging for Predicting the Therapeutic Effect of Magnetic Hyperthermia. *Open J. Med. Imaging* **2015**, *5*, 85–99. [CrossRef]
24. Kuboyabu, T.; Yabata, I.; Aoki, M.; Banura, N.; Nishimoto, K.; Mimura, A.; Murase, K. Magnetic Particle Imaging for Magnetic Hyperthermia Treatment: Visualization and Quantification of the Intratumoral Distribution and Temporal Change of Magnetic Nanoparticles in Vivo. *Open J. Med. Imaging* **2016**, *6*, 1–15. [CrossRef]
25. Tay, Z.W.; Chandrasekharan, P.; Chiu-Lam, A.; Hensley, D.W.; Dhavalikar, R.; Zhou, X.Y.; Conolly, S.M. Magnetic Particle Imaging-Guided Heating in Vivo Using Gradient Fields for Arbitrary Localization of Magnetic Hyperthermia Therapy. *ACS Nano* **2018**, *12*, 3699–3713. [CrossRef] [PubMed]
26. Lei, S.; He, J.; Huang, X.; Hui, H.; An, Y.; Tian, J. A Novel Local Magnetic Fluid Hyperthermia Based on High Gradient Field Guided by Magnetic Particle Imaging. *IEEE Trans. Biomed. Eng.* **2024**. *ahead of print*. [CrossRef]
27. Le, T.A.; Hadadian, Y.; Yoon, J. A prediction model for magnetic particle imaging-based magnetic hyperthermia applied to a brain tumor model. *Comput. Methods Programs Biomed.* **2023**, *235*, 107546. [CrossRef]
28. Carlton, H.; Weber, M.; Peters, M.; Arepally, N.; Lad, Y.S.; Jaswal, A.; Ivkov, R.; Attaluri, A.; Goodwill, P. HYPER: Pre-clinical device for spatially-confined magnetic particle hyperthermia. *Int. J. Hyperth.* **2023**, *40*, 2272067. [CrossRef]
29. Buchholz, O.; Sajjamark, K.; Franke, J.; Wei, H.; Behrends, A.; Münkel, C.; Hofmann, U.G. In situ theranostic platform combining highly localized magnetic fluid hyperthermia, magnetic particle imaging, and thermometry in 3D. *Theranostics* **2024**, *14*, 324–340. [CrossRef]

30. Behrends, A.; Wei, H.; Neumann, A.; Friedrich, T.; Bakenecker, A.C.; Franke, J.; Buzug, T.M. Integrable Magnetic Fluid Hyperthermia Systems for 3D Magnetic Particle Imaging. *Nanotheranostics* **2024**, *8*, 163–178. [CrossRef]
31. Paulides, M.M.; Stauffer, P.R.; Neufeld, E.; Maccarini, P.F.; Kyriakou, A.; Canters, R.A.M.; Diederich, C.J.; Bakker, J.F.; Van Rhoon, G.C. Simulation techniques in hyperthermia treatment planning. *Int. J. Hyperth.* **2013**, *29*, 346–357. [CrossRef]
32. Kok, H.P.; Crezee, J. Hyperthermia Treatment Planning: Clinical Application and Ongoing Developments. *IEEE J. Electromagn. RF Microw. Med. Biol.* **2021**, *5*, 214–222. [CrossRef]
33. Stalling, D.; Seebass, M.; Zöckler, M.; Hege, H.-C. *Hyperthermia Treatment Planning with HyperPlan—User's Manual*; Publication Server of Zuse Institute Berlin (ZIB): Berlin, Germany, 2000.
34. Gellermann, J.; Wust, P.; Stalling, D.; Seebass, M.; Nadobny, J.; Beck, R.; Hege, H.C.; Deuflhard, P.; Felix, R. Clinical evaluation and verification of the hyperthermia treatment planning system HyperPlan. *Int. J. Radiat. Oncol. Biol. Phys.* **2000**, *47*, 1145–1156. [CrossRef]
35. Sreenivasa, G.; Gellermann, J.; Rau, B.; Nadobny, J.; Schlag, P.; Deuflhard, P.; Felix, R.; Wust, P. Clinical use of the hyperthermia treatment planning system hyperplan to predict effectiveness and toxicity. *Int. J. Radiat. Oncol. Biol. Phys.* **2003**, *55*, 407–419. [CrossRef]
36. Schmid, G.; Überbacher, R.; Samaras, T.; Tschabitscher, M.; Mazal, P.R. The dielectric properties of human pineal gland tissue and RF absorption due to wireless communication devices in the frequency range 400–1850 MHz. *Phys. Med. Biol.* **2007**, *52*, 5457–5468. [CrossRef] [PubMed]
37. De Bruijne, M.; Wielheesen, D.H.M.; Van der Zee, J.; Chavannes, N.; Van Rhoon, G.C. Benefits of superficial hyperthermia treatment planning: Five case studies. *Int. J. Hyperth.* **2007**, *23*, 417–429. [CrossRef] [PubMed]
38. Kok, H.P.; Kotte, A.; Crezee, J. Planning, optimisation and evaluation of hyperthermia treatments. *Int. J. Hyperth.* **2017**, *33*, 593–607. [CrossRef]
39. Kok, H.P.; Crezee, J. Validation and practical use of Plan2Heat hyperthermia treatment planning for capacitive heating. *Int. J. Hyperth.* **2022**, *39*, 952–966. [CrossRef] [PubMed]
40. Chen, X.; Diederich, C.J.; Wootton, J.H.; Pouliot, J.; Hsu, I.C. Optimisation-based thermal treatment planning for catheter-based ultrasound hyperthermia. *Int. J. Hyperth.* **2010**, *26*, 39–55. [CrossRef]
41. Kandala, S.K.; Sharma, A.; Mirpour, S.; Liapi, E.; Ivkov, R.; Attaluri, A. Validation of a coupled electromagnetic and thermal model for estimating temperatures during magnetic nanoparticle hyperthermia. *Int. J. Hyperth.* **2021**, *38*, 611–622. [CrossRef]
42. Kandala, S.K.; Liapi, E.; Whitcomb, L.L.; Attaluri, A.; Ivkov, R. Temperature-controlled power modulation compensates for heterogeneous nanoparticle distributions: A computational optimization analysis for magnetic hyperthermia. *Int. J. Hyperth.* **2019**, *36*, 115–129. [CrossRef]
43. Banura, N.; Mimura, A.; Nishimoto, K.; Murase, K. Heat transfer simulation for optimization and treatment planning of magnetic hyperthermia using magnetic particle imaging. *arXiv* **2016**, arXiv:1605.08139.
44. Tang, Y.D.; Chen, M.; Flesch, R.C.C.; Jin, T. Extraction method of nanoparticles concentration distribution from magnetic particle image and its application in thermal damage of magnetic hyperthermia. *Chin. Phys. B* **2023**, *32*, 094401. [CrossRef]
45. Bender, P.; Fock, J.; Frandsen, C.; Hansen, M.F.; Balceris, C.; Ludwig, F.; Johansson, C. Relating Magnetic Properties and High Hyperthermia Performance of Iron Oxide Nanoflowers. *J. Phys. Chem. C* **2018**, *122*, 3068–3077. [CrossRef]
46. Hedayati, M.; Abubaker-Sharif, B.; Khattab, M.; Razavi, A.; Mohammed, I.; Nejad, A.; Ivkov, R. An optimised spectrophotometric assay for convenient and accurate quantitation of intracellular iron from iron oxide nanoparticles. *Int. J. Hyperth.* **2018**, *34*, 373–381. [CrossRef] [PubMed]
47. Carlton, H.; Ivkov, R. A new method to measure magnetic nanoparticle heating efficiency in non-adiabatic systems using transient pulse analysis. *J. Appl. Phys.* **2023**, *133*, 044302. [CrossRef] [PubMed]
48. Hergt, R.; Andra, W.; d'Ambly, C.G.; Hilger, I.; Kaiser, W.A.; Richter, U.; Schmidt, H.G. Physical limits of hyperthermia using magnetite fine particles. *IEEE Trans. Magn.* **1998**, *34*, 3745–3754. [CrossRef]
49. Andrä, W.; d'Ambly, C.G.; Hergt, R.; Hilger, I.; Kaiser, W.A. Temperature distribution as function of time around a small spherical heat source of local magnetic hyperthermia. *J. Magn. Magn. Mater.* **1999**, *194*, 197–203. [CrossRef]
50. Dutz, S.; Hergt, R. Magnetic particle hyperthermia-a promising tumour therapy? *Nanotechnology* **2014**, *25*, 28. [CrossRef]
51. Hergt, R.; Dutz, S. Magnetic particle hyperthermia-biophysical limitations of a visionary tumour therapy. *J. Magn. Magn. Mater.* **2007**, *311*, 187–192. [CrossRef]
52. Nagy, J.A.; DiDonato, C.J.; Rutkove, S.B.; Sanchez, B. Permittivity of ex vivo healthy and diseased murine skeletal muscle from 10 kHz to 1 MHz. *Sci. Data* **2019**, *6*, 37. [CrossRef] [PubMed]
53. National Institutes of Standards and Technology. Guidelines for Evaluating and Expressing the Uncertainty of NIST Measurement Results. Available online: http://physics.nist.gov/TN1297 (accessed on 15 October 2023).
54. Karpavicius, A.; Coene, A.; Bender, P.; Leliaert, J. Advanced analysis of magnetic nanoflower measurements to leverage their use in biomedicine. *Nanoscale Adv.* **2021**, *3*, 1633–1645. [CrossRef] [PubMed]

Disclaimer/Publisher's Note: The statements, opinions and data contained in all publications are solely those of the individual author(s) and contributor(s) and not of MDPI and/or the editor(s). MDPI and/or the editor(s) disclaim responsibility for any injury to people or property resulting from any ideas, methods, instructions or products referred to in the content.

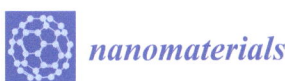

Article

Magnet-Guided Temozolomide and Ferucarbotran Loaded Nanoparticles to Enhance Therapeutic Efficacy in Glioma Model

Reju George Thomas [1,†], Subin Kim [2,†], Thi-Anh-Thuy Tran [3,4], Young Hee Kim [4], Raveena Nagareddy [1], Tae-Young Jung [4,5], Seul Kee Kim [1,6,*] and Yong Yeon Jeong [1,6,*]

1. Department of Radiology, Chonnam National University Hwasun Hospital, Hwasun 58128, Republic of Korea; regeth@gmail.com (R.G.T.)
2. Department of Biomedical Sciences, Chonnam National University Medical School, Gwangju 501190, Republic of Korea; soooo.bean@gmail.com
3. Biomedical Sciences Graduate Program (BMSGP), Chonnam National University, Hwasun 58128, Republic of Korea
4. Brain Tumor Research Laboratory, Chonnam National University Hwasun Hospital, Hwasun 58128, Republic of Korea; yung-ty@chonnam.ac.kr (T.-Y.J.)
5. Department of Neurosurgery, Chonnam National University Hwasun Hospital, Hwasun 58128, Republic of Korea
6. Department of Radiology, Chonnam National University Medical School, Gwangju 61469, Republic of Korea
* Correspondence: kimsk.rad@gmail.com (S.K.K.); yjeong@jnu.ac.kr (Y.Y.J.)
† These authors contributed equally to this work.

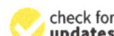

Citation: Thomas, R.G.; Kim, S.; Tran, T.-A.-T.; Kim, Y.H.; Nagareddy, R.; Jung, T.-Y.; Kim, S.K.; Jeong, Y.Y. Magnet-Guided Temozolomide and Ferucarbotran Loaded Nanoparticles to Enhance Therapeutic Efficacy in Glioma Model. *Nanomaterials* 2024, 14, 939. https://doi.org/10.3390/nano14110939

Academic Editor: James Chow

Received: 26 April 2024
Revised: 20 May 2024
Accepted: 22 May 2024
Published: 27 May 2024

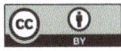

Copyright: © 2024 by the authors. Licensee MDPI, Basel, Switzerland. This article is an open access article distributed under the terms and conditions of the Creative Commons Attribution (CC BY) license (https:// creativecommons.org/licenses/by/ 4.0/).

Abstract: Background. The aim of the study was to synthesize liposomal nanoparticles loaded with temozolomide and ferucarbotran (LTF) and to evaluate the theranostic effect of LTF in the glioma model. **Methods.** We synthesized an LTF that could pass through the Blood Brain Barrier (BBB) and localize in brain tumor tissue with the help of magnet guidance. We examined the chemical characteristics. Cellular uptake and cytotoxicity studies were conducted in vitro. A biodistribution and tumor inhibition study was conduted using an in vivo glioma model. **Results.** The particle size and surface charge of LTF show 108 nm and −38 mV, respectively. Additionally, the presence of ferucarbotran significantly increased the contrast agent effect of glioma compared to the control group in MR imaging. Magnet-guided LTF significantly reduced the tumor size compared to control and other groups. Furthermore, compared to the control group, our results demonstrate a significant inhibition in brain tumor size and an increase in lifespan. **Conclusions.** These findings suggest that the LTF with magnetic guidance represents a novel approach to address current obstacles, such as BBB penetration of nanoparticles and drug resistance. Magnet-guided LTF is able to enhance therapeutic efficacy in mouse brain glioma.

Keywords: nanoparticle; glioma; theranostics; magnetic guidance

1. Introduction

Glioma is a highly aggressive primary central nervous system tumor with a low survival rate [1,2]. Surgery is the standard treatment for glioma with radiation and chemotherapy. However, the highly invasive growth pattern of glioma makes it impossible to completely remove the tumor by surgical resection without impairing the patient's brain function, which ultimately results in tumor recurrence and death of the patient [3]. Despite conventional treatment approaches, encompassing surgery, radiation, and chemotherapy, merely 3–5% of patients exhibit favorable prognoses. Furthermore, conventional chemotherapy exhibits several limitations, including suboptimal therapeutic efficacy and considerable systemic toxicity, stemming from its inadequate selectivity for malignant cells [4].

Temozolomide (TMZ) is a first-line chemotherapeutic option in the treatment of glioblastoma and functions as a DNA-alkylating agent. By methylating guanine and adenine bases, TMZ induces DNA single-strand or double-strand breaks, cell cycle arrest, and finally, cell death [5]. The anticancer effect of TMZ is achieved by its spontaneous hydrolysis into metabolite 3-methyl-(triazen-1-yl)imidazole-4-carboximide (MTIC), which subsequently decomposes into 5-aminoimidazole-4-carboxamide (AIC) and the methyl diazonium cation, both of which then alkylates DNA. TMZ, with its low molecular weight of 194 g/mol, can penetrate the BBB and be rapidly absorbed. However, the active metabolite of TMZ, MTIC, is reportedly unable to pass through cell membranes in general and the BBB in particular [6,7]. Therefore, while TMZ can cross the BBB due to its small size, its anticancer effect in the brain relies on the generation of MTIC within the brain tissue [6,8].

The BBB, which consists of microvascular endothelial cells, tight junctions, and nerves, forms a physical barrier to protect the brain tissue and maintain the environment [9]. However, it can also shield residual tumor cells that infiltrate the surrounding brain tissue and become resistant to chemotherapeutic drugs [10,11]. Thus, overcoming the BBB is a major challenge for chemotherapy in glioma treatment, and developing effective strategies to penetrate the BBB and target the tumor site is crucial for improving outcomes. There are also some limitations for TMZ, including hematological toxicity and acute cardiomyopathy, as well as poor solubility in physiological conditions that prevent drug uptake and dosage increase [12]. Additionally, the half-life of TMZ is about 1.8 h, which results in a short duration of action. This necessitates the administration of high doses of TMZ, which can cause bone marrow suppression [8,13]. To overcome these limitations, a TMZ-loaded nanoplatform has been developed to increase solubility and improve drug uptake for glioma.

Ferucarbotran (Resovist®, Bayer Healthcare, Berlin, Germany) is developed by Schering AG and is the second clinically approved superparamagnetic iron oxide (SPION) developed for contrast-enhanced MR imaging of the liver. Ferucarbotran, a type of SPION coated with carboxydextran, has been used as a T2 contrast agent [14,15]. The active particles are carboxydextrane-coated SPION, with a hydrodynamic diameter ranging between 45 and 60 nm. We have used the magnetofection method to enhance the accumulation of magnetic particle-loaded liposomes with TMZ in glioma. There are studies reported where in vivo magnetofection was performed. In this particular study, transportation of Tween-SPIONs, injected via the tail vein, through the intact blood-brain barrier in rats was subjected to an external magnetic field (EMF) [16,17]. The findings suggest that the Tween-SPIONs effectively traverse the blood-brain barrier (BBB) through an active penetration mechanism, which is facilitated by electromagnetic fields (EMF). A different strategy for the focused therapy of malignancies is magnetic hyperthermia (MH), which has been clinically introduced. In MH, an alternating magnetic field (AMF) is applied to magnetic nanoparticles (MNPs), which produce heat. Magnetofection can accumulate MNP to glioma, and MH can induce hyperthermia, causing tumor reduction. As demonstrated before, the ferucarbotran employed in our investigation likewise functions as a hyperthermia-generating nanoparticle.

In this study, we designed and synthesized a TMZ and ferucarbotran-loaded liposome to treat GL261 brain glioma. The liposome served as a nanoparticle to deliver TMZ and ferucarbotran across the BBB. By employing TMZ in conjunction with the SPION, we hypothesized that liposomal nanoparticles loaded with TMZ and ferucarbotran (LTF) have enhanced therapeutic effects as well as visualization of glioma on MR imaging. The aim of the study was to synthesize the LTF and to evaluate the theranostic effect in the glioma model.

2. Materials and Methods

2.1. Materials

The murine glioma cell line, GL261 was used for cell culture. Normal mouse fibroblast cell line (NIH3T3) and Microglial cells (BV2) were purchased from the American Type Culture Collection (ATCC, Virginia, VA, USA). 3-(4,5-dimethylthiazol-2-yl)-5-(3-carboxymethoxyphenyl)-2-(4-sulfophenyl)-2H-tetrazolium (MTS) was purchased from Promega (Promega Corporation, Wisconsin, WI, USA). Ferucarbotran (56 mg/mL) was ordered from Meito Sangyo Ltd. (Aichi, Japan). TMZ was purchased from Sigma Aldrich (Merck, Darmstadt, Germany). All other reagents were of analytical or chromatographic grade. Antibodies for immunohistochemistry were purchased from Abcam (Cambridge, UK).

2.2. Synthesis of Lipo-TMZ-Ferucarbotran (LTF)

Liposome was prepared using the film hydration method. Briefly 1, 2-Distearoyl-sn-glycero-3-phosphoethanolamine-Polyethylene glycol (DSPE-PEG), Dipalmitoylphosphatidylcholine (DPPC), and cholesterol were taken in a weight ratio of 1× (300 µg:300 µg:200 µg), 5× (1.5 mg:1.5 mg:1 mg), 10× (3 mg:3 mg:2 mg) and 15× (4.5 mg:4.5 mg:3 mg) and dissolved in their respective solvents (methanol for DSPE-PEG and DPPC, and chloroform for cholesterol). The mixture was vortexed for 2 min in a glass vial, and then a thin film was formed by evaporation of the solvents in a vacuum chamber at room temperature. The resulting film was hydrated with 1 mL of distilled water and heated in a glass vial for 30 min at 60 °C to promote the formation of multivesicular liposomes, which are heterogeneous in nature. To make LTF at 5×, 10× and 15× concentrations, 2.5, 5 mg, and 7.5 mg of TMZ and 3 mg, 6 mg and 9 mg of ferucarbotran were added to 1 mL of distilled water after the film hydration process, and the synthesis method was continued as per normal liposome synthesis. Lipo-TMZ (liposomal nanoparticle loaded only with TMZ) was synthesized using the same method except for the Ferucarbotran loading step. Purification was conducted using the dialysis method with Dialysis sacks MWCO 12,000 Da (Merck, Darmstadt, Germany) for 2 h.

2.3. Characterization of LTF

The LTF was characterized using several techniques. The hydrodynamic size and zeta potential of LTF were measured using a dynamic light scattering (Zetasizer Nano Z instrument, Malvern, UK), while the morphology of LTF was visualized using Field Emission Transmission Electron Microscopy (FE-TEM, Hitachi S3000H, Tokyo, Japan). The drug-loading and encapsulation efficiency were evaluated by thermogravimetric analyzer (TGA N-1000, Scinco, Seoul, Republic of Korea) and ICP-MS (820 ICP-MS Varian Bruker, Billerica, MA, USA) analyses, respectively. The release study was performed using a dialysis method. To do so, 3 mg/mL of LTF was dissolved in phosphate-buffered saline (PBS) and performed by oscillating shaker at a temperature of 37 °C. At different time points (0, 0.5, 1, 2, 4, 6, 8, 24, and 48 h), 1 mL samples were obtained and replaced with fresh PBS for high-performance liquid chromatography (HPLC) analysis.

2.4. In Vitro Study of LTF

The cytoviability study of LTF was evaluated by MTS assay in both BV2 neuronal and NIH3T3 mouse fibroblast cells. In a 96-well plate, 1×10^4 cells/well were seeded and maintained in Dulbecco's Modified Eagle Medium (DMEM) and incubated at 5% CO_2 and temperature of 37 °C for 24 h. After 24 h, the cell culture medium was removed, and a new medium containing TMZ, Lipo-TMZ, and LTF at a concentration range of 0 to 1000 µM [TMZ] was added to each well. Following a 24-h incubation period, 20 µL of MTS reagent was added to each well, and the plate was incubated for an additional 3 h. Finally, the absorbance was measured at 490 nm using a microplate reader.

Prussian blue staining is used in the detection of ferric iron in glioma cells. GL261 cells were plated at a density of 10^5 cells/well in an 8-well chamber and incubated overnight. After overnight incubation, a new medium containing LTF was treated at an equivalent Liposome concentration of 100 µg/mL for 6 h. The cells were washed with PBS three times and fixed with 4% paraformaldehyde. Then, the cells were stained with 100 µL of 10% potassium ferrocyanide and 2% hydrochloric acid at a 1:1 ratio for 20 min. After washing away the staining solution, the cells were counterstained with nuclear fast red stain for 5 min and observed under a bright field microscope.

The cytotoxicity study of TMZ and LTF was evaluated by MTS assay in GL261 cells. In a 96-well plate, 1×10^4 cells/well were seeded and maintained in Dulbecco's Modified Eagle Medium (DMEM) and incubated at 5% CO_2 and temperature of 37 °C for 24 h. After 24 h, the cell culture medium was removed, and a new medium containing TMZ and LTF at a concentration range of 0 to 1000 µM was added to each well. Neodymium (NdFeB) Disc Magnet was placed under 96 well plate for in vitro cytotoxicity analysis in GL261 cell line for 1 h and replaced with fresh media. After incubating for 24 h, 20 μL of MTS reagent was introduced into each well, and the plate was further incubated for 3 h. Subsequently, the absorbance was assessed at 490 nm utilizing a microplate reader.

For apoptosis analysis by caspase-3 assay (Caspase 3 Colorimetric Activity Assay Kit, DEVD, Chemicon, Massachusetts, MA, USA), GL261 cell was plated in a 12-well plate at a density of 5×10^5 cells/well and incubated overnight. After overnight incubation, a new medium containing free TMZ (62.5 μM) and LTF was treated at an equivalent TMZ concentration of 62.5 μM for 6 h. Next, the cells were washed with pre-cooled PBS and stained with caspase reagent for 30 min in the dark. After washing away the caspase reagent solution, the cells were observed under ZOE Fluorescent Cell Imager (Bio-Rad, California, CA, USA) bright field/Rhodamine B fluorescence filter.

Fluorescein diacetate (FDA) and propidium iodide (PI) staining was utilized to distinguish viable and dead cells in the LTF-treated GL261 cell line. This staining method detects live cells with FDA and dead cells with PI. We have incubated GL261 cells at a density of 5×10^5 cells/well. After 24 h, FDA/PI was added to 0.5 mL cell solution and incubated at 37 °C for 45 min. After washing away the FDA/PI solution, the cells were observed under ZOE Fluorescent Cell Imager (Bio-Rad, CA, USA) FITC/Rhodamine filter.

γ-H2AX is a marker of DNA damage and repair. It is formed when the Ser-139 residue of the H2AX histone variant is phosphorylated, indicating the presence of DNA double-strand breaks. Detecting γH2AX is a highly sensitive and specific way to monitor DNA damage and resolution. Quantifying γH2AX foci is a useful tool for evaluating the effectiveness of temozolomide in causing DNA damage. GL261 cells were cultured and seeded at 5×10^4 per well in 8 well Chamber. Once the cells were attached, the cells were incubated with free TMZ 62.5 μM, and LTF was treated at an equivalent TMZ concentration of 62.5 μM for 6 h. After incubation, the cells were given a media change and stained with mouse Anti-γ-H2AX overnight and Anti-mouse Flamma 594 for 1 h and fixed with Gold anti-phalloidin. Imaged in Zeiss Confocal Microscopy. Quantification was conducted using Image J Version 1.54g in different cells from the same image.

2.5. Release of TMZ from LTF

To conduct the drug release study, 10 mg of LTF was dispersed in 10 mL of PBS and added into a 12 kDa membrane (SpectraPor® Standard Grade RC Membrane, Fisher Scientific, Massachusetts, MA, USA). The sample was incubated at 37 °C, and 1 mL of the sample was taken in triplicates at different time points and replaced with fresh PBS. At the end of the study, the samples were dehydrated by freeze drying and dispersed in 90% methanol, then analyzed by UV-Vis.

2.6. Intracranial Glioma Mouse Model

The use of animals in this study was approved by the Chonnam National University Medical School Research Institutional Animal Care and Use Committee, and all procedures were conducted in accordance with the guidelines outlined in the National Institutes of Health Guide for the Care and Use of Laboratory Animals, under the approval reference CNU IACUC-H-2019-6. Six-week-old female C57BL/6 mice weighing 20–22 g were purchased from Orient-Bio (Seongnam-si, Republic of Korea). To establish the intracranial glioma model, 1×10^5 GL261 cells in 5 μL of PBS were stereotactically injected into the right striatum at a rate of 1 μL/min using a Harvard Apparatus Pump 11 Elite infusion syringe via a Hamilton syringe (Holliston, MA, USA). Injection sites were estimated by the following coordinates: 1 mm posterior, 2 mm lateral from bregma, and 4 mm deep from the cortical surface.

2.7. In Vivo MR Imaging and LTF Accumulation by Magnetic Guidance

GL261 cells were implanted into 6-week-old female C57BL/6 mice, and when the size of the brain tumor reached approximately 2 mm on MR imaging, the mice were divided into five groups, each receiving TMZ, Lipo-TMZ, or LTF according to a predetermined schedule. We divided the mice into five groups of four each; Group 1: control (0 mg/kg of TMZ), Group 2: free TMZ (11.3 mg/kg of TMZ), Group 3: Lipo-TMZ (11.3 mg/kg of TMZ), Group 4: LTF (magnet off) (11.3 mg/kg of TMZ) and Group 5: LTF (magnet on) (11.3 mg/kg of TMZ). All nanoparticles were administered intravenously 200 µL dose of LTF (8 mg/mL [1.4 mg of TMZ]) to each mouse four times on days 1, 2, 5, and 6. For group 5, after the LTF was injected, the animals were anesthetized with a combination of zoletil® and rompun® (zoletil: rompun: PBS ratio of 1 mL:0.5 mL:8.5 mL) 100 µL intraperitoneal injection in mice, and then neodymium magnets were placed on the heads of the mouse tumor models for 1 h.

MR imaging was performed using a preclinical 1T permanent magnet scanner (M7 system, Aspect Imaging, Shoham, Israel). To evaluate the contrast enhancement and tumor reduction efficacy of LTF, T2-weighted MR imaging was acquired using fast spin echo (FSE) sequences. The scan parameters T2WI included the following: echo time (TE) of 80 ms, repetition time (TR) of 7952 ms, slice thickness of 1 mm, field of view of 25 mm, 13 slices, and a matrix of 256 × 256. To evaluate the LTF contrast effect, the signal intensity was measured in the region of interest (ROI) area of the MR image to calculate the degree of contrast enhancement. In T2-weighted MR imaging, the signal intensity decreases proportionally as the contrast enhancement is increased by the LTF-loaded ferucarbotran.

2.8. Biodistribution of LTF

In the study, C57BL/6 mice with intracranial glioma were administered a 200 µL dose of LTF (2 mg/mL) intravenously. Following the LTF administration, a biodistribution study was conducted on the LTF (magnet-on) group. For the magnet-on group, after the injection of LTF, the mice were anesthetized using a combination of zoletil and rompun combination with 100 µL intraperitoneal injection in mice. The mice's heads were then positioned near a neodymium magnet for a duration of 1 h. This step aimed to facilitate the localization of LTF in the desired area, specifically the tumor region. When the tumor size reached 4 mm, we administered LTF. After 24 h of LTF administration, the mice were euthanized. Major organs (Heart, liver, spleen, lung, kidney, brain) and tumor were then harvested and subjected to Aqua regia (3 parts of Hydrochloric acid and 1 part of Nitric acid) treatment to break down the tissue and extract iron. The iron content of these organs was then investigated using inductively coupled plasma mass spectrometry (ICP-MS). This analysis aimed to determine the distribution and accumulation of iron, which serves as an indicator of the presence and localization of LTF in the organs and tumor tissues.

2.9. Glioma Reduction and Survival Study

Follow-up MR imaging was obtained daily until 7 days after the initial injection to observe changes in tumor volume. Tumor volume assessment using MR imaging was based on ROIs. In this study, ROIs were manually drawn on all image slices covering the majority of the tumor area. All image data were transferred in DICOM format through a picture archiving and transmission system (PACS), and tumor volumes were calculated using RadiAnt DICOM viewer (Medixant, Poland) and INFINITT PACS M6 image analysis software (Infinite Healthcare, Seoul, Republic of Korea).

The survival of the mice was tracked for 31 days, and surviving mice that were asymptomatic at the end of the trial were sacrificed. After 31 days, no mice from groups PBS, TMZ, and Lipo-TMZ survived. In LTF (MagOff) 2 mice and LTF (MagOn) 1 mouse survived after 31 days. Every mouse with a tumor was closely monitored daily and given proper care in the form of feed and water.

2.10. Immunohistochemistry

To observe the cellular damage due to LTF in the harvested organs, H&E imaging was performed using an optical microscope (Olympus). TUNEL assay was performed according to the manufacturer's instruction (DeadEnd™ Fluorometric TUNEL system, Promega, USA) and visualized with a microscopy (Zeiss Confocal Microscopy, Carl Zeiss,

Oberkochen, Baden-Württemberg, Germany). For Ki67 immunochemistry, tumor slides were deparaffinized and stained with a primary anti-mouse rabbit-originated Ki67 antibody (1:1000 dilution), followed by a secondary Alexa Fluor 488 goat-originated anti-rabbit antibody (1:250 dilution) and imaged using confocal microscopy (Zeiss Confocal Microscopy). The fluorescence intensities were quantified using ImageJ software from four randomly selected areas of equal size.

2.11. Statistical Analysis

All data represented either the mean ± standard error of the mean or mean ± standard deviation. The differences between the groups were evaluated with one-way analyses of variance (ANOVA) or Kruskal-Wallis, which was followed by Mann-Whitney U test or Tukey's multiple comparison tests or Student's t-test. A two-sided probability value (p) less than 0.05 was considered statistically significant. * indicates $p < 0.05$, † indicates $p < 0.01$. All measurements were taken by observers who were blinded to the individual treatments.

3. Results

3.1. Synthesis and Characterization of LTF

LTF was synthesized and analyzed for size, charge, and morphological characteristics. The morphology of LTF was determined in Field emission-transmission electron microscopy (TEM) (Figure 1A). Dynamic light scattering (DLS) showed a size of 108 ± 60 nm with polydispersity index (PDI) = 0.358 and a zeta potential value of −38 mV (Figure 1B). Elemental analysis by EDAX was conducted to check the percentage of iron (Fe) and oxygen (O) in LTF.11.05% of iron and 88.95% of oxygen were detected (Figure 1C). Encapsulation efficiency (%) of TMZ was 20.1%, 28.25%, and 24.03% for 5×, 10× and 15× of LTF and thermogravimetric analysis (TGA) of LTF of 42.91%, 40.19% and 38.09% for 5×, 10× and 15× of LTF. Based on the result from EE%, we can assume that LTF 10x concentration showed the best possible encapsulation of TMZ drug at 28.25%. TGA showed 40.19% iron oxide loading of ferucarbotran in LTF 10× concentration (Figure 1D). Therefore, based on the encapsulation value of the drug and the loading amount of iron oxide, we selected LTF 10× as the candidate for in vitro and in vivo analysis.

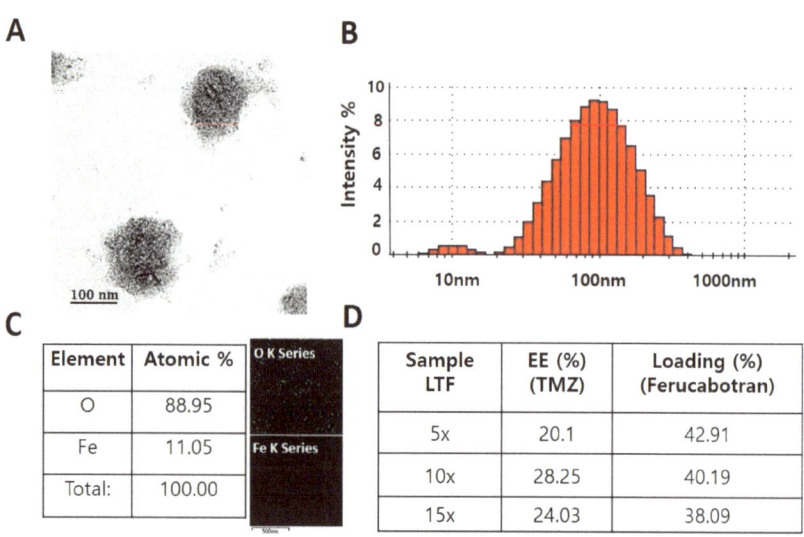

Figure 1. Characterization of Lipo-TMZ-Ferucarbotran. (**A**) Transmission electron microscope analysis of LTF (**B**). DLS of LTF nanoparticle. (inset figure show Size distribution from 10 nm to 1000 nm) (**C**) EDAX elemental analysis of LTF nanoparticle (**D**). Encapsulation efficiency and Thermogravimetric analysis of LTF nanoparticle.

3.2. In Vitro Characterization

The cell viability of LTF was analyzed using the MTS assay in BV2 and NIH3T3 cell lines, with a concentration range of up to 1000 µM [TMZ] and 24-h incubation. The cell viability was maintained and exhibited minimal toxicity even at 1000 µM (Figure 2A). Cell uptake analysis was performed using Prussian blue assay (Figure 2B). Ferucarbotran, which contains iron oxide nanoparticles, reacts with acidic ferrocyanide to produce a blue color. From the cell uptake data, it is clear that LTF is taken up into the cellular compartment, providing insights into cell toxicity.

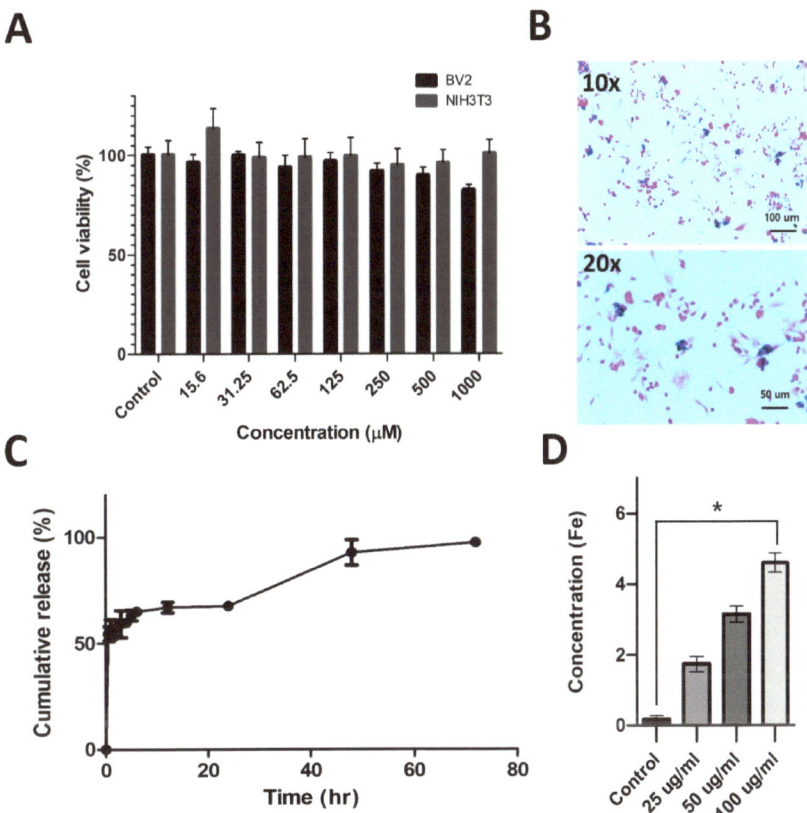

Figure 2. In vitro characterization of Lipo-TMZ-Ferucarbotran. (**A**) Cell viability study of Lipo-TMZ-Ferucarbotran in BV2 neuronal and NIH3T3 fibroblast cell line. (**B**) Cell uptake of Lipo-TMZ-Ferucarbotran in GL261 cell line by Prussian Blue assay. (**C**) Cumulative release profile of LTF. (**D**) ICP-AES accumulation analysis of LTF at different concentrations in GL261 cell line. The data are presented as the mean ± standard deviation control with a number of samples (* $p < 0.05$, n = 3). The Iron oxide (Fe) concentrations showed significant differences between 4 groups and in the post hoc analysis (Control vs. 25 µg/mL vs. 50 µg/mL vs. 100 µg/mL: $p = 0.01556$; Kruskal–Wallis test).

To analyze the drug release ability of TMZ from LTF, we conducted a drug release test with UV-Vis. The data showed a burst release of 50% of TMZ within 1 h of dialysis, indicating that the liposome is susceptible to body temperature and partially breaks down to release TMZ into the bloodstream. However, 70% of the release took almost 24 h, which is longer than the brain accumulation time of LTF. The 100% release took 76 h, supporting the sustained release claim of the nanoparticle [18] (Figure 2C). A quantitative level of uptake was conducted by ICP-AES on the cell incubated with LTF. Higher concentrations of the LTF accumulated in proportion to the concentration and were statistically significantly increased at 100 ug/mL compared to the control (Figure 2D).

The cell toxicity of LTF was analyzed using the MTS assay in the GL261 cell line in comparison with free TMZ, with a concentration range of up to 1000 µM [TMZ] and Neodymium (NdFeB) Disc Magnet was placed under 96 well plate for in vitro cytotoxicity analysis in GL261 cell line for 1 h and fresh media was added. Afterward, a 24-h incubation time was given. The cell viability progressively decreased from 15.6 µM for LTF, reaching a maximum of less than 30% at a concentration of 1000 µM, whereas TMZ exhibited minimal toxicity even at 1000 µM (Figure 3A). We performed a caspase-3 assay to detect apoptosis in LTF-treated cells and found an increase in caspase-3 activity as shown by red fluorescence in the LTF group compared to cells treated with TMZ alone and the control group. Apoptosis of glioma cells is more prominent in the LTF-treated group than in the TMZ group (Figure 3B). The live/dead assay using FDA/PI showed a similar trend to the caspase 3 assay. LTF-treated cells showed more cell death, with decreased green fluorescence in FDA staining and red fluorescence in PI staining (Figure 3B).

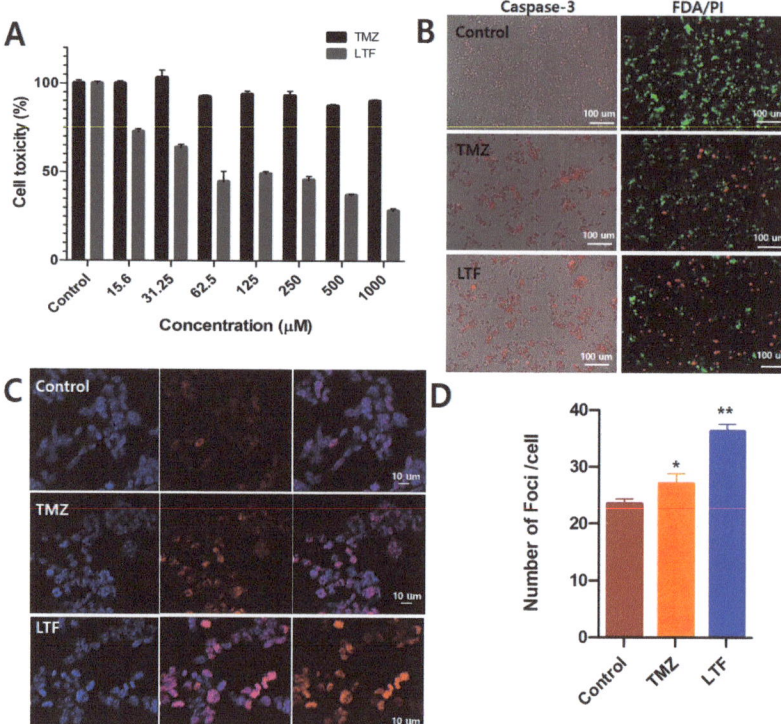

Figure 3. In vitro cytotoxicity of Lipo-TMZ-Ferucarbotran. (**A**) Cell toxicity study of TMZ and LTF in GL261 cell line by MTS assay with magnetofection. (**B**) Cell apoptosis study of Lipo-TMZ-Ferucarbotran in GL261 cell line by Caspase-3 assay (Red fluorescence indicates apoptotic cells). Cell death study of uptake of Lipo-TMZ-Ferucarbotran in GL261 cell line by FDA/PI staining (Green fluorescence-live cells; Red fluorescence—dead cells). (**C**) CLSM images of ɣ-H2AX (Scale bar 10 µm; Red fluorescence—double-strand break in DNA) and its (**D**) Quantification of ɣ-H2AX fluorescence. The data are presented as the mean ± standard error of the mean control (* $p < 0.05$; ** $p < 0.01$ when compared with the control group; Tukey post hoc test). The Number of Foci/Cell in the LTF group significantly increased compared with the Control or TMZ groups (Control vs. TMZ vs. LTF: $p = 0.00001$; one-way ANOVA test, TMZ vs. LTF: $p = 0.00008$; Control vs. LTF: $p = 0.00001$; Tukey post hoc test).

Double-stranded breaks (DSB) formation is an initial cellular response to radiation, and the detection of ɣ-H2AX foci serves as direct evidence to confirm the presence of DSBs. In our study, we investigated the impact of TMZ on the phosphorylation of ɣ-H2AX using CSLM imaging. As shown in (Figure 3C,D), the treated group exhibited a significant increase in the number of ɣ-H2AX foci compared to the control and TMZ group, indicating that LTF released TMZ-induced DSBs more than the TMZ group.

3.3. In Vivo MR Imaging and LTF Accumulation by Magnetic Guidance

In the LTF-treated groups, the decrease in MRI signal intensity of the glioma steadily decreased over time, especially in the magnet-on group (Figure 4A). The contrast effect of LTF (magnet-on) lasted until day 6, while the contrast effect of LTF (magnet-off) decreased significantly after day 2. On days 5, 6, and 7, the LTF (magnet-on) group had a statistically significant difference in contrast effect than the magnet-off group (Figure 4B). The decrease in signal intensity indicates that more LTFs are targeted and also that more TMZ accumulates in the glioma.

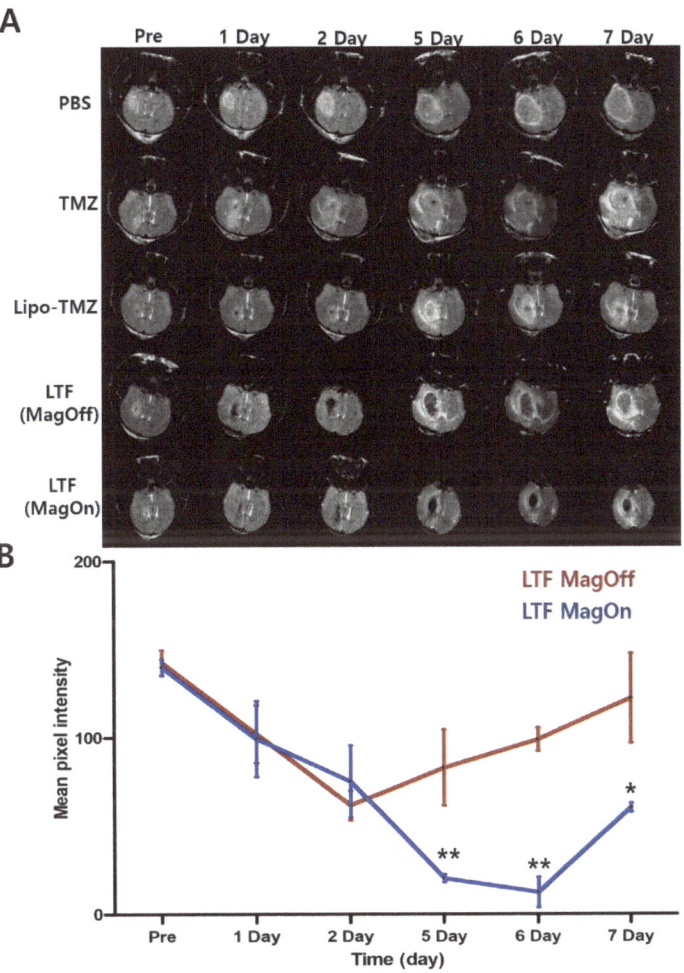

Figure 4. Tumor accumulation of LTF. (**A**) In vivo T2-weighted MR imaging of C57BL/6 mice injected with PBS, TMZ, Lipo-TMZ, LTF (Magnet-Off), LTF (Magnet-On) at different time points (Magnetofection

was conducted for one time after injection of LTF for one hour). (**B**) A quantitative graph shows changes in MR signal intensity over time. The average pixel intensity of the MR images shows a statistically significant difference between LTF (magnet on) and LTF (magnet off) using the one-way ANOVA test. The data are presented as the mean ± standard error of the mean control (* $p < 0.001$; ** $p < 0.01$) (n = 4). The MR signal intensity showed significant differences between 2 groups at different time points (LTF (Magnet-Off) vs. LTF (Magnet-On): $p = 0.0074$ at day 5, $p = 0.002$ at day 6 and $p = 0.0137$; One-way ANOVA).

3.4. Glioma Reduction and Survival Study

Glioma growth inhibition was observed in the LTF (Magnet-On) group from day 3 to day 7, with statistical significance (* $p < 0.01$) (Figure 5A). Lipo-TMZ also demonstrated significant tumor inhibition compared to the PBS and TMZ groups, which validates the ability of liposomes to penetrate the BBB. Lipo-TMZ and LTF (magnet off) groups exhibited a similar tumor inhibition profile, as expected, since Ferucarbotran does not contribute to any chemotherapeutic effect. Survival analysis of mice showed that the median survival duration for the LTF (magnet on) group was longer than the LTF (magnet off) group, likely attributable to a decrease in tumor growth and concomitant reduction in glioma volume (Figure 5B).

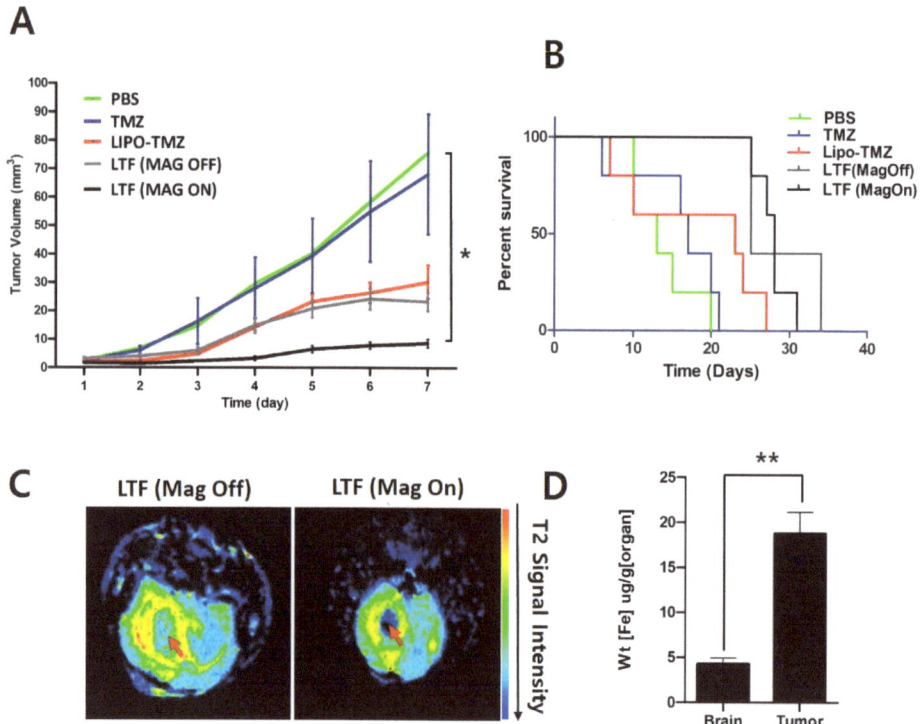

Figure 5. Tumor reduction study of LTF in GL261 tumor. (**A**) Tumor volume measurement after treatment of PBS, TMZ, Lipo-TMZ, LTF (mag off), and LTF (mag on). The data are presented as the mean ± standard error (* $p < 0.5$). The mean tumor size showed significant differences between the PBS, TMZ, LIPO-TMZ, LTF (MAG OFF), and LTF (MAG ON) as analyzed by the One-way ANOVA test on day 7 and Tukey post hoc test. (PBS vs. TMZ vs. LIPO-TMZ vs. LTF (MAG OFF) vs. LTF (MAG ON); One-way ANOVA: $p = 0.002$, PBS vs LTF (MAG OFF): $p = 0.03$, PBS vs. LTF (MAG ON): $p = 0.006$ and TMZ vs. LTF (MAG ON): $p = 0.016$: Tukey post hoc test). (**B**) Survival analysis of all groups after tumor reduction study was conducted using the Kaplan-Meir method. The data are

presented as the mean ± standard error (* $p < 0.5$). The survival curves are significantly different between the PBS, TMZ, LIPO-TMZ, LTF (MAG OFF), and LTF (MAG ON) as analyzed by the log-rank (Mantel-Cox) test ($p = 0.002$). (**C**) MR imaging of LTF accumulation in tumor. (**D**) ICP-MS analysis of LTF accumulation in brain and tumor. The data are presented as the mean ± standard deviation with a number of samples (n) = 4. ** indicates $p < 0.001$.

In contrast, LTF (magnet on) group accumulated more than LTF (magnet off) as shown by MRI data and ICP-MS data (Figure 5C,D).

3.5. Biodistribution and Immunohistochemistry

H and E staining on the organs and tumor assessed the potential toxic effects of TMZ but found no visible toxicity, including in the brain. H and E analysis depicted in (Figure 6A) also demonstrates that, following the treatment, the regrowth of the tumor tissue occurs with a reduced density of brain tissue. This suggests that the treatment has a suppressive effect on the growth and density of the tumor, contributing to the observed survival benefits. TUNEL analysis, which detects DNA fragmentation associated with apoptosis, investigates the presence of apoptotic cells in the tumor region of the brain. The TUNEL analysis showed green fluorescence, indicating the occurrence of apoptosis in that specific area (Figure 6B).

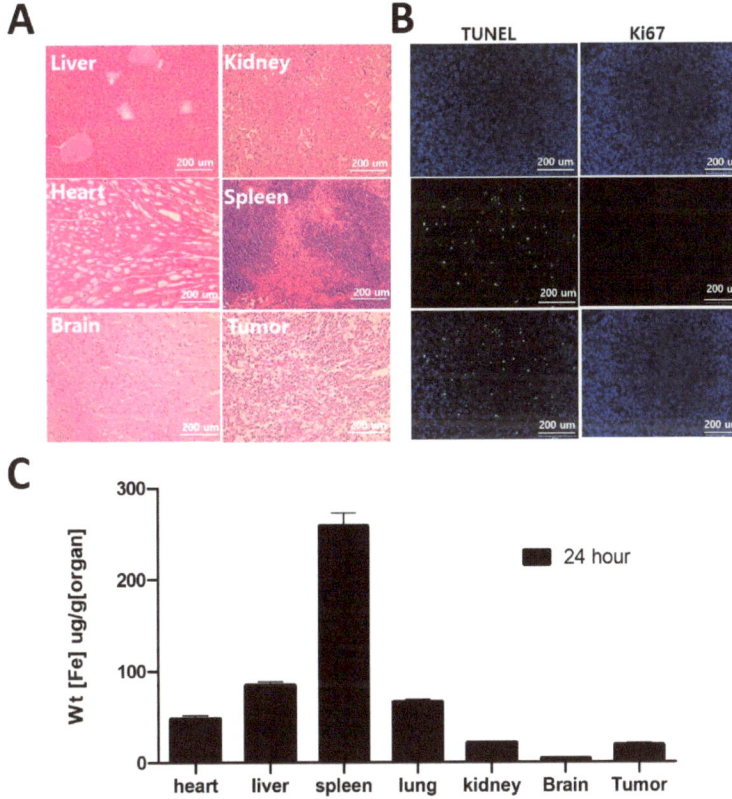

Figure 6. Histopathological analysis (**A**) H and E staining of tumor and organs. (**B**) TUNEL and Ki67 images of GL261 tumor extracted from brain (blue fluorescence: DAPI stain, green fluorescence: TUNEL/Ki67 stain). These findings indicate that the administration of LTF resulted in the initiation of apoptosis (cell death) in the tumor cells, accompanied by limited cell division or growth. (**C**) ICP-MS analysis of organs and tumor after 24 h of LTF administration and magnetofection.

Additionally, we employed Ki67 staining to identify proliferating cells, which are indicative of active cell division. Interestingly, the Ki67 staining did not show any proliferating cells in the tumor region, suggesting that the tumor cells had a very low proliferation index. These findings suggest that LTF treatment led to the induction of apoptosis in the tumor cells with minimal cell division or growth (Figure 6B). We can correlate H and E analysis of tumor tissue with reduced growth and density of the tumor to Ki67 staining data with a very low proliferation index and conclude that tumor growth is significantly affected by TMZ from LTF nanoparticles.

ICP-MS analysis in the LTF (magnet on) group revealed a significant accumulation of SPION in the tumor compared to the brain (Figure 6C). This suggests that the iron oxide specifically accumulated in the tumor region. Additionally, the study examined the distribution of LTF in various organs, and the results showed the highest accumulation of LTF in the spleen, which is known to serve as a storage organ for iron in the body [19].

Moreover, the study compared the accumulation of LTF in glioma tissue with that in normal brain tissue. The findings indicated that glioma tissue exhibited a higher accumulation of LTF than normal brain tissue, implying a potential targeting effect of LTF on the tumor. We can relate the effect of a higher accumulation of LTF nanoparticles in glioma tissue with the immunohistochemistry data, which shows that more TMZ accumulation can cause reduced tumor cell proliferation and thus inhibit glioma progression [20].

4. Discussion

To the best of our knowledge, this is the first report of targeted treatment of glioma under magnetic guidance by loading TMZ and SPION together in liposome nanoparticles. In our study, we successfully synthesized LTF nanoparticles loaded with TMZ and ferucarbotran and confirmed that the therapeutic effect of TMZ on glioma was increased by targeted delivery of TMZ to tumor cells. We also confirmed the contrast enhancement effect of glioma in MR imaging.

Treatment of glioma remains a challenge, largely due to the fast degradation of TMZ, the inability to deliver an effective dose of TMZ to tumors, and the lack of target specificity, which may cause systemic toxicity. Various attempts are being made to overcome this, especially targeted therapies using various nanoparticles. Similar to our study, previous studies reported that TMZ in liposomal formulation showed enhanced uptake by glioma cells compared to free TMZ, which relies only on passive diffusion for cellular uptake. The use of liposomal nanoparticles to enhance the delivery of TMZ across the BBB and improve the therapeutic efficacy of the drug [9,21].

Gliomas are characterized by endothelial proliferation by angiogenesis and the formation of tortuous, disorganized, and highly permeable vessels [22]. These excessive neovessels disrupt the BBB and cause contrast enhancement of the glioma on MR imaging [23]. Contrast agents such as gadolinium and spions do not cross the healthy BBB, but in tumors such as glioma, the BBB is physically destroyed by angiogenesis, allowing the contrast agent to leak into the tumor tissue, making the tumor visible on T1-weighted MR images [24]. So, in theory, intravenously administered nanoparticles could take advantage of this phenomenon in glioma for imaging and treatment. Optimum nanoparticle formulations were chosen according to particle size, TEM imaging, and higher encapsulation efficiency. The ideal nanoparticle formulation for localized brain delivery should be in a range of 10–200 nm and is preferred to be spherical [25]. In our study, the nanoparticles were 108 nm in size and passed through the BBB, allowing us to observe changes in tumor size in MR imaging. Based on the result from encapsulation efficiency, LTF 10x concentration showed the best possible loading of ferucarbotran and TMZ in liposomes used for in vitro and in vivo studies. Cumulative release data also show sustained release of TMZ over a period of 0 to 50 h, which allows LTF to get implanted in the tumor and release TMZ.

Cytotoxicity study revealed that the cell toxicity of LTF was significantly higher than that of free TMZ. This finding implies that the LTF system could offer enhanced therapeutic efficacy compared to conventional treatment methods. Previous studies have suggested that liposomal formulations of TMZ may have better uptake by glioma cells compared to TMZ taken up by cancer cells through passive diffusion alone [26,27]. In vitro uptake quantification by ICP-OES showed a concentration-mediated uptake profile of LTF in the GL261 cell line with the highest accumulation at 100 ug/mL concentration. Qualitative analysis by Prussian blue staining also shows significant uptake of LTF in GL261 cells.

Our study employed the LTF system, which demonstrated substantial nanoparticle accumulation in the magnetic guidance group in comparison to the non-magnetic guidance group, as evidenced by T2-weighed MR imaging. Even though BBB penetration is favored by positively charged nanoparticles, LTF exhibits negative zeta potential, which helps it to escape reticuloendothelial system (RES) phagocytosis. This result was attributed to the magnetic effect of ferucarbotran, a SPION agent. SPIONs are extensively investigated as standalone theranostic particles as well. The magnetic iron core can be visualized via MR imaging, allowing tracking of the particles and simultaneously presenting a way of directing the particles toward their goal via magnetic fields [28]. In addition, the attractive force of the external magnetic field can be utilized to guide the ferucarbotran toward the tumor site, thereby increasing the concentration of ferucarbotran in the tumor compared to the surrounding healthy tissue [29,30].

Our study demonstrated a significant inhibition of brain tumor size and an increase in lifespan compared to the control group. The targeted delivery of LTF to glioma is further facilitated by the application of an external magnetic field, and the therapeutic effect is further improved. These findings suggest that the LTF with magnetic guidance represents a promising approach to address current obstacles, such as BBB penetration of nanoparticles and drug resistance. The increased accumulation facilitated a significant reduction in tumor size, primarily due to the enhanced delivery of TMZ to the tumor site.

The ability to accurately visualize and quantify nanoparticle accumulation in tumor areas can greatly improve our understanding of biodistribution. ICP-MS analysis in the LTF (magnet on) group revealed a significant accumulation of SPION in the tumor compared to the normal brain. This finding suggests that magnetic guidance plays a crucial role in enhancing LTF accumulation within the tumor, resulting in improved therapeutic effect of the chemotherapeutic agent. Future studies should focus on optimizing the LTF system and magnetic guidance for enhanced drug delivery, as well as assessing the long-term safety and efficacy of this approach in preclinical and clinical settings.

In summary, our study showed to synthesize LTF is a promising drug delivery system for targeted glioma therapy. LTFs were loaded with TMZ and ferucarbotran so that more TMZ accumulated in glioma cells due to the magnetic effect of ferucarbotran. In vitro cytotoxicity studies showed that LTFs had a toxic effect on glioma cells. In an in vivo tumor reduction study, LTF reduced tumor size more effectively in the magnetic guidance group than TMZ or LTF without magnetic guidance.

In conclusion, this study provides a comprehensive characterization and evaluation of LTF as a targeted drug delivery system for glioma treatment. The combination of liposomal encapsulation and magnetic guidance has demonstrated improved therapeutic outcomes in a glioma mouse model. LTF may be a promising platform for further development and eventual clinical application.

Supplementary Materials: The following supporting information can be downloaded at: https://www.mdpi.com/article/10.3390/nano14110939/s1, Figure S1: (A) TEM image of LTF at higher magnification (B) Prussian blue staining of LTF at higher magnification (C) DLS size distribution of Ferucarbotran. Figure S2: Size of LTF at Day 1, Day 7 and Day 14. Figure S3: Cell viability study of Lipo-Ferucarbotran in NIH3T3 fibroblast cell line. Figure S4: Positioning of Neodymium (NdFeB) Disc Magnet (10 mm diameter and 5 mm thick) for in vitro and in vivo studies (A) Neodymium (NdFeB) Disc Magnet was placed under 96 well plate for in vitro cytotoxicity analysis in GL261 cell line (B) Neodymium (NdFeB) Disc Magnet was placed at axial plane relative to mice brain. Table S1: Size and Zeta potential values of LTF at $5\times$, $10\times$ and $15\times$ concentration.

Author Contributions: R.G.T., S.K., Y.Y.J. and S.K.K. wrote the manuscript, designed the experiments, and interpreted the results; R.G.T. and S.K. performed the in vitro experiments and animal studies; T.-A.-T.T., Y.H.K. and T.-Y.J. prepared glioblastoma tumor; R.N. performed FACS analysis and gamah2x study; Y.Y.J. and S.K.K. supervised all aspects of this work. All authors have read and agreed to the published version of the manuscript.

Funding: This study was financially supported by the Ministry of Science and ICT through the National Research Foundation of Korea (No. 2022R1A2C1003266) and Chonnam National University Hwasun Hospital Institute for Biomedical Science (HCRI 18008-1).

Data Availability Statement: Data are contained within the article and Supplementary Materials.

Conflicts of Interest: The authors have no conflicts to declare.

References

1. Lee, S.Y. Temozolomide resistance in glioblastoma multiforme. *Genes Dis.* **2016**, *3*, 198–210. [CrossRef] [PubMed]
2. Stupp, R.; Mason, W.P.; van den Bent, M.J.; Weller, M.; Fisher, B.; Taphoorn, M.J.; Belanger, K. Radiotherapy plus concomitant and adjuvant temozolomide for glioblastoma. *N. Engl. J. Med.* **2005**, *352*, 987–996. [CrossRef]
3. Giese, A.; Bjerkvig, R.; Berens, M.E.; Westphal, M. Cost of migration: Invasion of malignant gliomas and implications for treatment. *J. Clin. Oncol. Off. J. Am. Soc. Clin. Oncol.* **2003**, *21*, 1624–1636. [CrossRef] [PubMed]
4. Hoda, M. Potential Alternatives to Conventional Cancer Therapeutic Approaches: The Way Forward. *Curr. Pharm. Biotechnol.* **2021**, *22*, 1141–1148. [CrossRef] [PubMed]
5. Strobel, H.; Baisch, T.; Fitzel, R.; Schilberg, K.; Siegelin, M.D.; Karpel-Massler, G.; Debatin, K.-M.; Westhoff, M.-A. Temozolomide and Other Alkylating Agents in Glioblastoma Therapy. *Biomedicines* **2019**, *7*, 69. [CrossRef]
6. Newlands, E.S.; Blackledge, G.R.; Slack, J.A.; Rustin, G.J.; Smith, D.B.; Stuart, N.S.; Quarterman, C.P.; Hoffman, R.; Stevens, M.F.G.; Brampton, M.H.; et al. Phase I trial of temozolomide (CCRG 81045: M&B 39831: NSC 362856). *Br. J. Cancer* **1992**, *65*, 287–291.
7. Baker, S.D.; Wirth, M.; Statkevich, P.; Reidenberg, P.; Alton, K.; Sartorius, S.E.; Dugan, M.; Cutler, D.; Batra, V.; Grochow, L.B.; et al. Absorption, metabolism, and excretion of 14C-temozolomide following oral administration to patients with advanced cancer. *Clin. Cancer Res. Off. J. Am. Assoc. Cancer Res.* **1999**, *5*, 309–317.
8. Lam, F.C.; Morton, S.W.; Wyckoff, J.; Vu Han, T.L.; Hwang, M.K.; Maffa, A.; Balkanska-Sinclair, E.; Yaffe, M.B.; Floyd, S.R.; Hammond, P.T. Enhanced efficacy of combined temozolomide and bromodomain inhibitor therapy for gliomas using targeted nanoparticles. *Nat. Commun.* **2018**, *9*, 1991. [CrossRef] [PubMed]
9. Zhao, M.; van Straten, D.; Broekman, M.L.D.; Préat, V.; Schiffelers, R.M. Nanocarrier-based drug combination therapy for glioblastoma. *Theranostics* **2020**, *10*, 1355–1372. [CrossRef]
10. Gregory, J.V.; Kadiyala, P.; Doherty, R.; Cadena, M.; Habeel, S.; Ruoslahti, E.; Lowenstein, P.R.; Castro, M.G.; Lahhan, J. Systemic brain tumor delivery of synthetic protein nanoparticles for glioblastoma therapy. *Nat. Commun.* **2020**, *11*, 5687. [CrossRef]
11. Fang, C.; Wang, K.; Stephen, Z.R.; Mu, Q.; Kievit, F.M.; Chiu, D.T.; Press, O.W.; Zhang, M. Temozolomide nanoparticles for targeted glioblastoma therapy. *ACS Appl. Mater. Interfaces* **2015**, *7*, 6674–6682. [CrossRef] [PubMed]
12. Nordling-David, M.M.; Yaffe, R.; Guez, D.; Meirow, H.; Last, D.; Grad, E.; Salomon, S.; Sharabi, S.; Levi-Kalisman, Y.; Golomb, G.; et al. Liposomal temozolomide drug delivery using convection enhanced delivery. *J. Control. Release Off. J. Control. Release Soc.* **2017**, *261*, 138–146. [CrossRef] [PubMed]
13. Jiang, G.; Li, R.; Tang, J.; Ma, Y.; Hou, X.; Yang, C.; Guo, W.; Xin, Y.; Liu, Y. Formulation of temozolomide-loaded nanoparticles and their targeting potential to melanoma cells. *Oncol. Rep.* **2017**, *37*, 995–1001. [CrossRef] [PubMed]
14. Chung, T.-H.; Hsiao, J.-K.; Yao, M.; Hsu, S.-C.; Liu, H.-M.; Huang, D.-M. Ferucarbotran, a carboxydextran-coated superparamagnetic iron oxide nanoparticle, induces endosomal recycling, contributing to cellular and exosomal EGFR overexpression for cancer therapy. *RSC Adv.* **2015**, *5*, 89932–89939. [CrossRef]
15. Hamm, B.; Staks, T.; Taupitz, M.; Maibauer, R.; Speidel, A.; Huppertz, A.; Frenzel, T.; Lawaczeck, R.; Wolf, K.J.; Lange, L. Contrast-enhanced MR imaging of liver and spleen: First experience in humans with a new superparamagnetic iron oxide. *J. Magn. Reson. Imaging* **1994**, *4*, 659–668. [CrossRef]
16. Huang, Y.; Zhang, B.; Xie, S.; Yang, B.; Xu, Q.; Tan, J. Superparamagnetic Iron Oxide Nanoparticles Modified with Tween 80 Pass through the Intact Blood–Brain Barrier in Rats under Magnetic Field. *ACS Appl. Mater. Interfaces* **2016**, *8*, 11336–11341. [CrossRef]
17. Thomsen, L.B.; Thomsen, M.S.; Moos, T. Targeted drug delivery to the brain using magnetic nanoparticles. *Therapeutic Delivery* **2015**, *6*, 1145–1155. [CrossRef]
18. Yoo, J.; Won, Y.-Y. Phenomenology of the Initial Burst Release of Drugs from PLGA Microparticles. *ACS Biomater. Sci. Eng.* **2020**, *6*, 6053–6062. [CrossRef] [PubMed]
19. Kolnagou, A.; Michaelides, Y.; Kontoghiorghe, C.N.; Kontoghiorghes, G.J. The importance of spleen, spleen iron, and splenectomy for determining total body iron load, ferrikinetics, and iron toxicity in thalassemia major patients. *Toxicol. Mech. Methods* **2013**, *23*, 34–41. [CrossRef]

20. Erthal, L.C.S.; Shi, Y.; Sweeney, K.J.; Gobbo, O.L.; Ruiz-Hernandez, E. Nanocomposite formulation for a sustained release of free drug and drug-loaded responsive nanoparticles: An approach for a local therapy of glioblastoma multiforme. *Sci. Rep.* **2023**, *13*, 5094. [CrossRef]
21. Amarandi, R.M.; Ibanescu, A.; Carasevici, E.; Marin, L.; Dragoi, B. Liposomal-Based Formulations: A Path from Basic Research to Temozolomide Delivery Inside Glioblastoma Tissue. *Pharmaceutics* **2022**, *14*, 308. [CrossRef]
22. Dubois, L.G.; Campanati, L.; Righy, C.; D'Andrea-Meira, I.; Leite de Sampaio e Spohr, T.C.; Porto-Carreiro, I.; Pereira, C.M.; Balca-Silva, J.; Kahn, S.A.; DosSantos, M.F.; et al. Gliomas and the vascular fragility of the blood brain barrier. *Front. Cell. Neurosci.* **2014**, *8*, 418. [CrossRef] [PubMed]
23. Holodny, A.I.; Nusbaum, A.O.; Festa, S.; Pronin, I.N.; Lee, H.J.; Kalnin, A.J. Correlation between the degree of contrast enhancement and the volume of peritumoral edema in meningiomas and malignant gliomas. *Neuroradiology* **1999**, *41*, 820–825. [CrossRef] [PubMed]
24. Heye, A.K.; Culling, R.D.; del C. Valdés Hernández, M.; Thrippleton, M.J.; Wardlaw, J.M. Assessment of blood-brain barrier disruption using dynamic contrast-enhanced MRI. A systematic review. *NeuroImage Clin.* **2014**, *6*, 262–274. [CrossRef] [PubMed]
25. Brown, T.D.; Habibi, N.; Wu, D.; Lahann, J.; Mitragotri, S. Effect of Nanoparticle Composition, Size, Shape, and Stiffness on Penetration Across the Blood–Brain Barrier. *ACS Biomater. Sci. Eng.* **2020**, *6*, 4916–4928. [CrossRef] [PubMed]
26. Zou, Y.; Wang, Y.; Xu, S.; Liu, Y.; Yin, J.; Lovejoy, D.B.; Zheng, M.; Liang, X.-J.; Park, J.B.; Efremov, Y.M.; et al. Brain Co-Delivery of Temozolomide and Cisplatin for Combinatorial Glioblastoma Chemotherapy. *Adv. Mater.* **2022**, *34*, 2203958. [CrossRef] [PubMed]
27. Barenholz, Y. Liposome application: Problems and prospects. *Curr. Opin. Colloid Interface Sci.* **2001**, *6*, 66–77. [CrossRef]
28. Gobbo, O.L.; Sjaastad, K.; Radomski, M.W.; Volkov, Y.; Prina-Mello, A. Magnetic Nanoparticles in Cancer Theranostics. *Theranostics* **2015**, *5*, 1249–1263. [CrossRef]
29. Kritika; Roy, I. Therapeutic applications of magnetic nanoparticles: Recent advances. *Mater. Adv.* **2022**, *3*, 7425–7444. [CrossRef]
30. Ravikanth, R. Advanced Magnetic Resonance Imaging of Glioblastoma Multiforme. *J. Neurosci. Rural Pract.* **2017**, *8*, 439–440. [CrossRef]

Disclaimer/Publisher's Note: The statements, opinions and data contained in all publications are solely those of the individual author(s) and contributor(s) and not of MDPI and/or the editor(s). MDPI and/or the editor(s) disclaim responsibility for any injury to people or property resulting from any ideas, methods, instructions or products referred to in the content.

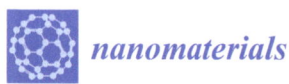

Article

Physico-Chemical Properties of CdTe/Glutathione Quantum Dots Obtained by Microwave Irradiation for Use in Monoclonal Antibody and Biomarker Testing

M. A. Ruiz-Robles [1], Francisco J. Solís-Pomar [1,*], Gabriela Travieso Aguilar [2], Maykel Márquez Mijares [3], Raine Garrido Arteaga [4], Olivia Martínez Armenteros [4], C. D. Gutiérrez-Lazos [1], Eduardo G. Pérez-Tijerina [1] and Abel Fundora Cruz [3]

[1] Centro de Investigación en Ciencias Físico Matemáticas, Facultad de Ciencias Físico Matemáticas, Universidad Autónoma de Nuevo León, Av. Universidad s/n, San Nicolás de Los Garza 66455, Nuevo León, Mexico; mitchel.ruizrb@uanl.edu.mx (M.A.R.-R.); claudio.gutierrezl@uanl.edu.mx (C.D.G.-L.); eduardo.pereztj@uanl.edu.mx (E.G.P.-T.)

[2] Instituto de Ciencia y Tecnología de Materiales (IMRE), Universidad de La Habana, La Habana 10400, Cuba; gabriela.travieso@imre.uh.cu

[3] Instituto Superior de Ciencias y Tecnologías Aplicadas (InSTEC), Universidad de La Habana, La Habana 10400, Cuba; mmarquez@instec.cu (M.M.M.); abel.fundora@instec.cu (A.F.C.)

[4] Grupo de Análisis, Instituto Finlay de Vacunas, Avenida 21 No. 19810, Atabey, Playa, La Habana 10400, Cuba; rgarrido@finlay.edu.cu (R.G.A.); omartinez@finlay.edu.cu (O.M.A.)

* Correspondence: francisco.solispm@uanl.edu.mx

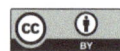

Citation: Ruiz-Robles, M.A.; Solís-Pomar, F.J.; Travieso Aguilar, G.; Márquez Mijares, M.; Garrido Arteaga, R.; Martínez Armenteros, O.; Gutiérrez-Lazos, C.D.; Pérez-Tijerina, E.G.; Fundora Cruz, A. Physico-Chemical Properties of CdTe/Glutathione Quantum Dots Obtained by Microwave Irradiation for Use in Monoclonal Antibody and Biomarker Testing. *Nanomaterials* 2024, *14*, 684. https://doi.org/10.3390/nano 14080684

Academic Editors: Yurii K. Gun'ko and Igor Nabiev

Received: 23 February 2024
Revised: 3 April 2024
Accepted: 10 April 2024
Published: 16 April 2024

Copyright: © 2024 by the authors. Licensee MDPI, Basel, Switzerland. This article is an open access article distributed under the terms and conditions of the Creative Commons Attribution (CC BY) license (https:// creativecommons.org/licenses/by/ 4.0/).

Abstract: In this report, we present the results on the physicochemical characterization of cadmium telluride quantum dots (QDs) stabilized with glutathione and prepared by optimizing the synthesis conditions. An excellent control of emissions and the composition of the nanocrystal surface for its potential application in monoclonal antibody and biomarker testing was achieved. Two samples (QDYellow, QDOrange, corresponding to their emission colors) were analyzed by dynamic light scattering (DLS), and their hydrodynamic sizes were 6.7 nm and 19.4 nm, respectively. Optical characterization by UV-vis absorbance spectroscopy showed excitonic peaks at 517 nm and 554 nm. Photoluminescence spectroscopy indicated that the samples have a maximum intensity emission at 570 and 606 nm, respectively, within the visible range from yellow to orange. Infrared spectroscopy showed vibrational modes corresponding to the functional groups OH-C-H, C-N, C=C, C-O, C-OH, and COOH, which allows for the formation of functionalized QDs for the manufacture of biomarkers. In addition, the hydrodynamic radius, zeta potential, and approximate molecular weight were determined by dynamic light scattering (DLS), electrophoretic light scattering (ELS), and static light scattering (SLS) techniques. Size dispersion and the structure of nanoparticles was obtained by Transmission Electron Microscopy (TEM) and by X-ray diffraction. In the same way, we calculated the concentration of Cd^{2+} ions expressed in mg/L by using the Inductively Coupled Plasma Atomic Emission Spectrometry (ICP-OES). In addition to the characterization of the nanoparticles, the labeling of murine myeloid cells was carried out with both samples of quantum dots, where it was demonstrated that quantum dots can diffuse into these cells and connect mostly with the cell nucleus.

Keywords: quantum dots; murine myeloid cells; glutathione; cadmium telluride; microwave

1. Introduction

Quantum dots' (QDs) emission wavelengths span over UV and IR spectra ensuring high quantum yield, high photostability, and high molar extinction coefficients [1–3]. Among the most prolific applications they can have in nanotechnology is nanobiotechnology, responsible for creating and using this type of material in diagnosis, treatment and monitoring in biological systems, as well as in the release of drugs [4], reducing side effects in benign areas and increasing the efficiency of signaling or monitoring of a specific site of the organism [5]. Among the various types of QDs, those synthesized in aqueous solutions [6] with relatively small sizes (2–6 nm) are employed as biomarkers owing to their size properties, specifically luminescence [7,8], and their biocompatibility [9–12], enabling them to be ideal candidates for biotechnological and medical applications. These luminescent nanoparticles have been the subject of much research in recent years. In addition, the ease of synthesis of these nanoparticles from almost any inorganic precursor and in aqueous solution provides the biotechnology industry with the opportunity to take advantage of their luminescent properties for various purposes, including their use as cellular biomarkers [13–15].

Compared to conventional organic fluorophores, QDs, specifically glutathione-stabilized CdTe-QDs, exhibit advantageous properties, including tunable emissions, photostability and high brightness [16,17]. These unique properties make different types of quantum dots highly desirable for certain biological applications and provide new possibilities for biological imaging and protein conjugations to detect polysaccharides [18,19]. QDs widely used in biolabeling were initially synthesized in the organic phase using high-boiling solvents and stabilizers such as trioctylphosphine oxide (TOPO) or reducers such as trioctylphosphine (TOP) [20,21]. Generally, these nanocrystals are capped with hydrophobic ligands. Therefore, to obtain biofunctional QDs, it is necessary to realize a change-phase process to transfer them to an aqueous solution and make them soluble in water [22,23]. Weller et al. pioneered the aqueous-based preparation of thiol-capped QDs [24]. So far, water-based synthesis with thiols as protective ligands has been developed as an interesting alternative [20,25]. Compared to conventional organometallic approaches, wet solution preparation is cost-effective and convenient, but generally results in a low quantum yield (QY) of 1 to 10% [26]. Of all the QDs reported to date, CdTe exhibits comparable optical properties to its organometallic analogs when prepared in water [20,25,26]. In the present research, glutathione (GSH) was chosen as a ligand to synthesize high-quality CdTe-QDs in an aqueous solution [27,28].

Highly stabilized CdTe quantum dots can be obtained taking advantage of the structure of the glutathione molecule [29]. The first advantage is the fact that glutathione contains the thiol group (R-SH), which is widely demonstrated to exhibit a strong chemical affinity with transition metals, such as cadmium. Consequently, the synthesis employs a majority cadmium precursor with respect to telluride precursor to favor the formation of a nanocrystal surface rich in cadmium ions. Then, the valence levels will be passivated by the thiol group, supplying the stabilization [30–32]. This surface is a natural mono-thiol compound that exists in most organs at the mM level and has no cytotoxicity [33]. In addition, surface modifications of GSH-coated QDs with biomolecules are relatively easy, because GSH has two functional groups, two carboxyl and one primary amino group, which can be conjugated to a biological compound such as an antibody [34]. Precisely, this property defines the other two advantages that the glutathione structure offers. The second advantage that the glutathione molecule offers is that it contains the carboxyl group (COOH) at its ends, which provides solubility in an aqueous medium, and the third advantage refers to the amine group site (NH_2), which can interact with cysteine receptors present on myeloid cells. On the other hand, the COOH group of glutathione can bind to scavenger-like receptors (SRs) present on the surface of myeloid cells. Therefore, once bound to the receptors, glutathione-stabilized quantum dots and the molecules to which they have been bound are internalized by myeloid cells through a process of endocytosis. The labeling process of myeloid cells with glutathione has been used for the development of vaccines and cancer therapies. The COOH and NH_2 functional groups of glutathione play a fundamental role in the labeling of myeloid cells. These groups allow glutathione to bind to specific receptors on the surface of myeloid cells, internalize, and activate the immune response. Glutathione can also modulate the immune response, depending on the concentration and the type of myeloid cell [35].

On the other hand, the advantages of preparing quantum dots with synthesis assisted by microwave irradiation are widely known [36–38]. This favors a thermal treatment directly on the nanocrystals by using a relatively simple method that requires shorter heating times with controlled vapor pressure in nearly inert conditions. This has allowed the preparation of a wide variety of compounds, including CdTe with a wide variety of organic stabilizants [39,40]; however, in the literature, it is not possible to find references to the microwave-assisted synthesis of CdTe quantum dots stabilized with glutathione. In this work, we have analyzed the synthesis and optical, structural and chemical characterization of CdTe/GSH-QDs. The novelty and advancements accomplished in this work are the study of the physico-chemical properties of CdTe/GSH-QDs and the use of microwave irradiation in their synthesis. These nanocrystals are used in biology and medicine to achieve cellular and biomarker testing [12,41–46].

2. Experimental Procedure

2.1. Materials

All reagents used, listed here, were from Sigma-Aldrich and used as received without further purification: Cadmium chloride ($CdCl_2$, anhydrous $\geq$ 99%), Trisodium citrate dihydrate, L-glutathione (GSH, $\geq$98%), sodium borohydride ($NaBH_4$, $\geq$96%), sodium tellurite (Na_2TeO_3, -100 mesh, 99%).

2.2. Synthesis of CdTe-GSH Quantum Dots

Luminescent CdTe/GSH-QDs were obtained from a precursor solution synthesized at room temperature following a facile one-pot method reported previously [47]. Briefly, a $CdCl_2$ solution (0.04 M) was prepared in 40 mL of deionized water. This solution was added to 250 mL of deionized water under mechanical agitation. Then, 1000 mg of trisodium citrate dihydrate was added to the solution, maintaining the mechanical agitation; then, 500 mg of L-glutathione was added until a homogeneous solution was reached. Next, 10 mL of Na_2TeO_3 solution (0.01 M) was added to the mixture, and finally, 500 mg of $NaBH_4$ was added until its complete dissolution.

To activate the fluorescence of CdTe/GSH-QDs, a post-synthesis treatment was realized by a microwave irradiation-assisted hydrothermal method, employing an Anton Paar Monowave 300 microwave reactor. Here, 20 mL of QDs solution was placed in a 30 mL G30 reactor followed by rapid heating with Monowave-300 up to 90 °C (for QDYellow) and 110 °C (QDOrange) and was maintained for 10 min. Thereafter, the reactor was rapidly cooled down to 50 °C.

The quantum dots were stored at 4 °C where the agglomeration of the nanocrystals was avoided, as well as possible cases of suspension, since the autoxidation of the thiol group was reduced, or where enzymatic reduction occurred of disulfides. This meant that the R-HS thiol group could derive into a disulfide, decreasing the stability of the QDs [48].

Although reports with glutathione establish a pH of 8 as optimal for the synthesis of CdTe-QDs, a general rule for establishing chemical bridges with other organic materials is not reported. Through studies prior to characterization, it was possible to determine that for the quantum dots analyzed, the optimal pH to develop a subsequent conjugation process should be in a range between 5 and 6. In this way, a high surface charge can be guaranteed and, with it, there is a greater possibility of anchoring to biomolecules. Due to this, and to guarantee that the QDs were bioconjugable, a surface charge of the nanoparticle greater than -20 mV was achieved, reducing the pH from 8 to 5. In this way, it is guaranteed that there is a greater number of functional groups on the surface with a negative charge that can bind to other functional groups that proteins have [49,50].

In this case, quantum dots show a molecular weight–particle size relationship, since a lower weight implies better purification. This is explained by the fact that the smaller this value is with respect to proteins, the greater the probability that the peaks of effectiveness of the conjugations will be narrower and more defined. Furthermore, a smaller size implies a lower number of ions and, therefore, a lower molecular weight of the nanocrystal [51].

2.3. Optical Absorbance Spectroscopy

For the optical absorbance measurements of QDs, aliquots of samples were added in a 10 mm quartz cuvette (Hellma Analytics, Müllheim. Germany) and placed in an Ultrospec 9000PC UV–Visible Spectrophotometer (Biochrom, Cambridge, UK). The Resolution CFR (Biochrom, version 3.2.0) software was used to collect and analyze the data.

2.4. Dynamic, Static and Electrophoretic Light Scattering

Dynamic Light Scattering (DLS), Electrophoretic Light Scattering (ELS) and Static Light Scattering (SLS) measurements were taken with an Anton Paar Litesizer^{TM} (Anton Paar ShapeTec GmbH, Wundschuh, Austria) 500 equipped with a 658 nm He–Ne laser operating at an angle of 90°. Scattering light detected at 90° was automatically adjusted by laser attenuation filters. The particle size distribution and molecular weight were measured in a 3 mm low-volume quartz cuvette (Hellma Analytics). The determination of zeta potential of the samples was carried out using an omega cuvette (Anton Paar). For data analysis, the viscosity, refractive index (RI) and relative permittivity of water (at 25 °C) were used. The Kalliope Professional (Anton Paar, version 2.18) software was used to collect and analyze the data. Each sample was characterized by DLS and ELS techniques using a concentration of 0.5 mg/mL. For the SLS measurements, each sample was prepared with a concentration of 3–9 mg/mL.

2.5. Transmission Electron Microscopy (TEM) and X-ray Diffraction (XRD)

CdTe/GSH-QDs were analyzed to determine their morphology, size dispersion and structure using a TEM JEOL-JEM-2010, with an acceleration voltage of 120 kV. Initially, the sample was cleaned by 5 cycles of centrifugation at 3000 rpm for 5 min in a 1:1 solution of ethanol and deionized water, and then 30 µL/mL aqueous solution was put on a mesh #200 TEM cupper grid.

X-ray diffraction (XRD) pattern was obtained on a PNalytical X'Pert^3 Powder diffractometer with Cu κ_α radiation (λ = 1.5405 Å).

2.6. Photoluminescence Spectroscopy

The photoluminescence spectra were measured with a Hellma spectro fluorimeter FP-8200 (Hellma Analytics), where Hellma quartz cuvettes of the type 105.202-QS were used. The measurement was performed under an excitation wavelength of 466 nm. The detector was set to low sensitivity, and it was unnecessary to dilute the sample since the obtained spectra fit the desired intensity range.

2.7. FT-IR Spectroscopy

Surface composition analysis of samples was performed by Shimadzu IR Prestige 21 (Shimadzu, Tokyo, Japan). Aliquots of 5 mL of samples were deposited in a porcelain capsule and placed in an oven at room temperature for five days until the water content evaporated completely. Once the product was dried, 100 mg of crushed potassium bromide was taken and spread throughout the capsule to drag the microparticles of the solid and thus form the tablet that would be placed in the IR equipment. The FT-IR spectra of the sample were acquired in the wavelength range of 4000–600 cm^{-1}.

2.8. Atomic Emission Spectroscopy (AES)

The AES analysis was realized in an Ultima Expert ICP-OES spectrophotometer with induction-coupled plasma, coupled to a polychromator with argon gas. Its optical system was thermally stabilized, with a 1 m focal length lens, 2400 g/mm and grating used in the 1st and 2nd order with an optical resolution less than 6 pm for 120–450 nm and less than 11 pm for 450–800 nm.

The spectral line used for Cd was 226.5 nm, which is free from interference. The water method (2023), which contains 25 elements placed in 50 mL volumetric containers with initial concentrations of 1000 mg/L, was used.

3. Results and Discussion

3.1. Particle Size

DLS is an optical method for the characterization of suspensions and emulsions. Analysis of the fluctuations of the scattered light gives information about the suspended particles. Fluctuations in the intensity of the scattered radiation are characterized by calculating the intensity compensation function, which ultimately allows for the evaluation of the diffusion coefficients of the particles. The quality of the result essentially depends on the quality of the data and the parameter settings. Modern dynamic light scattering devices automatically perform an intensity analysis of the compensation function and calculate the diffusion coefficient [33].

The diffusion coefficient D is related to the radius of the nanoparticles using Equation (1):

$$R_h = \frac{k_B T}{6\pi\eta D} \tag{1}$$

where R_h is the hydrodynamic radius, k_B is the Boltzmann constant, T is the absolute temperature, η is the mean viscosity, and D is the translational diffusion coefficient [52].

The hydrodynamic radius of the samples prepared via both methods is given in Table 1. The radius of QDYellow was 6.70 nm and it was 19.4 nm for QDOrange.

Table 1. Hydrodynamic radius is determined by DLS. The size reported is derived from the volume graph.

	DLS	
	QDYellow	QDOrange
R_h (nm)	6.70	19.37

Figure 1a,b show distributions of the hydrodynamic radius value for the analyzed samples with the intensity and the volume graphs. We can see that one of the size populations seen on the intensity graph disappeared in the volume graph. We consider that the particles are dispersed and have minimal agglomeration in the solution. This measurement includes the hydrodynamic size of the compound in which the nanoparticle itself (nucleus/shell) is included and a part of the ionic atmosphere that moves with it [53]. Likewise, the notable difference in nanoparticle size between the QDYellow and QDOrange samples could be due to the binding of glutathione molecules with the shell of the same stabilizer deposited on the surface of the quantum dot.

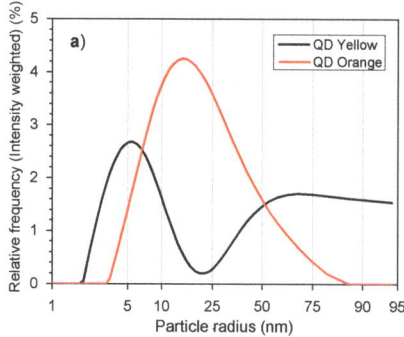
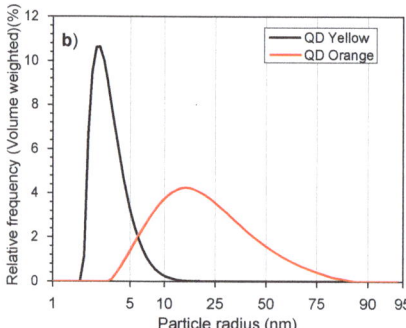

Figure 1. Average size distribution of QD samples. (**a**) Intensity distribution, (**b**) volume distribution.

During the measurements, nanocrystals can absorb some of the transmitted frequencies, mainly the larger ones, which do not exhibit luminescence. But due to this absorption, it is possible to record variations in the intensity of the scattered laser light, which is why the large size is predominant for the QDOrange sample. It should be noted that the recorded size not only includes the solid phase of the nanocrystal but also absorption sites of the organic shell and the ionic environment of the nanocrystal itself.

3.2. Transmission Electron Microscopy and X-ray Diffraction

The morphology and structural properties of the CdTe/GSH-QD samples were inspected by TEM at 800,000×. Despite the fact that the micrographs exhibited a slight agglomeration of nanocrystals, a homogeneous mean size distribution was obtained after measuring 100 nanoparticles for each sample with a mean size of 2.5 nm for the QDYellow sample and 3.4 nm for the QDOrange sample. The crystallinity of the CdTe/GSH-QDs was indexed with the same fcc crystal phase of CdTe for both samples as previously reported [43]. The insets of the TEM images show a spacing of 4 Å of the (200) plane family for the QDYellow sample (Figure 2a) and a 3.55 Å spacing of the (111) plane family for the QDOrange sample (Figure 2b). Figure 2c contains the XRD patterns of both samples. The two down-right insets show the fast Fourier transform (FFT) of the selected zone in red, and indicate the excellent crystallinity of both samples. In Figure 2c, the XRD patterns of QDYellow and QDOrange are shown. The nanocrystals exhibited diffraction peaks at 25.5°, 28.5° and 45.7°, which are slightly shifted with respect to the position of the diffraction peaks belonging to the most stable crystalline phase of CdTe [44]. Various reports indicate that this shift is due to induced stresses by the GSH stabilization, possibly due to the incorporation of sulfide ions into the CdTe nanocrystals [24,54,55].

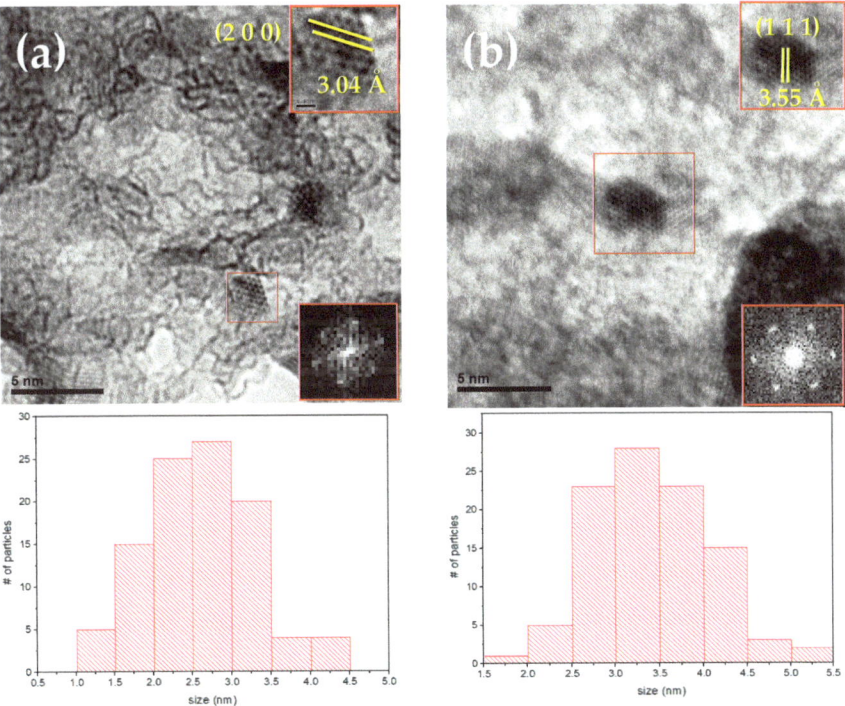

Figure 2. Cont.

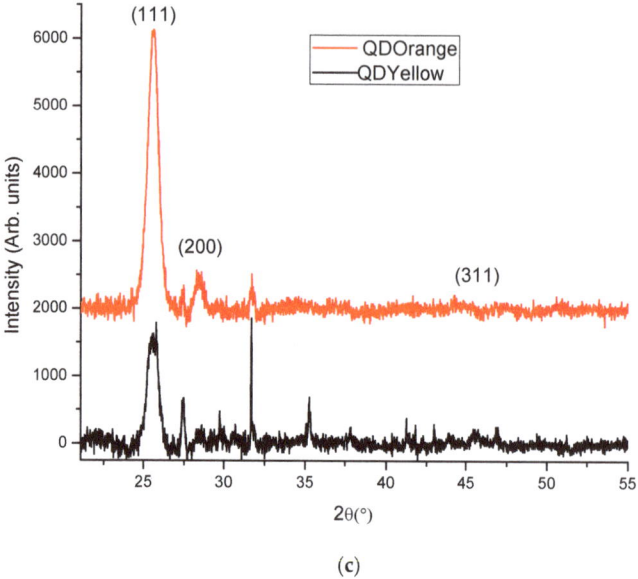

(c)

Figure 2. HRTEM images and size distribution of (**a**) QDYellow sample, (**b**) QDOrange sample, (**c**) XRD patterns of both samples (ICSD-093942).

3.3. Molecular Weight

Static Light Scattering allows us to determine the molecular mass and the second coefficient of the virial of solid phases dispersed in solution, such as colloidal systems. In this technique, the intensity of the scattered light is directly related to the molecular weight.

In a Litesizer system, the scattering intensity is measured in solutions with different concentrations and a Debye diagram is generated. The intercept of which at zero concentration provides the molecular weight (Zimm equation of the Rayleigh–Debye–Gans Model (Equation (2))) [56]. On the other hand, the second coefficient of the virial is a thermodynamic parameter that describes the interaction of the dissolved molecules with each other and with the molecules of the solvent. It is possible to determine this parameter from the Debye Diagram with Equation (2). Here, the second coefficient of the virial is the slope of the graph.

$$\frac{KC}{R(\theta)} = \frac{1}{M_W P(\theta)} + 2A_2 C \qquad (2)$$

where M_W is the mean molecular weight, A_2 is the second virial coefficient, $P(\theta)$ is a corrective shape factor for large particles/molecules with respect to the laser wavelength, $R(\theta)$ is the Rayleigh relation, C is the concentration of particles and K is an optical constant.

The results obtained, shown in Table 2, indicate a first positive virial coefficient for QDYellow, which shows that the molecules of the QD tend to have a higher affinity for the molecules of solvents. That is, they are preferably surrounded by molecules of solvents and not by other segments of QDs. Whereas in the case of QDOrange, a negative coefficient was obtained, ascribing a greater affinity for other segments of quantum dots than between them and the molecules of solvents. This causes a structural rearrangement of the QD, becoming more compact and draining the solvent molecules. The difference in molecular weight values is owed to the presence of agglomeration in the sample and their own synthesis conditions. This difference in the molecular weight of the two samples is consistent with the results previously analyzed by light scattering, since the size of the nanocrystal is practically 3 times larger for QDOrange with respect to QDYellow, which means that the QDOrange sample contains a greater number of ions and therefore a higher molecular weight.

Table 2. Results obtained by static light scattering.

Aspects	Debye Method	
	QDYellow	QDOrange
M_w (Da)	314	969
A_2 (mol × mL/g^2)	7.44×10^{-1}	-8.44×10^{-3}

3.4. Fourier-Transform Infrared Spectroscopy (FT-IR)

The FT-IR spectra of the analyzed samples is given in Figure 3. The vibrational modes corresponding to functional groups of glutathione molecule are listed in Table 3. From the analysis, it is possible to determine the functional group that is coordinating the surface of QDs. It turned out to be the COOH group in equilibrium with the carboxylates, whose ionization makes the two C-O bonds equivalent [57]. On the other hand, when we used a stabilizer on the structure such as GSH, it was possible to determine that the functional group would be coordinating the core/shell of the internal structure of the QD [51].

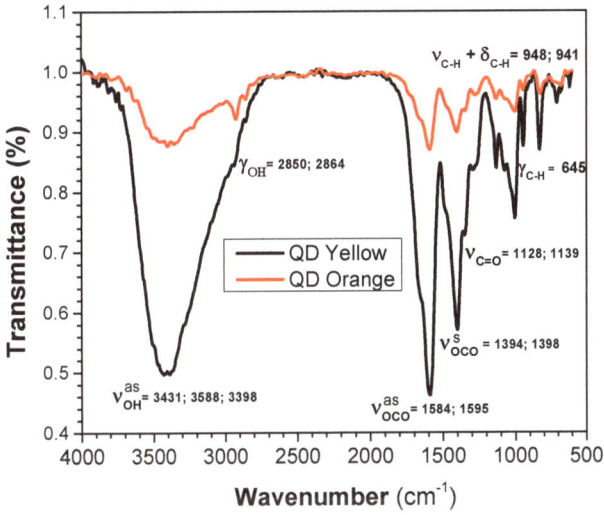

Figure 3. FT-IR spectra for CdTe/GSH-QDs.

Table 3. Assignment of the bands corresponding to GSH molecule shown in the IR.

Assignment	Wavenumber (cm^{-1})	
	QDYellow	QDOrange
ν_{OH}	3431; 3388; 2935	3508; 3398; 2922
ν_{C-N}	1280	1267
ν_{C-O}	1128; 1074; 1001	1139; 1001
$\nu_{C-H} + \delta_{C-H}$	2850	2864
ν_{OCO}^{as} ν_{OCO}^{s}	1595; 1394	1584; 1398
γ_{NH}	835	821
γ_{OH}	948	941
γ_{C-H}	703	675

With these results, it is verified that glutathione binds to the surface of the QD through the thiol group. When the thiol has been deprotonated, an R-S$^-$ radical bonds strongly to the Cd^{2+} majority surface, although it still not accepted that a CdS shell is formed; this bond provides stability to CdTe-QDs against aggregation. In addition, the molar ratio between CdCl$_2$ and Na$_2$TeO$_3$ is 4:1. It is expected that the surface of the QDs will have mostly Cd^{2+} ions, and the solubility of the nanocrystal will depend on the carboxyl groups. The amine bonds are terminals that allow the functionalization of the quantum dots with other anions (molecules, proteins, enzymes, etc.).

3.5. Zeta Potential

Electrophoretic Light Scattering (ELS) is a method used to measure electrophoretic mobility through Doppler shifts in scattered light. The electrophoretic mobility μ_E is defined in Equation (3)

$$\mu_E = \frac{\nu}{E} \tag{3}$$

where ν is the particle electrophoretic velocity, and E is the applied electric field.

The zeta potential of particles in suspensions ζ is derived from the measured electrophoretic mobility, using Equation (4) (Henry equation with Smoluchowski approximation).

$$\zeta = \frac{3\eta\mu_E}{2\varepsilon} \tag{4}$$

where ε is the relative permittivity and η is the dynamic viscosity [58].

The results of ζ potential measurements are presented in Figure 4. Infrared spectroscopy demonstrates that the carboxyl group is responsible for the negative charge of QDs in the solution due to it dissociating into carboxylate ions. Therefore, it remains outside the coordination sphere and free for conjugation. Simultaneously, inside the nanocrystals, the R-SH$^-$ group is found coordinating with the S^{2-} ions generated possibly from the rupture of Cd-S. Consequently, zeta potential values were obtained for the QDYellow sample of -6.6 mV and -16.8 Mv for QDOrange. The charge concentration for both samples is due to the difference in charge existing between the surface, i.e., the solvation layer, and the interior of the nanocrystals [58]. The negative values indicate the excess of negative charges that exist on the surface of both samples, which can be associated with the presence of the conjugated form of the carboxyl: COOH $\rightleftarrows$ COO$^-$.

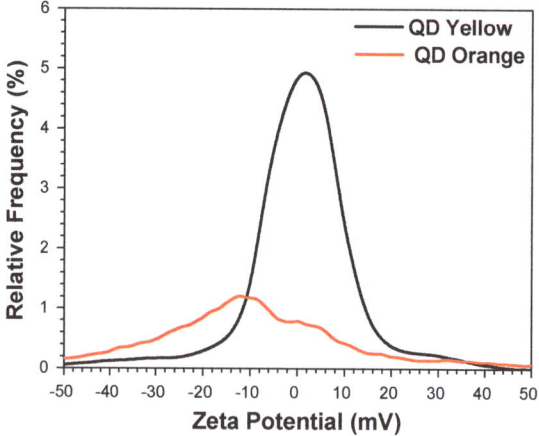

Figure 4. Determination of the average zeta potential.

The presence of negative charges associated with the strong coupling of oscillators between the resonant structures constitutes a crucial factor for future chemical to biomolecular bonds, such as the union with an NH_2 group of proteins such as antibodies to form an amide bond.

3.6. Optical Absorbance Spectroscopy (UV-Vis)

Figure 5 shows the absorbance spectra of both CdTe/GSH-QDs samples. The slight separation in the position of the excitonic peak is due to the difference in nanocrystal size, and the widening of the excitonic peak is related to their size dispersion [59].

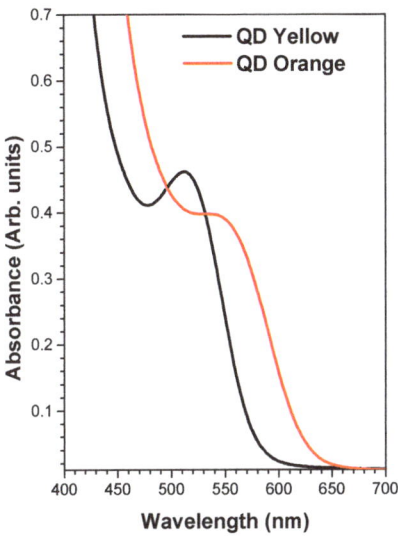

Figure 5. Absorbance spectrum of QDYellow (black line), of which the maximum excitonic peak is localized around 517 nm, and of QDOrange (red line), of which the maximum of the excitonic peak is localized around to 554 nm.

The relationship between the maximum of the excitonic peak with the size of quantum dots [60] helps us to understand the coating extension of the glutathione shell on the QD surface. The very close position between the maxima of the excitonic peaks of the QDOrange sample and QDYellow suggests the formation of an extensive glutathione shell in the QDOrange sample, since the nanocrystal size measurement by DLS was 19.4 nm.

3.7. Photoluminescence

The ability of CdTe-QDs to be strongly luminescent lies in their ability to absorb UV radiation, which means that they are excellent absorbers in the UV spectral range [61]. The normalized photoluminescence spectra in Figure 6 unveil the emission properties of the QDs and corroborate the maximum emission wavelengths for each of the samples.

It exhibits a well-defined peak, within the interval of 570–590 nm (corresponding to the yellow color) and 590–620 nm (orange) [62]. The maximum intensity peaks are at 570 nm and 606 nm, respectively, which produces an emission very close to orange. The photoluminescence spectra are a characteristic measure of the quality of the synthesis and size distribution of the prepared nanocrystals [59].

For both samples, the maximum peak of luminescence is shifted to a higher wavelength with respect to the maximum peak of the excitation source, which was 473 nm. So, any contribution of the excitation source in the emission spectrum obtained can be neglected.

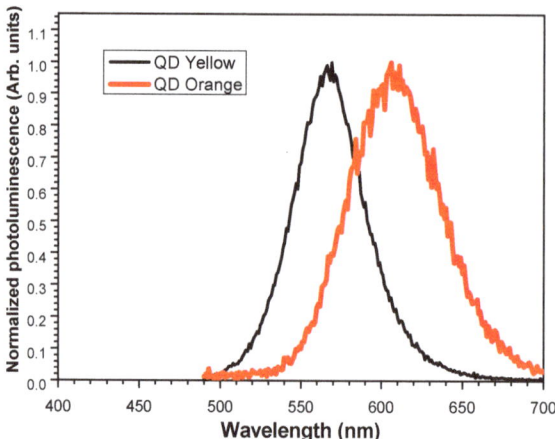

Figure 6. Normalized emission spectra corresponding to analyzed samples. For QDYellow, the maximum wavelength of emission was 570 nm, under an excitation wavelength of 472 nm. For QDOrange, the maximum wavelength of emission was 606 nm, under an excitation wavelength of 473 nm.

3.8. Inductively Coupled Plasma–Atomic Emission Spectrometry (ICP-OES)

To perform the ICP-OES measurements, four standard solutions of known concentrations were prepared in a volume of 100 mL, to which the cadmium standard substance was added in concentrations of 0.5; 1.5; 3.0; 6.0 mg/L, respectively. The working dilution was 1:100 by adding distilled water starting from 500 µL up to 50 mL for each QD. The final concentrations of Cd^{2+} obtained in both samples are summarized in Table 4.

Table 4. Results of the analysis by ICP of the samples analyzed.

Sample	Size	Cd^{2+} (mg/L)
QDYellow	6.70 nm	5.246
QDOrange	19.37 nm	5.198

For the synthesis of CdTe quantum dots, a nominal concentration of cadmium chloride $[CdCl_2]$ = 0.04 M, with a molecular weight of MW = 183.32 g/mol, was used. If we subtract the mass of the two chlorine atoms, we have MW = 112.414 g/mol of Cd^{2+} alone. This represents a nominal mass in the CdTe synthesis of

$$\left[Cd^{2+}\right] = 0.04 \text{ mol } 112.414 \text{ g/molL} = 4.49 \text{ g/L}$$

A nominal content of 4.49 mg/mL of cadmium was applied to the synthesis; for 40 mL of solution in deionized water, a nominal total of 179.6 mg was used.

Given the considerable values obtained, the presence of Cd^{2+} in both samples is confirmed. Furthermore, the appearance of the analytical signal for Cd^{2+}, as well as the calibration curve obtained, was suitable for the analysis, with a correlation coefficient higher than 0.99 as elaborated in Figure 7a,b. Thus, the presence of Cd^{2+} ions is verified by the high concentration values obtained.

Table 5 summarizes the main results obtained for the measurements taken.

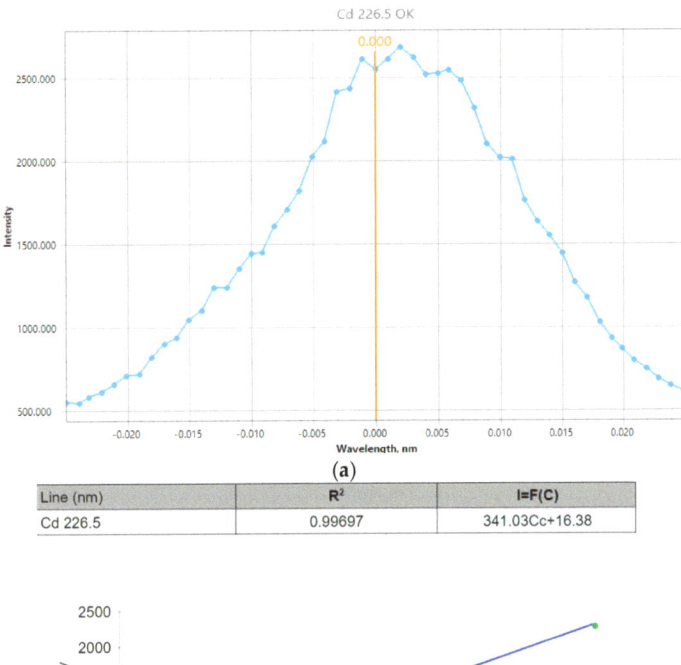

Figure 7. (a) Analytical signal for Cd^{2+}, (b) calibration curve for Cd^{2+}.

Table 5. Main results.

Aspects	QDYellow	QDOrange
Particle Size (DLS)	6.70 nm	19.4 nm
Particle Size (QELS)	9.30 nm	19.6 nm
Molecular Weight (Debye Method)	314 Da	969 Da
2nd Virial coefficient (Debye Method)	7.44×10^{-1} mol × mL/g^2	-8.44×10^{-3} mol × mL/g^2
Mean zeta Potential	−6.6 mV	−16.8 mV
Emission, excitation and absorption wavelength	$\lambda_{em.} = 570$ nm $\lambda_{ex.} = 472$ nm $\lambda_{abs.} = 517$ nm	$\lambda_{em.} = 606$ nm $\lambda_{ex.} = 473$ nm $\lambda_{abs.} = 554$ nm
Main functional groups	3431 cm^{-1} (ν_{OH}^{asoc}), 1595 cm^{-1} (ν_{oco}^{as}), 1394 cm^{-1} (ν_{oco}^{s})	3508 cm^{-1} (ν_{OH}^{asoc}), 1584 cm^{-1} (ν_{oco}^{as}), 1398 cm^{-1} (ν_{oco}^{s})
Cd^{2+} concentration	5.246 mg/L	5.198 mg/L

According to the particle size obtained by the DLS and QELS techniques within a range of 6–20 nm, the values of the emission, excitation and absorption wavelengths correspond to quantum dots with emissions of yellow and orange, according to what is reported by the literature [59]. Furthermore, the low molecular weight determined by the SLS technique is proportional to the nominal concentrations of Cd^{2+} ions and those determined by atomic emission spectrometry. It is considerably feasible to establish possible conjugation strategies with different proteins such as monoclonal antibodies, since it would be possible to apply a method of purification and separation of excesses in a simple way, due to the considerable difference between the molecular weight of the antibodies (~180 kDa), which is higher than that of the QDs.

Additionally, the results of the valence vibrations and the characteristic bands obtained in the IR spectrum correspond to the negative values of zeta potential recorded through electrophoretic light scattering. This is strongly associated with the intense coupling of oscillators due to the COO- ⇌ COOH resonant structures coming from glutathione. Since there is a free carboxylate group in the coordination sphere of the nanoparticle, the possibilities of conjugations are not restricted, but rather the probability of forming chemical bonds with other biomolecules is considerably high.

On the other hand, once the samples were characterized, the design, preparation and testing of the labeling of murine myeloid cells with quantum dots was carried out. To obtain the high-resolution images shown in Figure 8, a fluorescence optical microscope was used. The cells were placed on a glass slide fixed in cold acetone for 30 min. For their preparation, the electroporation internalization method was used fixed in acetone to permeabilize them with 30% of cold methanol for 30 min. Two washes were performed with 1X PBS before and after their permeabilization. The incubation time was 2 h at a temperature of 27 °C.

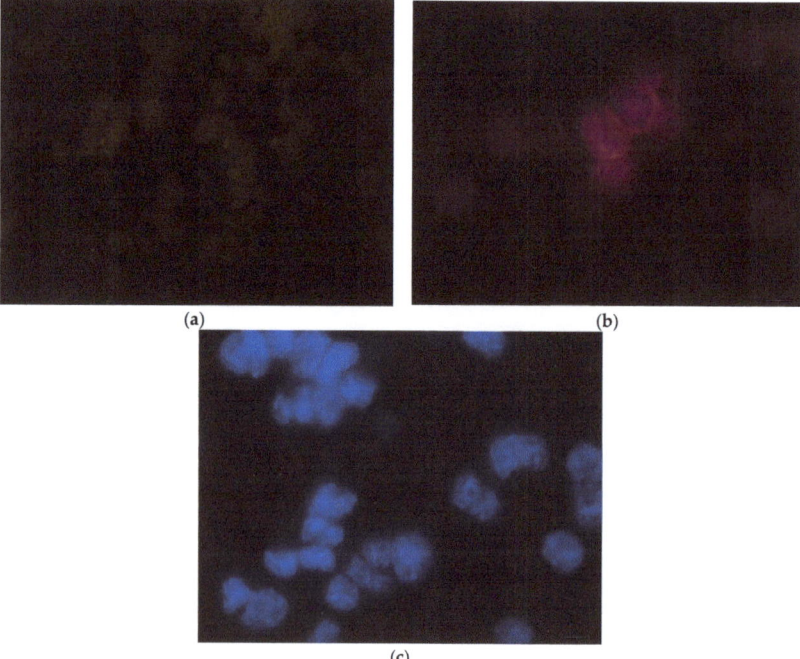

Figure 8. Micrographs of murine myeloid cells labeled with quantum dots. (**a**) Myeloid cells labeled with CdTe/GSH/Yellow with 40× green filter. (**b**) Myeloid cells labeled with CdTe/GSH/Orange with 40× red filter. (**c**) Myeloid cells labeled with DAPI 100×.

The quantum dots were added drop by drop into each of the circular regions that contain the cells. In Figure 8a,b, images taken of one of the fields of these cells marked with each type of quantum dot are shown. One of these regions, which was prepared only with 4′,6-diamidino-2-phenylindole or DAPI, was taken as a positive control (Figure 8c). This nuclear contrast dye is commonly used as a colored fluorescent nucleic acid blue stain which binds strongly to the regions rich in adenine and thymine in the minor groove of the double-stranded DNA molecule to localize the position and shape of the nuclei [63] and at the same time serves as a contrast with the respective emission colors of quantum dots.

Once the luminescent nanoparticles are in the cells, they will be in contact with multiple and widely varied biomolecules, including proteins, lipids, saccharides, etc., which will immediately adhere to the surface of these nanoparticles (forming a commonly corona-named structure), giving it a totally different biological identity. This causes the interaction with the cell membrane (CM) to be influenced by variations on the specificity of the nanoparticles, modifying the internalization mechanisms and/or activating different intercellular signaling pathways [64].

Quantum dots, once internalized, can take different routes within the cell. For example, when interacting with human macrophages, they are rapidly endocytosed, and subsequently they are directed by active cytoplasmic transport to the nucleus, which they enter through the nuclear pore complexes until they reach the nucleosome, where they accumulate [65].

In general, it was observed that both the nucleus and the cytoplasm of the cells were marked with quantum dots, since these act as a visual indicator for the hybridization of the complementary DNA sequences with the target of the quantum dot. Furthermore, DNA binding molecules are capable of targeting and binding nanomaterials to DNA in cell nuclei. The above could be explained because glutathione is the organic molecule that binds to DNA either by binding to the major and/or minor groove, intercalation, binding to the main phosphate chain and/or DNA alkylation. The different DNA binding agents each target the nanomaterial to DNA, but the affinity of the DNA binding agent determines the staining profile of DNA in the nucleus [66]. In the part that joins the cytoplasm, it stains irregularly due to the appearance of small RNA inclusions and the accumulation of waste substances. Furthermore, DNA is contained in a specific region of the cytoplasm, called the nucleoid, in most cases without being separated by the membrane [67].

Another fact that could explain this labeling is due to the nanometric size of QDs, allowing the nanocrystals to cross the cell membrane and the organelle membranes, where once internalized, their presence can be detected, as shown in Figure 8a,b, which shows similarity with the previously stated results, since these show great affinity with molecules such as DNA and RNA, joining through strong interactions. Their size directly affects the effectiveness of the internalization mechanism and its kinetics, without leaving aside their chemical nature. Their very small dimensions initially accumulate on the cell membrane and subsequently enter the cell gradually [65].

In general, quantum dots are encapsulated in vesicles and internalized either by active mechanisms or by passive penetration into the inner cell. However, internalization is not the only way in which these nanoparticles exert an effect inside the cell since their interaction with different membrane receptors can trigger very different and varied intricellular signaling pathways [68]. Furthermore, they contribute to defining the nucleus, delineating its boundary and establishing its morphology.

4. Conclusions

The physicochemical properties of glutathione-stabilized quantum dots analyzed in this research indicate that nanocrystals can be useful for the detection of tissues and malignant tumors smaller than 1 cm in size. The hydrodynamic radius of CdTe-QDs was reported with higher values than that reported by TEM microscopy, possibly due to the agglomeration of glutathione molecules on the nanocrystal surface. Additionally, glutathione tends to crystallize and then the diffraction patterns of the samples exhibit highly intense peaks due this organic phase, making it necessary to subtract this signal to appreciate the diffraction of the inorganic phase of CdTe. The Inductively Coupled Plasma–Atomic Emission Spectrometry results allow us to verify that glutathione-stabilized CdTe quantum dots not only internalize into the cells but also mark the cytoplasmic, nuclear and surrounding regions in the cytoplasmic membrane. This was shown through a strong interaction between the DNA and RNA present in the cells with the quantum dots, constituting an example of their effectiveness as cellular biomarkers, when observing their luminescence by fluorescence optical microscopy. According to the presented data from this report, we can conclude that CdTe-QDs are stabilized with glutathione, whose synthesis is assisted by microwave irradiation; they can be applied in both nuclear and cytoplasmic labeling, which could allow a more precise diagnosis of diseases such as leukemia, lymphoma and other myeloproliferative disorders. Additionally, they could be used to target specific drugs or therapeutic agents to myeloid cells, which would increase the effectiveness of the treatment and reduce side effects.

Author Contributions: Conceptualization, F.J.S.-P., C.D.G.-L., E.G.P.-T. and A.F.C.; Methodology, M.A.R.-R., F.J.S.-P., G.T.A., R.G.A., O.M.A., C.D.G.-L. and A.F.C.; Formal analysis, F.J.S.-P., R.G.A., O.M.A., C.D.G.-L., E.G.P.-T. and A.F.C.; Investigation, M.A.R.-R., F.J.S.-P., G.T.A., M.M.M. and C.D.G.-L.; Writing—original draft, M.A.R.-R., F.J.S.-P., G.T.A. and A.F.C.; Writing—review & editing, F.J.S.-P., C.D.G.-L., E.G.P.-T. and A.F.C.; Supervision, E.G.P.-T. All authors have read and agreed to the published version of the manuscript.

Funding: Programas de Estancias Posdoctorales por México 2020 y 2021(2), del Consejo Nacional de Humanidades, Ciencia y Tecnología (CONAHCyT), a través de los apoyos bajo los convenios I1200/94/2020 MOD.ORD./10/2020. Programa Nacional de Nanociencias y Nanotecnología "Efectividad de los puntos cuánticos para aplicaciones Biológicas", Proyecto PN211LH008-038.

Data Availability Statement: All data are available as part of the article.

Conflicts of Interest: The authors declare no competing interests.

References

1. Vassiltsova, O.; Jayez, D.; Zhao, Z.; Carpenter, M.; Petrukhina, M. Synthesis of nanocomposite materials with controlled structures and optical emissions: Application of various methacrylate polymers for CdSe quantum dots encapsulation. *J. Nanosci. Nanotechnol.* **2010**, *10*, 1635–1642. [CrossRef] [PubMed]
2. Zhou, Y.; Zhao, H.; Ma, D.; Rosei, F. Harnessing the properties of colloidal quantum dots in luminescent solar concentrators. *Chem. Soc. Rev.* **2018**, *47*, 5866–5890. [CrossRef] [PubMed]
3. Morselli, G.; Villa, M.; Fermi, A.; Critchley, K.; Ceroni, P. Luminescent copper indium sulfide (CIS) quantum dots for bioimaging applications. *Nanoscale Horiz.* **2021**, *6*, 676–695. [CrossRef] [PubMed]
4. Chaturvedi, V.K.; Singh, A.; Singh, V.K.; Singh, M.P. Cancer nanotechnology: A new revolution for cancer diagnosis and therapy. *Curr. Drug Metab.* **2019**, *20*, 416–429. [CrossRef] [PubMed]
5. Barbosa, M.E.M.; Montembault, V.; Cammas-Marion, S.; Ponchel, G.; Fontaine, L. Synthesis and characterization of novel poly(γ-benzyl-L-glutamate) derivatives tailored for the preparation of nanoparticles of pharmaceutical interest. *Polym. Int.* **2007**, *56*, 317–324. [CrossRef]
6. Valencia, C.A.Z.; Valderrama, M.I.R.; Carbajal, A.D.J.H.; Rodríguez, E.S.; Lugo, V.R. Evaluación de la lumiscencia de puntos cuánticos de carbono sintetizados mediante el método hidrotermal a partir de triticum. *Pädi Boletín Científico De Cienc. Básicas E Ing. Del ICBI* **2019**, *7*, 19–22. [CrossRef]
7. Farzin, M.A.; Abdoos, H. A critical review on quantum dots: From synthesis toward applications in electrochemical biosensors for determination of disease-related biomolecules. *Talanta* **2021**, *224*, 121828. [CrossRef] [PubMed]
8. Sobhanan, J.; Rival, J.V.; Anas, A.; Shibu, E.S.; Takano, Y.; Biju, V. Luminescent Quantum Dots: Synthesis, Optical Properties, Bioimaging and Toxicity. *Adv. Drug Deliv. Rev.* **2023**, *197*, 114830. [CrossRef] [PubMed]
9. Chinen, A.B.; Guan, C.M.; Ferrer, J.R.; Barnaby, S.N.; Merkel, T.J.; Mirkin, C.A. Nanoparticle probes for the detection of cancer biomarkers, cells, and tissues by fluorescence. *Chem. Rev.* **2015**, *115*, 10530–10574. [CrossRef]
10. Li, P.; Liu, S.; Yan, S.; Fan, X.; He, Y. A sensitive sensor for anthraquinone anticancer drugs and hsDNA based on CdTe/CdS quantum dots fluorescence reversible control. *Colloids Surfaces A Physicochem. Eng. Asp.* **2011**, *392*, 7–15. [CrossRef]
11. Norris, D.J.; Nirmal, M.; Murray, C.B.; Sacra, A.; Bawendi, M.G. Size dependent optical spectroscopy of II–VI semiconductor nanocrystallites (quantum dots). *Eur. Phys. J. D* **1993**, *26*, 355–357. [CrossRef]
12. Minelli, C.; Lowe, S.B.; Stevens, M.M. Engineering nanocomposite materials for cancer therapy. *Small* **2010**, *6*, 2336–2357. [CrossRef]

13. Rojas-Valencia, O.G.; Díaz-Santiago, D.L.; Casas-Espínola, J.L.; Reza-San-Germán, C.M.; Estrada-Flores, M.; Torres-Santillán, E. Síntesis de partículas luminiscentes de carbono a partir de la carbonización de Beta Vulgaris (betabel). *Pädi Boletín Científico De Cienc. Básicas E Ing. Del ICBI* **2023**, *10*, 80–84. [CrossRef]
14. Chang, Q.; Meng, T.; Tan, H. Preparation and fluorescence characteristics of CdTe/CdS and CdTe/ZnS core-shell semiconductor quantum dots. *Infrared Laser Eng.* **2021**, *50*, 1–7. [CrossRef]
15. Triana, M.A.; López, A.F.; Camargo, R.J. Síntesis, Caracterización y Evaluación Fotocatalítica de Puntos cuánticos de CdSe cubiertos con 2 tipos de Tioles. *Inf. Tecnol.* **2015**, *26*, 121–134. [CrossRef]
16. Díaz González, M.; de la Escosura Muñiz, A.; Fernandez Argüelles, M.T.; Alonso, F.J.G.; Costa Fernandez, J.M. Quantum dot bioconjugates for diagnostic applications. In *Surface-Modified Nanobiomaterials for Electrochemical and Biomedicine Applications*; Springer: Cham, Switzerland, 2020; pp. 133–176. [CrossRef]
17. Dos Santos, G.A.; Capelo, R.G.; Liu, C.; Manzani, D. In-situ synthesis of luminescent CdS quantum dots embedded in phosphate glass. *J. Non-Cryst. Solids* **2022**, *587*, 121599. [CrossRef]
18. Kairdolf, B.A.; Smith, A.M.; Stokes, T.H.; Wang, M.D.; Young, A.N.; Nie, S. Semiconductor quantum dots for bioimaging and biodiagnostic applications. *Annu. Rev. Anal. Chem.* **2013**, *6*, 143–162. [CrossRef] [PubMed]
19. Zhang, L.-J.; Xia, L.; Xie, H.-Y.; Zhang, Z.-L.; Pang, D.-W. Quantum dot based biotracking and biodetection. *Anal. Chem.* **2018**, *91*, 532–547. [CrossRef]
20. Zhou, J.; Pu, C.; Jiao, T.; Hou, X.; Peng, X. A two-step synthetic strategy toward monodisperse colloidal CdSe and CdSe/CdS core/shell nanocrystals. *J. Am. Chem. Soc.* **2016**, *138*, 6475–6483. [CrossRef]
21. Chen, P.E.; Anderson, N.C.; Norman, Z.M.; Owen, J.S. Tight binding of carboxylate, phosphonate, and carbamate anions to stoichiometric CdSe nanocrystals. *J. Am. Chem. Soc.* **2017**, *139*, 3227–3236. [CrossRef]
22. Luo, D.; Han, R.; Chen, Y.; Zheng, Q.; Wang, L.; Hong, Y.; Sha, Y. Design and Fabrication of a Geometrically Ordered Hydrophobic Interlayer to Prepare High-Quality QD/SiO2 for Cell Imaging. *J. Biomed. Nanotechnol.* **2017**, *13*, 1344–1353. [CrossRef]
23. Karaagac, Z.; Gul, O.T.; Ildiz, N.; Ocsoy, I. Transfer of hydrophobic colloidal gold nanoparticles to aqueous phase using catecholamines. *J. Mol. Liq.* **2020**, *315*, 113796. [CrossRef]
24. Silva, F.O.; Carvalho, M.S.; Mendonça, R.; Macedo, W.A.; Balzuweit, K.; Reiss, P.; Schiavon, M.A. Effect of surface ligands on the optical properties of aqueous soluble CdTe quantum dots. *Nanoscale Res. Lett.* **2012**, *7*, 536. [CrossRef] [PubMed]
25. Monrás, J.P.; Díaz, V.; Bravo, D.; Montes, R.A.; Chasteen, T.G.; Osorio-Román, I.O.; Vásquez, C.C.; Pérez-Donoso, J.M. Enhanced glutathione content allows the in vivo synthesis of fluorescent CdTe nanoparticles by Escherichia coli. *PLoS ONE* **2012**, *7*, e48657. [CrossRef] [PubMed]
26. Subramanian, S.; Ganapathy, S.; Rajaram, M.; Ayyaswamy, A. Tuning the optical properties of colloidal quantum dots using thiol group capping agents and its comparison. *Mater. Chem. Phys.* **2020**, *249*, 123127. [CrossRef]
27. Wang, L.; Xu, D.; Gao, J.; Chen, X.; Duo, Y.; Zhang, H. Semiconducting quantum dots: Modification and applications in biomedical science. *Sci. China Mater.* **2020**, *63*, 1631–1650. [CrossRef]
28. Dogar, A.H.; Ullah, S.; Qayyum, H.; Rehman, Z.U.; Qayyum, A. Characterization of charge and kinetic energy distribution of ions emitted during nanosecond pulsed laser ablation of several metals. *J. Phys. D Appl. Phys.* **2017**, *50*, 385602. [CrossRef]
29. Ju, J.; Zhang, R.; Chen, W. Photochemical deposition of surface-clean silver nanoparticles on nitrogen-doped graphene quantum dots for sensitive colorimetric detection of glutathione. *Sensors Actuators B Chem.* **2016**, *228*, 66–73. [CrossRef]
30. Baig, M.S.; Suryawanshi, R.M.; Zehravi, M.; Mahajan, H.S.; Rana, R.; Banu, A.; Subramanian, M.; Kaundal, A.K.; Puri, S.; Siddiqui, F.A.; et al. Surface decorated quantum dots: Synthesis, properties and role in herbal therapy. *Front. Cell Dev. Biol.* **2023**, *11*, 1139671. [CrossRef]
31. Wang, Z.; Xing, X.; Yang, Y.; Zhao, R.; Zou, T.; Wang, Z.; Wang, Y. One-step hydrothermal synthesis of thioglycolic acid capped CdS quantum dots as fluorescence determination of cobalt ion. *Sci. Rep.* **2018**, *8*, 8953. [CrossRef]
32. Al Rifai, N.; Desgranges, S.; Le Guillou-Buffello, D.; Giron, A.; Urbach, W.; Nassereddine, M.; Charara, J.; Contino-Pépin, C.; Taulier, N. Ultrasound-triggered delivery of paclitaxel encapsulated in an emulsion at low acoustic pressures. *J. Mater. Chem. B* **2020**, *8*, 1640–1648. [CrossRef]
33. Gil, H.M.; Price, T.W.; Chelani, K.; Bouillard, J.-S.G.; Calaminus, S.D.; Stasiuk, G.J. NIR-quantum dots in biomedical imaging and their future. *iScience* **2021**, *24*, 102189. [CrossRef]
34. Jeong, S.; Jung, Y.; Bok, S.; Ryu, Y.; Lee, S.; Kim, Y.; Song, J.; Kim, M.; Kim, S.; Ahn, G.; et al. Multiplexed In Vivo Imaging Using Size-Controlled Quantum Dots in the Second Near-Infrared Window. *Adv. Health Mater.* **2018**, *7*, e1800695. [CrossRef] [PubMed]
35. Gautier, J.; Monrás, J.; Osorio-Román, I.; Vásquez, C.; Bravo, D.; Herranz, T.; Marco, J.; Pérez-Donoso, J. Surface characterization of GSH-CdTe quantum dots. *Mater. Chem. Phys.* **2013**, *140*, 113–118. [CrossRef]
36. Gerbec, J.A.; Magana, D.; Washington, A.; Strouse, G.F. Microwave-enhanced reaction rates for nanoparticle synthesis. *J. Am. Chem. Soc.* **2005**, *127*, 15791–15800. [CrossRef]
37. Hu, M.Z.; Zhu, T. Semiconductor Nanocrystal quantum dot synthesis approaches towards large-scale industrial production for energy applications. *Nanoscale Res. Lett.* **2015**, *10*, 469. [CrossRef] [PubMed]
38. Singh, S.; Sabri, Y.M.; Jampaiah, D.; Selvakannan, P.; Nafady, A.; Kandjani, A.E.; Bhargava, S.K. Easy, one-step synthesis of CdTe quantum dots via microwave irradiation for fingerprinting application. *Mater. Res. Bull.* **2017**, *90*, 260–265. [CrossRef]
39. Zhu, J.; Palchik, O.; Chen, S.; Gedanken, A. Microwave assisted preparation of CdSe, PbSe, and $Cu_{2-x}Se$ nanoparticles. *J. Phys. Chem. B* **2000**, *104*, 7344–7347. [CrossRef]

40. Ziegler, J.; Merkulov, A.; Grabolle, M.; Resch-Genger, U.; Nann, T. High-Quality ZnS Shells for CdSe Nanoparticles: Rapid Microwave Synthesis. *Langmuir* **2007**, *23*, 7751–7759. [CrossRef]
41. Kagan, C.R.; Bassett, L.C.; Murray, C.B.; Thompson, S.M. Colloidal quantum dots as platforms for quantum information science. *Chem. Rev.* **2020**, *121*, 3186–3233. [CrossRef] [PubMed]
42. Lai, L.; Li, S.-J.; Feng, J.; Mei, P.; Ren, Z.-H.; Chang, Y.-L.; Liu, Y. Effects of surface charges on the bactericide activity of Cdte/Zns quantum dots: A cell membrane disruption perspective. *Langmuir* **2017**, *33*, 2378–2386. [CrossRef]
43. Antony, J.V.; Pillai, J.J.; Kurian, P.; Nampoori, V.P.N.; Kochimoolayil, G.E. Photoluminescence and optical nonlinearity of CdS quantum dots synthesized in a functional copolymer hydrogel template. *New J. Chem.* **2017**, *41*, 3524–3536. [CrossRef]
44. Rabadanov, M.K.; Verin, I.A.; Ivanov, Y.M.; Simonov, V.I. Refinement of the atomic structure of CdTe single crystals. *Crystallogr. Rep.* **2001**, *46*, 636–641. [CrossRef]
45. Belenkii, D.I.; Averkin, D.V.; Vishnevetskii, D.V.; Khizhnyak, S.D.; Pakhomov, P.M. Development and Creation of a Zeta Potential Reference Material of Particles in a Liquid Medium. *Meas. Technol.* **2021**, *64*, 328–332. [CrossRef]
46. Gómez-Piñeros, B.S.; Granados-Oliveros, G. Síntesis y caracterización de las propiedades ópticas de puntos cuánticos de CdSe y CdSe/ZnS. *Rev. Colomb. De Química* **2018**, *47*, 57–63. [CrossRef]
47. Silva-Vidaurri, L.G.; Ruiz-Robles, M.A.; Gutiérrez-Lazos, C.D.; Solis-Pomar, F.; Fundora, A.; Meléndrez, M.F.; Pérez-Tijerina, E. Study of the influence of microwave irradiation under controlled conditions on the optical and structural properties of CdTe quantum dots synthesized by one-pot synthesis. *Chalcogenide Lett.* **2019**, *16*, 241–248.
48. Pan, J.; Zheng, Z.; Yang, J.; Wu, Y.; Lu, F.; Chen, Y.; Gao, W. A novel and sensitive fluorescence sensor for glutathione detection by controlling the surface passivation degree of carbon quantum dots. *Talanta* **2017**, *166*, 1–7. [CrossRef] [PubMed]
49. Qu, Z.; Li, N.; Na, W.; Su, X. A novel fluorescence "turn off–on" nanosensor for sensitivity detection acid phosphatase and inhibitor based on glutathione-functionalized graphene quantum dots. *Talanta* **2019**, *192*, 61–68. [CrossRef] [PubMed]
50. Wang, Y.; Feng, M.; He, B.; Chen, X.; Zeng, J.; Sun, J. Ionothermal synthesis of carbon dots from cellulose in deep eutectic solvent: A sensitive probe for detecting Cu^{2+} and glutathione with "off-on" pattern. *Appl. Surf. Sci.* **2022**, *599*, 153705. [CrossRef]
51. Chen, X.; Guo, Z.; Miao, P. One-pot synthesis of GSH-Capped CdTe quantum dots with excellent biocompatibility for direct cell imaging. *Heliyon* **2018**, *4*, e00576. [CrossRef]
52. Ruiz-Robles, M.A.; Solis-Pomar, F.; Gutiérrez-Lazos, C.D.; Fundora-Cruz, A.; Mayoral, Á.; Pérez-Tijerina, E. Synthesis and characterization of polymer/silica/QDs fluorescent nanocomposites with potential application as printing toner. *Mater. Res. Express* **2018**, *6*, 025314. [CrossRef]
53. Kini, S.; Kulkarni, S.D.; Ganiga, V.; Nagarakshit, T.K.; Chidangil, S. Dual functionalized, stable and water dispersible CdTe quantum dots: Facile, one-pot aqueous synthesis, optical tuning and energy transfer applications. *Mater. Res. Bull.* **2019**, *110*, 57–66. [CrossRef]
54. Qian, H.; Dong, C.; Weng, J.; Ren, J. Facile One-Pot Synthesis of Luminescent, Water-Soluble, and Biocompatible Glutathione-Coated CdTe Nanocrystals. *Small* **2006**, *2*, 747–751. [CrossRef] [PubMed]
55. Wansapura, P.T.; Díaz-Vásquez, W.A.; Vásquez, C.C.; Pérez-Donoso, J.M.; Chasteen, T.G. Thermal and photo stability of glutathione-capped cadmium telluride quantum dots. *J. Appl. Biomater. Funct. Mater.* **2015**, *13*, 248–252. [CrossRef] [PubMed]
56. Kim, C.; Deratani, A.; Bonfils, F. Determination of the refractive index increment of natural and synthetic poly(*cis*-1,4-isoprene) solutions and its effect on structural parameters. *J. Liq. Chromatogr. Relat. Technol.* **2009**, *33*, 37–45. [CrossRef]
57. Li, X.; Wang, C.; Ma, L.; Liu, U. Ellipsometry-transmission measurement of the complex refractive indices for a series of organic solvents in the 200–1700 nm spectral range. *Infrared Phys. Technol.* **2022**, *125*, 104313. [CrossRef]
58. Alibolandi, M.; Abnous, K.; Ramezani, M.; Hosseinkhani, H.; Hadizadeh, F. Synthesis of AS1411-aptamer-conjugated CdTe quantum dots with high fluorescence strength for probe labeling tumor cells. *J. Fluoresc.* **2014**, *24*, 1519–1529. [CrossRef] [PubMed]
59. Rogach, A.L.; Franzl, T.; Klar, T.A.; Feldmann, J.; Gaponik, N.; Lesnyak, V.; Shavel, A.; Eychmüller, A.; Rakovich, Y.P.; Donegan, J.F. Aqueous Synthesis of Thiol-Capped CdTe Nanocrystals: State-of-the-Art. *J. Phys. Chem. C* **2007**, *111*, 14628–14637. [CrossRef]
60. Spittel, D.; Poppe, J.; Meerbach, C.; Ziegler, C.; Hickey, S.G.; Eychmüller, A. Absolute energy level positions in CdSe nanostructures from potential-modulated absorption spectroscopy (EMAS). *ACS Nano* **2017**, *11*, 12174–12184. [CrossRef]
61. Pietryga, J.M.; Park, Y.-S.; Lim, J.; Fidler, A.F.; Bae, W.K.; Brovelli, S.; Klimov, V.I. Spectroscopic and device aspects of nanocrystal quantum dots. *Chem. Rev.* **2016**, *116*, 10513–10622. [CrossRef]
62. Zhang, M.; Yue, J.; Cui, R.; Ma, Z.; Wan, H.; Wang, F.; Dai, H. Bright quantum dots emitting at ~1600 nm in the NIR-IIb window for deep tissue fluorescence imaging. *Proc. Natl. Acad. Sci. USA* **2018**, *115*, 6590–6595. [CrossRef]
63. Sidiqi, A.M.; Wahl, D.; Lee, S.; Cao, S.; Cui, J.Z.; To, E.; Beg, M.; Sarunic, M.; Matsubara, J.A. In vivo imaging of curcumin labeled amyloid beta deposits in retina using fluorescence scanning laser ophthalmoscopy in an Alzheimer mouse model. *Investig. Ophthalmol. Vis. Sci.* **2018**, *59*, 6065.
64. Rodríguez-Hernández, A.G.; Aguilar Guzmán, J.C.; Vázquez-Duhalt, R. Membrana celular y la inespecificidad de las nanopartículas. ¿Hasta dónde puede llegar un nanomaterial dentro de la célula? *Mundo nano. Rev. Interdiscip. Nanociencias Nanotecnología* **2018**, *11*, 43–52. [CrossRef]
65. Li, W.; Schierle, G.S.K.; Lei, B.; Liu, Y.; Kaminski, C.F. Fluorescent nanoparticles for super-resolution imaging. *Chem. Rev.* **2022**, *122*, 12495–12543. [CrossRef] [PubMed]

66. Ma, B.; Fan, Y.; Zhang, D.; Wei, Y.; Jian, Y.; Liu, D.; Wang, Z.; Gao, Y.; Ma, J.; Chen, Y.; et al. De Novo Design of an Androgen Receptor DNA Binding Domain-Targeted peptide PROTAC for Prostate Cancer Therapy. *Adv. Sci.* **2022**, *9*, e2201859. [CrossRef] [PubMed]
67. Brown, T.A.; Tkachuk, A.N.; Shtengel, G.; Kopek, B.G.; Bogenhagen, D.F.; Hess, H.F.; Clayton, D.A. Superresolution fluorescence imaging of mitochondrial nucleoids reveals their spatial range, limits, and membrane interaction. *Mol. Cell. Biol.* **2011**, *31*, 4994–5010. [CrossRef]
68. Shang, L.; Nienhaus, K.; Nienhaus, G.U. Engineered nanoparticles interacting with cells: Size matters. *J. Nanobiotechnol.* **2014**, *12*, 5. [CrossRef]

Disclaimer/Publisher's Note: The statements, opinions and data contained in all publications are solely those of the individual author(s) and contributor(s) and not of MDPI and/or the editor(s). MDPI and/or the editor(s) disclaim responsibility for any injury to people or property resulting from any ideas, methods, instructions or products referred to in the content.

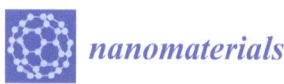 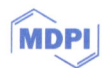

Article

An Optimized Method for Evaluating the Potential Gd-Nanoparticle Dose Enhancement Produced by Electronic Brachytherapy

Melani Fuentealba [1,2,3], Alejandro Ferreira [4], Apolo Salgado [5], Christopher Vergara [1,2], Sergio Díez [3,6] and Mauricio Santibáñez [1,2,*]

1 Departamento de Cs. Físicas, Universidad de La Frontera, Temuco 4811230, Chile
2 Laboratorio de Radiaciones Ionizantes, Universidad de La Frontera, Temuco 4811230, Chile
3 Departamento de Fisiología, Universitat de València, 46010 Valencia, Spain
4 Facultad de Medicina y Ciencia, Universidad San Sebastián, Santiago 7510602, Chile
5 IORT, Santiago 7500833, Chile
6 Medical Physics Department, Hospital Clínico Universitario de Valencia, 46010 Valencia, Spain
* Correspondence: mauricio.santibanez@ufrontera.cl; Tel.: +56-452325320

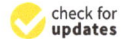

Abstract: This work reports an optimized method to experimentally quantify the Gd-nanoparticle dose enhancement generated by electronic brachytherapy. The dose enhancement was evaluated considering energy beams of 50 kVp and 70 kVp, determining the Gd-nanoparticle concentration ranges that would optimize the process for each energy. The evaluation was performed using delaminated radiochromic films and a Poly(methyl methacrylate) (PMMA) phantom covered on one side by a thin 2.5 µm Mylar filter acting as an interface between the region with Gd suspension and the radiosensitive film substrate. The results for the 70 kVp beam quality showed dose increments of $6 \pm 6\%$, $22 \pm 7\%$, and $9 \pm 7\%$ at different concentrations of 10, 20, and 30 mg/mL, respectively, verifying the competitive mechanisms of enhancement and attenuation. For the 50 kVp beam quality, no increase in dose was recorded for the concentrations studied, indicating that the major contribution to enhancement is from the K-edge interaction. In order to separate the contributions of attenuation and enhancement to the total dose, measurements were replicated with a 12 µm Mylar filter, obtaining a dose enhancement attributable to the K-edge of $29 \pm 7\%$ and $34 \pm 7\%$ at 20 and 30 mg/mL, respectively, evidencing a significant additional dose proportional to the Gd concentration.

Keywords: dose enhancement; delaminated EBT3 films; Gd nanoparticles

Citation: Fuentealba, M.; Ferreira, A.; Salgado, A.; Vergara, C.; Díez, S.; Santibáñez, M. An Optimized Method for Evaluating the Potential Gd-Nanoparticle Dose Enhancement Produced by Electronic Brachytherapy. *Nanomaterials* **2024**, *14*, 430. https://doi.org/10.3390/nano14050430

Academic Editor: James Chow

Received: 8 December 2023
Revised: 8 January 2024
Accepted: 11 January 2024
Published: 27 February 2024

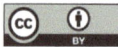

Copyright: © 2024 by the authors. Licensee MDPI, Basel, Switzerland. This article is an open access article distributed under the terms and conditions of the Creative Commons Attribution (CC BY) license (https://creativecommons.org/licenses/by/4.0/).

1. Introduction

It is widely known that high-atomic-number nanoparticle infusion within biological tissue presents multiple benefits in diagnostic and therapeutic terms, as is the case for teletherapy and brachytherapy [1?–3]. This is due to the localized deposition of energy by photoelectrons and Auger electrons produced by photoelectric interaction augmentation between primary radiation and the high-Z nanoparticle infused into the tissue. This effect is denominated as dose enhancement and has the characteristics of being highly localized and restricted exclusively to the infusion area, increasing the dose solely in the region of interest without affecting the surrounding tissue [5–7].

There are several radiotherapy modalities that can potentially produce a relevant dose enhancement, such as: electronic brachytherapy (eBx) [8–10], intraoperative radiotherapy (IORT) [11–13], and superficial radiation therapy (SRT) [14,15] by low-energy X-rays. These treatment modalities, using new equipment, promise to replace the traditional sources of conventional brachytherapy treatments based on radioactive isotopes (typically ^{192}Ir, ^{60}Co, and the obsolete ^{137}Cs) by the new generations of mini-X-ray tubes with energies in the range of 35–100 kVp [16,17].

The production of nanoparticle agents with high internalization, biocompatibility, and the ability to be incorporated inside malignant cells at a higher concentration compared to normal tissue cells has been studied in detail for metallic nanoparticles such as gold (GNPs). Functionalization through bonding to lipids [18,19], peptides [20? ,21], proteins [23,24], and antibodies associated with over-expression in tumoral cells [6,25–28] is the path explored to achieve high tumor concentrations. Even though GNPs have been researched the most, gadolinium nanoparticles (GdNPs) are receiving more attention (given their long-standing history in clinical imagenology as safe MRI contrast agents), with experimental studies demonstrating great biocompatibility and internalization capabilities for in vitro and in vivo applications [29,30]. The first investigations that explored the viability of Gd as a dose enhancer assessed its use in treating brain tumors via the application of microbeams [31,32]. GdNPs such as AGuIX® NPs (NH TherAguix SA, Meylan, France) have been used for human studies in MRI-guided radiotherapy [29], as well as phase-I clinical trials [33,34] as dose enhancers.

Even though the photoelectric absorption process reaches its maximum probability when the excitation occurs at energies just above the absorption edge, in certain high-Z elements the maximum dose enhancement would not be close to these energies. This is explained by the need to find an energy that simultaneously maximizes the ratio of the mass energy absorption coefficients and the ratio of the mass absorption coefficients of the enhancing element with respect to the tissue to be doped [14,35]. In particular, in the case of gold, the maximum dose enhancement has been obtained at photon energies of 40 keV [36], which is considerably below its K-edge (80.7 keV). Nevertheless, in the case of iodine with a K-edge of 33.3 keV, the optimal energy has been determined both theoretically and empirically to be 50 keV [14]. In the particular case of gadolinium, unlike gold or iodine, the optimal energy described in the literature is 60 keV [14] or 65 keV [31], slightly above its absorption K-edge of 50.2 keV.

The determination of the Dose Enhancement Factor (DEF) has been addressed by different Monte Carlo (MC) simulations, as in the work of Zygmanski et al., 2013 [37], who performed a comprehensive study using the GEANT4 MC code with GNPs, testing different monoenergetic beams between 11 keV and 1 MeV and applying a water phantom with NPs located at a 2 cm depth. This work evaluated the dependence on the distance from the source to the GNP, beam size, NP size, and NP clustering, concluding that the DEF is sensitive to specific irradiation geometries and source types and essentially depends on the X-ray beam energy, which for energies under 20 keV resulted in beam attenuation rather than dose enhancement. Spiga et al., 2019 [38], using the same code, investigated the dose distribution of an X-ray beam slightly above the absorption edge of metal-based compounds (gadolinium and iodine) at several concentrations in a water-equivalent phantom. For monochromatic energies between 30 and 140 keV, comparing Monte Carlo data with the experimental results, strong agreement was obtained with differences of less than 5% for depths <60 mm. Regarding iodine dose enhancement, for 10 mg/mL concentrations and 35 keV spectra, increases of up to 150% in the dose were reported, reaching maximum enhancement for the 45 keV spectrum with a dose enhancement of 190%. In the case of gadolinium, at the same concentration, maximum enhancement was obtained for the 55–75 keV spectral range, with a difference of 40% at 21 mm and 20% at 54 mm compared to iodine. Another study reporting on Gd with monochromatic beams between 51 and 100 keV showed the existence of the DEF for energies above the K-edge, with a maximum DEF in the 58–65 keV range and a marked decrease for higher energies [29,31].

On the other hand, experimental quantification still presents important challenges, the main difficulty being the ability to record the contribution of low-energy photoelectrons and Auger electrons, which do not manage to pass through the walls that cover traditional dosimeters and be recorded by the radiosensitive region. Dose enhancement measurements obtained through Gafchromic model EBT2 and EBT3 radiochromic films (specially designed for "External Beam Therapy (EBT)" and commercially known as EBT2 and EBT3 films) have already been reported some years ago [39,42? ? ,43]. The EBT3 film possesses a 30 μm radiosensitive substrate placed between two 125 μm transparent polyester films, barriers not penetrable by electrons with energies <90 keV, making it difficult to directly measure the DEF for energy beams close to the Gd absorption edge. A feasible alternative is film delamination on one of the faces, exposing the polymeric substrate to the medium and the photon beam. The delamination process has been suggested and assessed for different beam types and qualities, such as alpha particles [44], medium-energy X-rays [45], and low-energy heavy-ion dosimeters [46], removing the energy constraint of the detectable particles. However, in these studies, EBT3 films were not submerged in water since the active substrate is highly sensitive and is easily damaged when in contact with water. This limits the dosimetric determination of dose enhancement at different concentrations since the experimental conditions are different from an actual clinical scenario. Consequently, interventions are limited to delamination followed by the application of a new waterproof element with a thickness that enhances the detection of low-energy electrons. Recently, the possibility of altering EBT3 dosimetric films by delaminating and resealing them using materials with thicknesses of 12 μm to maintain their water immersion properties has been reported [47]. The dosimeters evaluated after the intervention maintained their dosimetric properties unaltered, allowing the recording of photoelectrons of energies greater than 25 keV, generated by a ^{192}Ir brachytherapy source in a phantom with Gd suspensions and dose enhancement values of 15%, compatible with Monte Carlo simulations and previous measurements.

The aim of this work was to find a method to optimize Gd-nanoparticle dose enhancement measurement, allowing one to record the dose contribution of photoelectrons with energies below 20 keV (typically produced in irradiation with electronic brachytherapy equipment). The use of delaminated and non-resealed EBT3 films and filters sufficiently thin to let through the generated photoelectrons, maintaining the property of being a barrier between the radiosensitive substrate and the water with the Gd suspension, is promising.

2. Materials and Methods

2.1. EBT3 Radiochromic Film Processing and Reading

Gafchromic® EBT3 films (Ashland Advanced Materials, Bridgewater, NJ, USA) were meticulously delaminated based on the method described by [47]. The opening of the first 125 μm layer of polyester was carried out employing a surgical scalpel and applying a constant traction force achieved through the use of a controlled mechanical device.

From the delaminated EBT3 film sheets, 30 mm square fragments were obtained in order to be used as dosimetric elements adaptable to the implemented setup. All the delaminated EBT3 films used during the experiments were characterized in terms of their optical transmittance by pre- and post-irradiation readings, performed using an EPSON Perfection V370 (Seiko Epson Corporation, Suwa, Nagano, Japan) transmittance scanner, configured at 48 bits (16 bits per color) and 144 dpi. Additionally, since any interference with the film (including radiation exposure and mechanical stress) would alter the active substrate, producing polymerization reactions, a stabilization time of at least 16 h had to be allowed before any reading. Thus, the pre-irradiation reading was executed 24 h after the mechanical intervention (i.e., delamination and cutting), while a 24 h post-irradiation reading was chosen.

The data acquired with the scanner were processed with ImageJ software (Version 1.54), utilizing exclusively the red channel, since it has been widely reported that this channel provides the dose–response curve with the highest sensitivity for doses lower than 8 Gy. In view of the possible inherent measurement fluctuations that may have been registered in each pixel of the digital image, the same region of interest (ROI) size of 50 × 50 square pixels was defined for all the images analyzed. For this ROI, the "Measurement" function was used, which provided statistical data such as: maximum pixel value, minimum value, average, and standard deviation. In all measurements, the selected reading value was the average. To establish the change in the dosimeter transmittance due to the absorbed dose effect, the figure of merit used was the optical density (OD), as follows:

$$D.O. = log\left(\frac{I_0}{I}\right); \qquad \Delta D.O. = \frac{1}{ln_{10}} \cdot \sqrt{\frac{\Delta I_0^2}{I_0^2} + \frac{\Delta I^2}{I^2}} \qquad (1)$$

where I_0 is the average pixel intensity of an ROI of the pre-irradiation transmission image, and I is the post-irradiation reading averaged in the same ROI.

2.2. PMMA Phantom Manufacturing and Setup

A phantom that simulated a tumoral volume doped with a Gd suspension was designed, which allowed direct adaptation to the clinical electronic brachytherapy equipment applicator and the superficial irradiation of the volume. A second feature of the designed phantom was that one of its sides allowed the adherence of films of different thicknesses, without experiencing the leakage of the water with the Gd suspension. In this way, the phantom could be positioned directly on a delaminated EBT3 film, without the need to dip the film directly into the dose-enhancing medium.

The phantom was manufactured as a square prism with an external geometry of 4.5 cm for the square face side and 1.5 cm in height. Its interior was formed by two concentric cylinders, the first cylinder being 2.8 cm in diameter, which completely crossed the prism, enabling the phantom to be opened on both ends (Figure 1), and the second being 3.5 cm in diameter and 5.0 mm deep. The measurements were adapted to the D30-5 surface applicator diameter, permitting the applicator to rest on the phantom and keeping a constant distance of 1.0 cm from the irradiation surface to the other prism external face, where the EBT3 film would be placed behind the insulating film of the water with the Gd suspension (measured at a 1.0 cm depth in water) (Figure 1).

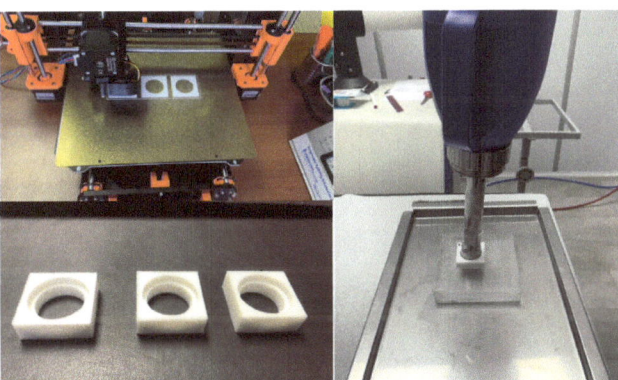

Figure 1. (**Left**) Design of PMMA phantoms by means of 3D printer. (**Right**) Applicator inserted into phantom.

PMMA in the form of 3D printer filament, 1.75 mm in diameter, was selected as the fabrication material for the phantom walls. Thus, the phantom was directly printed using a PRUSA 3D printer model i3 MK3S (Figure 1). For the printing parameters, a 100% infill was selected in order to reduce the leakage of the water with the Gd suspension through the walls, maximizing the measurement time without damaging the delaminated EBT3 film on which the phantom was positioned. Multiple phantoms with the same geometrical characteristics but different extruder and bed temperature conditions were manufactured to evaluate the imperfections in the geometry and tolerances in the measurements considering the requirement of containing the clinical applicator and the Mylar film with the EBT3.

The fabricated phantoms were sealed on one side with a Spectro Film thin Mylar film marketed by SPI supplies (West Chester, PA, USA), presenting thicknesses of 2.5 and 12 microns. This allowed them to contain a total volume of 6.15 cm^3, which was filled with Gd suspensions in concentration ranges of 0–30 mg/mL, simulating a tumor undoped and doped with Gd, and the Mylar films acted as two different energy barrier thicknesses for the photoelectrons produced by the Gd, which were recorded on the other side by the delaminated EBT3 film. Subsequent to the manufacture of the PMMA phantom, the entire structure was completed with a set of PMMA slabs ($15 \times 15 \times 0.5 \times 0.5$) cm^3 to achieve the backscattering component (see Figure 1).

Given that the Mylar film acted as a thin interface between the region with water containing the Gd suspension and the region with the radiosensitive substrate of the EBT3 dosimeters (which is highly affected in its dosimetric and structural properties by direct water contact), and given the inherent porosities that exist in 3D printing machining, it was necessary to evaluate the degree of phantom sealing. The implemented criteria considered maximum times without filtration under static conditions (time taken for the filter and the walls of the phantom to leak the suspension onto the EBT3 film while resting on it) and dynamic conditions (time taken for the filter and the phantom walls to leak the suspension onto the EBT3 film after the successive positioning and removal of the phantom on the film—conditions more similar to the required measurement process, which generated micro-tears in the Mylar film that would allow the leakage of water with the Gd suspension onto the EBT3 film in a shorter times).

2.3. Irradiation System

Clinical treatment equipment consisting of a WoMed model IORT-50 mobile surface radiotherapy and intraoperative radiotherapy system was used (Figure 2). This equipment allows irradiation with 3 beam qualities, 35, 50, and 70 kVp, and maximum surface dose rates of 1–1.5 Gy/min. The system has a set of collimators that permit the formation of circular fields 1–3 cm in diameter on the surface for surface irradiation and a set of spherical applicators 3–5 cm in diameter for intra-operative treatments. Depending on the type of applicator, the system configures a kVp and a current for which it has dosimetric calibration tables at different water depths. In this way, the irradiation time is selected exclusively according to the dose to be prescribed in the treatment. Given the need to minimize radiation penetration for surface treatments, the equipment in its treatment mode allows the use of energies of 35 and 50 kVp exclusively, limiting the beam quality to 70 kVp for intra-operative treatment only.

When employing EBT3 films as dosimeters, it is imperative to generate a flat irradiation on them in order to use the information from the largest number of pixels. This creates the need to exclusively implement the surface applicator (which is why it was necessary to design the phantom to be compatible with this accessory, as described in the previous subsection) and operate the equipment in "Service" mode, for the purpose of removing the kVp restriction, allowing a 70 kVp beam quality to be used with this applicator. However, since the equipment does not have depth dose tables for this beam quality, it was necessary to first perform dosimetric measurements to determine the dose rate delivered at that energy with the applicator. Dosimetric determination was performed following the TG-61 code of practice for the 50 kVp (HVL: 3.38 mm Al) and 70 kVp (HVL: 4.70 mm Al) beam qualities [48], whose kV were verified according to routine quality-control equipment using a RadCal Accu-kV (40–160 kVp) kV meter with a valid calibration certificate. The dosimetric protocol involves obtaining the dose from in-air kerma measurements taken within a small-volume parallel-plate ionization chamber calibrated under these conditions. A PTW model TN34013 chamber with a sensitive volume of 0.005 cm^3, designed for measurements in the 10–70 kVp range, and a PTW model Unidos E electrometer were used for the measurements.

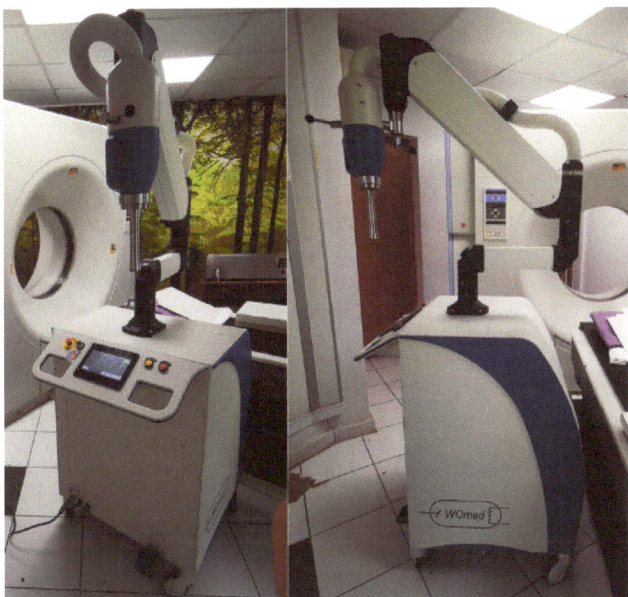

Figure 2. WOmed ioRT-50 clinical surface radiotherapy equipment used in the measurements.

2.4. EBT3 Film Calibration Curve

The determination of dose enhancement by the dosimetric use of EBT3 films requires the prior acquisition of a calibration curve that relates the change in optical density to different absorbed doses in the ranges of interest and under the same conditions as the experimental procedure: at the prescription depth (1 cm) and placing the radiochromic film under a PMMA phantom with water. Reproducing the same reference conditions for calibration and measurement is fundamental for the range of kV energies, since unlike MV beams, the former drastically change their quality at different depths in a medium. The calibration curve was obtained considering 6 measurement points in the dose range of 1.5–5.5 Gy, with each measurement in triplicate (18 total measurements), in order to consider both the uncertainties of the procedure and the heterogeneity inherent to the EBT3 film. The resulting curve was obtained by fitting a polynomial function, using the R^2 parameter as a goodness-of-fit criterion.

2.5. Dose Enhancement Evaluation

Dose enhancement was measured in an initial stage considering two available beam qualities: one with an energy below the K absorption edge of Gd (50.2 kV) of 50 kVp, for which it was feasible to generate dose enhancement in the L and M layers of the Gd exclusively; and one with an energy of 70 kVp, above the K absorption edge, which could additionally generate dose enhancement in the K layer. Two concentrations of water with a Gd suspension at 10 and 20 mg/mL were prepared and injected into the PMMA-fabricated tumor phantom. A set of 10 measurements was performed for each concentration and for each beam quality to account for possible fluctuations in the film. The prescription in each measurement was 3.0 Gy in water at the depth of the EBT3 film (1.0 cm), which was achieved by adjusting only the irradiation time, since for both configurations (50 kVp and 70 kVp) a fixed current of 7 mA was used. As a barrier between the Gd suspension and the active substrate of the delaminated EBT3 film, a 2.5 micron Mylar filter was placed on the tumor phantom, which limited the penetration of photoelectrons with an energy less than 10 keV. The dose enhancement was evaluated from the DEF defined as a function of the beam quality E (in this case, kVp) and the percentage of Gd (concentration in mg/mL), presenting uncertainty values of one SD for all measurements:

$$DEF_{(E,\%Gd)} = \frac{\text{Dose readout in EBT3 for beam quality } E \text{ and phantom with Gd}}{\text{Dose readout in EBT3 for beam quality } E \text{ and phantom without Gd}} \quad (2)$$

Considering that beam qualities slightly above the absorption edge (such as that of 70 kVp emitted by the studied clinical equipment) allow one to achieve a dose enhancement at greater depths than lower energies, it was decided to study the concentration at which the competitive phenomenon of dose decrease due to self-attenuation (the attenuation of the incident radiation by the high Gd concentration) would offset the increase in dose due to the enhancement phenomenon, in order to determine the range of useful concentrations. Additionally, given that there will always be a sub-quantification of the net dose enhancement, given the inherent restriction of photoelectrons with a lower energy imposed by the Mylar coating necessary to isolate the delaminated EBT3 film from direct contact with the water containing the Gd suspension, we proceeded to evaluate the dose achieved by the different concentrations for two Mylar film thicknesses: 2.5 µm and 12 µm. The latter thickness corresponds to a barrier that restricts the detection of all the photoelectrons produced by the K-edge, since it imposes an energy barrier of 25 keV.

Three different concentrations of water with a Gd suspension were prepared: 10, 20, and 30 mg/mL. A volume of 6.15 cm^3 of each concentration was infused inside 3 PMMA phantoms, closed at one end with a 2.5 µm Mylar film (minimum thickness available as a barrier for the generated photoelectrons). Similarly, a volume of 6.15 cm^3 of each concentration was infused into 3 PMMA phantoms that were closed at one end by a 12 µm Mylar film (a thickness that would not allow the penetration of photoelectrons with energies less than 25 keV). A prescription of 3.0 Gy in water was delivered at a depth of 1.0 cm (the position of the delaminated EBT3 film), with the equipment configured at 70 kV and 7 mA and an irradiation time of 1 min and 6 s. Differences in the doses recorded for the same beam quality and for the same Gd concentration, but with a phantom equipped with different Mylar thicknesses, were associated exclusively with the dose enhancement component, which was recorded as significantly higher in the measurements of the 2.5 µm Mylar film than those of the 12 µm Mylar film, allowing at first order the separation of the dose enhancement from the attenuation components of the total dose measured.

3. Results

3.1. PMMA Phantom Manufacturing and Evaluation

Following the defined geometries and the tolerances given by the clinical equipment used, it was possible to manufacture by the additive deposition of PMMA filaments multiple versions of the phantom adaptable to the surface applicator to contain the Gd suspension (Figure 3). Given the particular characteristics of the PMMA material in filament form, it was necessary to evaluate the results of the final prints of the phantom in terms of geometry imperfections and tolerances in the final measurements obtained for different temperature values of the printer extruder, in the range of 230–250 °C, indicating that the optimum temperature was 250 °C. Additionally, the same criteria were compared for different printed phantoms depending on the temperature of the printing surface, in the range of 90–110 °C, indicating that the best results were achieved for 100 °C.

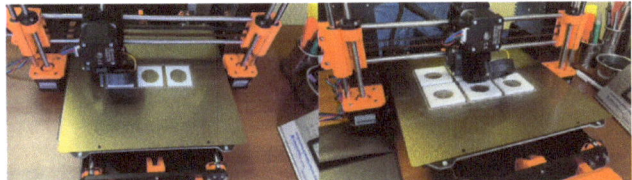

Figure 3. Manufacturing of multiple phantoms with the same geometry but different temperature parameters for the nozzle extruder and printing surface.

From the passive and active tightness criteria defined for the PMMA phantom sealed with 2.5 μm or 12 μm Mylar filters (Figure 4), it was determined that for the case of phantoms configured with a 12 μm Mylar film, the passive tightness reached average times of up to 30 min without filtering, with the first affected area being the edges of the EBT3 film. Likewise, phantoms configured with a 2.5 μm Mylar film resisted for average times of 25–30 min. A relevant aspect to consider is that, in real measurement conditions, the phantoms are repeatedly positioned on different films for shorter irradiation times, with the actions of positioning and removing inducing more damage on the thin film, resulting in the generation of micro-cracks capable of causing the leakage of the water with the Gd suspension. When implementing the active sealing evaluations, it was evidenced that the average sealing time was effectively reduced by half, and the first leaks for both Mylar thicknesses occurred after only 15 min. However, given the equipment dose rate, the irradiation times required for the calibration curves and dose enhancement measurements were lower than the active sealing times, ensuring that the phantom configuration used was adequate for the required measurement.

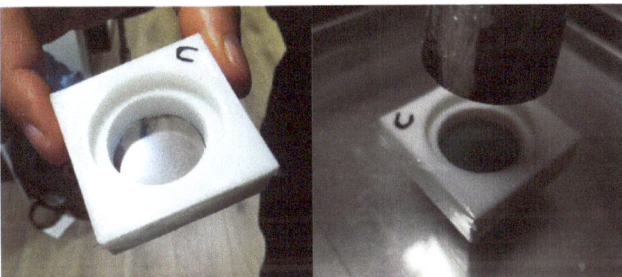

Figure 4. PMMA phantoms sealed with 2.5 μm and 12 μm Mylar films to contain a 6.15 cm^3 suspension volume deposited on delaminated EBT3 film dosimeters.

3.2. Dose Enhancement Measurements

3.2.1. Calibration Curve

Figure 5 displays the calibration curve obtained from fitting the dose-optical density response of the delaminated films read 24 h post-irradiation to a second-degree polynomial function. The fit quality achieved for the dose range of 1.5–5.5 Gy was $R^2 = 0.9821$. The error bars correspond to the dispersion value obtained in triplicate for each point on the curve. The indicated uncertainties correspond to one SD level.

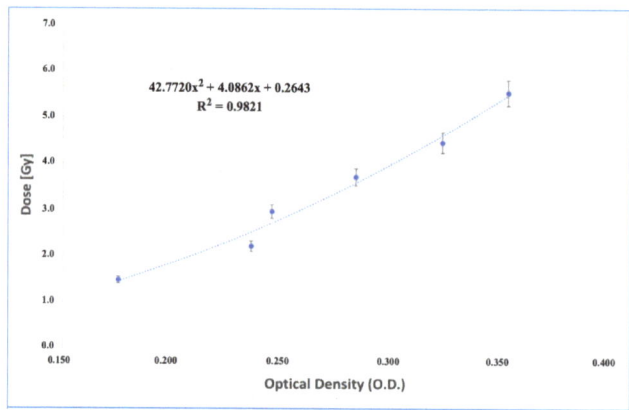

Figure 5. Delaminated EBT3 film dose–response curve in terms of optical density achieved at different dose values in the range of 1.5–5.5 Gy.

Is important to note that the OD–dose relationship is not linear in EBT3 films, and better results are achieved through empirical models with variable coefficients or polynomial fits. Besides, the OD values are only valid for a specific wavelength of light analyzed [49] and can vary according to the scanner and parameters like the scanner orientation and reading conditions [50].

3.2.2. Dose Enhancement Evaluation as a Function of Beam Quality

For the first evaluation of the DEF, in terms of beam quality and a dose prescription of 3.0 Gy at a 1.0 cm depth, it was found that for irradiations with 50 kVp at concentrations of 10 mg/mL Gd, there was a decrease in the prescribed dose, while the same behavior was exhibited for the higher concentration of 20 mg/mL, as shown in Table 1. This phenomenon could be explained given that the 50 kVp beam was not able to excite the K-edge of Gd (50.2 keV edge), so it only had the option of generating enhancement in the L layer. However, the greater beam attenuation achieved when propagating in a medium with a higher attenuation coefficient than water generated a more substantial effect compared to dose enhancement, which was accentuated at higher concentrations, not allowing dose enhancement to be achieved at the concentration and depth studied.

Table 1. Dose and DEF achieved for 50 and 70 kVp beam quality with 10 and 20 mg/mL Gd concentrations.

Medium	50 kVp		70 kVp	
	Dose (Gy)	DEF	Dose (Gy)	DEF
Water	3.00	–	3.00	–
10 mg/mL	2.84 ± 0.12	−5 ± 4%	3.16 ± 0.18	+6 ± 6%
20 mg/mL	2.32 ± 0.18	−23 ± 6%	3.67 ± 0.21	+22 ± 7%

For the 70 kVp beam quality, a slightly higher dose was obtained for irradiations at 10 mg/mL Gd concentrations. On the other hand, for the 20 mg/mL Gd concentration, an increase of a 22 ± 7% DEF was achieved (Table 1). For this beam quality, it was observed that the contribution of photoelectrons generated in the photoelectric absorption processes with the K layer was more significant than the contribution to the dose from interactions with the L layer, although only photoelectrons with energies greater than 10 keV were recorded with the 2.5 μm film. For this reason, only the limited spectral region between 60 and 70 keV of the radiation beam contributed to the dose enhancement in the dosimeter. Additionally, the higher energy decreased the self-attenuation generated by the higher-absorption-coefficient medium, allowing, at least at the tumor depth studied, the enhancement phenomenon to be greater than the attenuation, achieving an effective DEF.

3.2.3. Dose Enhancement Evaluation as a Function of Gd Concentration for the Most Energetic Clinical Beam Quality

The results obtained from the readings of the new film set (considering a 70 kVp energy and a Gd concentration range between 10 and 30 mg/mL), which were transformed to dose via the calibration curve previously obtained, once again showed dose values equivalent to those previously obtained for 10 and 20 mg/mL Gd concentrations of 3.17 ± 0.17 Gy and 3.67 ± 0.22 Gy, respectively. For the newly evaluated concentration of 30 mg/mL, an average DEF of $9 \pm 7\%$ was recorded (Table 2), which was slightly above the experimental uncertainty, possibly marking the concentration limit at which dose enhancement would generate a net dose increase at the studied depth, and thus the optimal concentration value to use would be around 20 mg/mL.

Table 2. Dose and DEF achieved for 70 kVp beam quality with 10, 20, and 30 mg/mL Gd concentrations.

Concentration (mg/mL Gd)	Prescribed Dose (Gy)	Measured Dose (Gy)	DEF (%)
10	3.00	3.17 ± 0.17	$+6.0 \pm 6\%$
20	3.00	3.67 ± 0.22	$+22.0 \pm 7\%$
30	3.00	3.26 ± 0.20	$+9.0 \pm 7\%$

As mentioned, there is a point in a dosimeter where the dose enhancement does not predominate and the dose begins to fall due to the attenuation produced by the high concentrations of the enhancement material. With the purpose of evaluating, at first order, the percentage of attenuation and the percentage of dose enhancement contribution separately with respect to the net dose recorded, the delaminated EBT3 films with a 12 µm Mylar barrier (which completely eliminated the enhancement component of the K-edge) were assessed. A dose of 2.84 ± 0.15 Gy was obtained for the 20 mg/mL concentration of Gd, equivalent to a decrease of $6 \pm 5\%$ in the prescribed dose (a consequence of the higher attenuation with respect to water), while for the 30 mg/mL concentration a dose of 2.43 ± 0.18 Gy was obtained, corresponding to a decrease of $19 \pm 6\%$ in the prescribed dose (Table 3).

Table 3. Dose recorded for Mylar films that prevented enhancement recording (12 µm) and Mylar films that allowed enhancement recording (2.5 µm) for a beam quality of 70 kVp at Gd concentrations of 20–30 mg/mL.

Concentration (mg/mL Gd)	Prescribed Dose (Gy)	Measured Dose with a 12 µm Film (Gy)	Measured Dose with a 2.5 µm Film (Gy)	Relative DEF (%) 2.5 µm/12 µm
20	3.00	2.84 ± 0.15	3.67 ± 0.22	$+29.0 \pm 7\%$
30	3.00	2.43 ± 0.18	3.26 ± 0.20	$+34.0 \pm 7\%$

The results obtained showed more significantly that although the concentration increase generated a strong attenuation, the dose enhancement component of the K-layer was responsible for generating a significant additional dose proportional to the concentration, which in the case of the 20 mg/mL Gd concentration produced an additional dose increase of $29 \pm 7\%$ and for the 30 mg/mL concentration an increase of $34 \pm 7\%$ (Table 3).

4. Discussion

Previously reported methods found in the literature that involve the delamination and subsequent resealing of EBT3 films limited the dosimetry measurement in water of the dose enhancement produced by nanoparticles to exclusively gamma photons and medium-energy X-rays (>80 kV according to the IAEA TRS-398 protocol), which were capable of generating photoelectrons of energies greater than 25 keV that managed to pass through the thin film used in the resealing process (10-times thinner than the original laminate) [47], preventing the use of this methodology for the low-energy beams (<80 kV) employed by eBT and IORT units. The method proposed in this work used a filter that was five-times thinner (2.5 µm) than that of the previous procedure, since its function was limited to being a waterproof barrier between the radiosensitive substrate present in the film and the water that contained the Gd suspension, thus removing the mechanical strength and elasticity that was required of the filters, in both the resealing process and the subsequent immersion of the film in water, damaging the latter due to the entry of water into the active substrate and resulting in a greater dispersion and uncertainty in its reading. In this way, by reducing the thickness of the film, the photoelectron detection range was increased to energies of 10 keV and higher, and the mechanical stress effects that occur due to resealing and submerging the film in water were removed.

The assays performed using PMMA phantoms manufactured by 3D printing with infill percentages of 99% and a 2.5 µm Mylar film accession showed an adequate ability to hold water with a Gd suspension at a volume of 6.15 cm^3 without leakages for 15 min, considering rise and fall movements. In addition, it should be noted that the existence of 3D-printed filaments of dosimetrically useful materials such as PMMA permits the fast, customized, and economical generation of phantoms adaptable to unconventional requirements such as dose enhancement measurements.

For the clinical equipment and beam quality used (70 kVp, HVL 4.70 mm Al), the greatest dose enhancement for the gadolinium suspension was obtained for a 20 mg/mL concentration, with an increase of up to $22 \pm 7\%$ with respect to the prescribed dose, while for 30 mg/mL concentrations only a $9 \pm 7\%$ enhancement was achieved, due to the existence of a critical competitive process between concentration and dose enhancement. For lower concentrations, it was not possible to discriminate the enhancement from the experimental uncertainties.

The evaluation of how the dose increase was modified as a function of the Mylar film thickness imposed onto the EBT3 dosimeter showed that by implementing a thickness that blocked the totality of the photoelectrons generated from the Gd K-edge, the doses for the 20 mg/mL concentration decreased by $6 \pm 5\%$, while for 30 mg/mL concentrations the decrease in the dose reached $19 \pm 6\%$. This shows that the photoelectrons contributed by the K-layer that managed to pass through a 2.5 µm thick Mylar film promoted dose increases of $28 \pm 7\%$ and $34 \pm 7\%$ for 20 and 30 mg/mL Gd concentrations, respectively. Thus, it is expected that implementing Mylar films of smaller thicknesses or dosimeters without these limitations would result in much higher dose enhancement measurements than those reported in this work.

Even though the obtained results were a sub-estimation of the actual dose enhancement, since we were not able to detect photoelectrons of an energy lower than 10 keV, increasing the energetic recording range has shown a significant advancement in the feasibility of measuring dose enhancement at first order produced by the K-edge of Gd in a series of existing electronic brachytherapy and intraoperative radiotherapy clinical units, approaching values reported by Monte Carlo simulations.

5. Conclusions

It is feasible to implement delaminated EBT3 films without resealing by manufacturing adequate phantoms that can contain the necessary volume of water with a Gd suspension and adding films of reduced thickness that act as walls and prevent the leakage of the content.

The set of printed PMMA phantoms and the access to Mylar filters of smaller thicknesses open up the possibility of implementing these measurements in different clinical systems, in order to evaluate optimal configurations for various beam qualities and high-Z agents.

We performed an experimental determination of the Dose Enhancement Factor for a 70 kVp beam quality produced by a clinical electronic brachytherapy system, showing a maximum dose enhancement for a gadolinium suspension concentration of around 20 mg/mL, while a decrease was observed for higher concentrations due to the self-shielding effect that the same Gd nanoparticles generated in the incident radiation spectra.

Author Contributions: Conceptualization, M.S.; methodology, M.F., A.F. and A.S.; software, C.V.; validation, A.F., A.S. and S.D.; formal analysis, M.F.; investigation, M.S., C.V., M.F. and A.F.; resources, A.S. and M.S.; data curation, C.V.; writing—original draft preparation, M.S., M.F. and S.D.; supervision, M.S.; project administration, M.S., A.F. and A.S.; funding acquisition, M.S. All authors have read and agreed to the published version of the manuscript.

Funding: This research was funded by the ANID program through FONDECYT regular grant No. 1221000 and the Research Division of the UNIVERSIDAD DE LA FRONTERA through DIUFRO grants DI21-0072 and DIM23-0014. The author C. Vergara would like to thank ANID for the scholarship support, No. 22220168.

Data Availability Statement: Data are contained within the article.

Conflicts of Interest: The authors declare that this study received funding from ANID by FONDECYT Regular grant 1221000. The funder was not involved in the study design, collection, analysis, interpretation of data, the writing of this article or the decision to submit it for publication.

References

1. Penninckx, S.; Heuskin, A.-C.; Michiels, C.; Lucas, S. Gold Nanoparticles as a Potent Radiosensitizer: A Transdisciplinary Approach from Physics to Patient. *Cancers* **2020**, *12*, 2021. [CrossRef] [PubMed]
2. Siddique, S.; Chow, J.C.L. Application of Nanomaterials in Biomedical Imaging and Cancer Therapy. *Nanomaterials* **2020**, *10*, 1700. [CrossRef] [PubMed]
3. Kakade, N.R.; Kumar, R.; Sharma, S.D.; Datta, D. Equivalence of silver and gold nanoparticles for dose enhancement in nanoparticle-aided brachytherapy. *Biomed. Phys. Eng. Express* **2019**, *5*, 055015. [CrossRef]
4. Santibáñez, M.; Saavedra, R.; Vedelago, J.; Malano, F.; Valente, M. Optimized EDXRF system for simultaneous detection of gold and silver nanoparticles in tumor phantom. *Rad. Phys. Chem.* **2019**, *165*, 108415. [CrossRef]
5. Rasouli, F.S.; Masoudi, S.F. Monte Carlo investigation of the effect of gold nanoparticles' distribution on cellular dose enhancement. *Rad. Phys. Chem.* **2019**, *158*, 6–12. [CrossRef]
6. Hainfeld, J.F.; Smilowitz, H.M.; O'Connor, M.J.; Dilmanian, F.A.; Slatkin, D.N. Gold nanoparticle imaging and radiotherapy of brain tumors in mice. *Nanomedicine* **2013**, *8*, 1601–1609. [CrossRef]
7. Ngwa, W.; Kumar, R.; Sridhar, S.; Korideck, H.; Zygmanski, P.; Cormack, R.A.; Berbeco, R.; Makrigiorgos, G.M. Targeted radiotherapy with gold nanoparticles: Current status and future perspectives. *Nanomedicine* **2014**, *9*, 1063–1082. [CrossRef]
8. Shahhoseini, E.; Ramachandran, P.; Patterson, W.R.; Geso, M. Determination of dose enhancement caused by AuNPs with Xoft® Axxent® Electronic (eBx™) and conventional brachytherapy: In vitro study. *Int. J. Nanomed.* **2018**, *13*, 5733–5741. [CrossRef]
9. Mesbahi, A.; Rajabpour, S.; Smilowitz, H.M.; Hainfeld, J.F. Accelerated brachytherapy with the Xoft electronic source used in association with iodine, gold, bismuth, gadolinium, and hafnium nano-radioenhancers. *Brachytherapy* **2022**, *21*, 968–978. [CrossRef]
10. Cifter, G.; Chin, J.; Cifter, F.; Altundal, Y.; Sinha, N.; Sajo, E.; Ngwa, W. Targeted radiotherapy enhancement during electronic brachytherapy of accelerated partial breast irradiation (APBI) using controlled release of gold nanoparticles. *Phys. Med.* **2015**, *31*, 1070–1074. [CrossRef]
11. Alyani Nezhad, Z.; Geraily, G.; Hataminia, F.; Parwaie, W.; Ghanbari, H.; Gholami, S. Bismuth oxide nanoparticles as agents of radiation dose enhancement in intraoperative radiotherapy. *Med. Phys.* **2021**, *48*, 1417–1426. [CrossRef] [PubMed]
12. Baghani, H.R.; Nasrollahi, S. Efficacy of various nanoparticle types in dose enhancement during low energy X-ray IORT: A Monte Carlo simulation study. *Rad. Phys. Chem.* **2021**, *183*, 109432. [CrossRef]
13. Moradi, F.; Sani, S.A.; Khandaker, M.U.; Sulieman, A.; Bradley, D.A. Dosimetric evaluation of gold nanoparticle aided intraoperative radiotherapy with the Intrabeam system using Monte Carlo simulations. *Rad. Phys. Chem.* **2021**, *178*, 108864. [CrossRef]
14. Abd Rahman, W.N.W. Gold Nanoparticles: Novel Radiobiological Dose Enhancement Studies for Radiation Therapy, Synchrotron Based Microbeam and Stereotactic Radiotherapy. Ph.D. Thesis, RMIT University, Melbourne, VIC, Australia, 2010.

15. Kim, S.R.; Kim, E.H. Gold nanoparticles as dose-enhancement agent for kilovoltage X-ray therapy of melanoma. *Int. J. Radiat. Biol.* **2017**, *93*, 517–526. [CrossRef]
16. Garcia-Martinez, T.; Chan, J.P.; Perez-Calatayud, J.; Ballester, F. Dosimetric characteristics of a new unit for electronic skin brachytherapy. *J. Contemp. Brachyther.* **2014**, *6*, 45–53. [CrossRef] [PubMed]
17. Dickler, A.; Dowlatshahi, K. Xoft Axxent electronic brachytherapy™. *Expert Rev. Med. Devices* **2009**, *6*, 27–31. [CrossRef] [PubMed]
18. Bromma, K.; Rieck, K.; Kulkarni, J.; O'Sullivan, C.; Sung, W.; Cullis, P.; Schuemann, J.; Chithrani, D.B. Use of a lipid nanoparticle system as a Trojan horse in delivery of gold nanoparticles to human breast cancer cells for improved outcomes in radiation therapy. *Cancer Nanotechnol.* **2019**, *10*, 1–17. [CrossRef]
19. Yang, C.; Bromma, K.; Di Ciano-Oliveira, C.; Zafarana, G.; Van Prooijen, M.; Chithrani, D.B. Gold nanoparticle mediated combined cancer therapy. *Cancer Nanotechnol.* **2018**, *9*, 1–14. [CrossRef]
20. Albertini, B.; Mathieu, V.; Iraci, N.; Van Woensel, M.; Schoubben, A.; Donnadio, A.; Greco, S.M.; Ricci, M.; Temperini, A.; Wauthoz, N.; et al. Tumor targeting by peptide-decorated gold nanoparticles. *Mol. Pharm.* **2019**, *16*, 2430–2444. [CrossRef]
21. Chen, G.; Xie, Y.; Peltier, R.; Lei H.; Wang, P.; Chen, J.; Hu, Y.; Wang, F.; Yao, X.; Sun, H. Peptide-decorated gold nanoparticles as functional nano-capping agent of mesoporous silica container for targeting drug delivery. *ACS Appl. Mater. Interfaces* **2016**, *8*, 11204–11209. [CrossRef]
22. Grüner, F.; Blumendorf, F.; Schmutzler, O.; Staufer, T.; Bradbury, M.; Wiesner, U.; Rosentreter, T.; Loers, G.; Lutz, D.; Hoeschen, C.; et al. Localising functionalised gold-nanoparticles in murine spinal cords by X-ray fluorescence imaging and background-reduction through spatial filtering for human-sized objects. *Sci. Rep.* **2019**, *8*, 16561. [CrossRef] [PubMed]
23. Liu, J.; Peng, Q. Protein-gold nanoparticle interactions and their possible impact on biomedical applications. *Acta Biomater.* **2017**, *55*, 13–27. [CrossRef] [PubMed]
24. Wangoo, N.; Bhasin, K.K.; Mehta, S.K.; Suri, C.R. Synthesis and capping of water-dispersed gold nanoparticles by an amino acid: Bioconjugation and binding studies. *J. Colloid Interface Sci.* **2008**, *323*, 247–254. [CrossRef] [PubMed]
25. Reuveni, T.; Motiei, M.; Romman, Z.; Popovtzer, A.; Popovtzer, R. Targeted gold nanoparticles enable molecular CT imaging of cancer: An in vivo study. *Int. J. Nanomed.* **2011**, *6*, 2859–2864.
26. Hainfeld, J.F.; O'Connor, M.J.; Dilmanian, F.A.; Slatkin, D.N.; Adams, D.J.; Smilowitz, H.M. Micro-CT enables microlocalisation and quantification of Her2-targeted gold nanoparticles within tumour regions. *Br. J. Radiol.* **2011**, *84*, 526–533. [CrossRef]
27. Ahn, S.; Jung, S.Y.; Lee, S.J. Gold Nanoparticle Contrast Agents in Advanced X-ray Imaging Technologies. *Molecules* **2013**, *18*, 5858–5890. [CrossRef] [PubMed]
28. Hainfeld, J.F.; Slatkin, D.N.; Focella, T.M.; Smilowitz, H.M. Gold nanoparticles: A new X-ray contrast agent. *Br. J. Radiol.* **2006**, *79*, 248–253. [CrossRef]
29. Delorme, R.; Taupin, F.; Flaender, M.; Ravanat, J.L.; Champion, C.; Agelou, M.; Elleaume, H. Comparison of gadolinium nanoparticles and molecular contrast agents for radiation therapy-enhancement. *Med. Phys.* **2017**, *44*, 5949–5960. [CrossRef]
30. Miladi, I.; Aloy, M.T.; Armandy, E.; Mowat, P.; Kryza, D.; Magné, N.; Tillement, O.; Lux, F.; Billotey, C.; Janier, M.; et al. Combining ultrasmall gadolinium-based nanoparticles with photon irradiation overcomes radioresistance of head and neck squamous cell carcinoma. *Nanomed. Nanotechnol. Biol. Med.* **2015**, *11*, 247–257. [CrossRef]
31. Prezado, Y.; Fois, G.; Le Duc, G.; Bravin, A. Gadolinium dose enhancement studies in microbeam radiation therapy. *Med. Phys.* **2009**, *36*, 3568–3574. [CrossRef]
32. Zhang, D.G.; Feygelman, V.; Moros, E.G.; Latifi, K.; Zhang, G.G. Monte Carlo study of radiation dose enhancement by gadolinium in megavoltage and high dose rate radiotherapy. *PLoS ONE* **2014**, *9*, e109389. [CrossRef]
33. Verry, C.; Dufort, S.; Barbier, E.L.; Montigon, O.; Peoc'h, M.; Chartier, P.; Lux, F.; Balosso, J.; Tillement, O.; Sancey, L.; et al. MRI-guided clinical 6-MV radiosensitization of glioma using a unique gadolinium-based nanoparticles injection. *Nanomedicine* **2016**, *11*, 2405–2417. [CrossRef] [PubMed]
34. Bort, G.; Lux, F.; Dufort, S.; Crémillieux, Y.; Verry, C.; Tillement, O. EPR-mediated tumor targeting using ultrasmall-hybrid nanoparticles: From animal to human with theranostic AGuIX nanoparticles. *Theranostics* **2020**, *10*, 319–1331. [CrossRef] [PubMed]
35. Berger, M.J. XCOM: Photon cross sections database. *NIST* **1998**, *8*, 3587. Available online: https://physics.nist.gov/PhysRefData/Xcom/html/xcom1.html (accessed on 18 July 2023).
36. Rahman, W.N.; Corde, S.; Yagi, N.; Abdul Aziz, S.A.; Annabell, N.; Geso, M. Optimal energy for cell radiosensitivity enhancement by gold nanoparticles using synchrotron-based monoenergetic photon beams. *Int. J. Nanomed.* **2014**, *19*, 22459–22467. [CrossRef] [PubMed]
37. Zygmanski, P.; Liu, B.; Tsiamas, P.; Cifter, F.; Petersheim, M.; Hesser, J.; Sajo, E. A stochastic model of cell survival for high-Z nanoparticle radiotherapy. *Phys. Med. Biol.* **2013**, *58*, 7961–7977. [CrossRef] [PubMed]
38. Spiga, J.; Pellicioli, P.; Manger, S.P.; Duffy, J.A.; Bravin, A. Experimental benchmarking of Monte Carlo simulations for radiotherapy dosimetry using monochromatic X-ray beams in the presence of metal-based compounds. *Phys. Med.* **2019**, *66*, 45–54. [CrossRef] [PubMed]
39. Sisin, N.N.T.; Rashid, R.A.; Abdullah, R.; Razak, K.A.; Geso, M.; Akasaka, H.; Sasaki, R.; Tominaga, T.; Miura, H.; Nishi, M.; et al. Gafchromic™ EBT3 Film Measurements of Dose Enhancement Effects by Metallic Nanoparticles for 192Ir Brachytherapy, Proton, Photon and Electron Radiotherapy. *Radiation* **2022**, *2*, 130–148. [CrossRef]
40. Santibáñez, M.; Fuentealba, M. Experimental determination of Gd dose enhancement and Gd dose sparing by ^{192}Ir brachytherapy source with Gafchromic EBT3 dosimeter. *Appl. Radiat. Isot.* **2021**, *175*, 5109787. [CrossRef]

41. Santibáñez, M.; Fuentealba, M.; Torres, F.; Vargas, A. Experimental determination of the gadolinium dose enhancement in phantom irradiated with low energy X-ray sources by a spectrophotometer-Gafchromic-EBT3 dosimetry system. *Appl. Radiat. Isot.* **2019**, *154*, 108857. [CrossRef]
42. Cho, J.; Gonzalez-Lepera, C.; Manohar, N.; Kerr, M.; Krishnan, S.; Cho, S.H. Quantitative investigation of physical factors contributing to gold nanoparticle-mediated proton dose enhancement. *Phys. Med. Biol.* **2016**, *61*, 562–2581. [CrossRef] [PubMed]
43. Ahmad, R.; Royle, G.; Lourenço, A.; Schwarz, M.; Fracchiolla, F.; Ricketts, K. Investigation into the effects of high-Z nano materials in proton therapy. *Phys. Med. Biol.* **2016**, *61*, 4537–4550. [CrossRef] [PubMed]
44. Ng, C.Y.P.; Chun, S.L.; Yu, K.N. Quality assurance of alpha-particle dosimetry using peeled-off Gafchromic EBT3® film. *Rad. Phys. Chem.* **2016**, *125*, 176–179. [CrossRef]
45. Kakade, N.R.; Das, A.; Kumar, R.; Sharma, S.D.; Chadha, R.; Maiti, N.; Kapoor, S. Application of unlaminated EBT3 film dosimeter for quantification of dose enhancement using silver nanoparticle-embedded alginate film. *Biomed. Phys. Eng. Express* **2022**, *8*, 035014. [CrossRef]
46. Yuri, Y.; Narumi, K.; Yuyama, T. Characterization of a Gafchromic film for the two-dimensional profile measurement of low-energy heavy-ion beams. *Nucl. Instrum. Methods Phys. Res. Sect. A Accel. Spectrometers Detect. Assoc. Equip.* **2016**, *828*, 515–521. [CrossRef]
47. Fuentealba, M.; Santibañez, M.; Bodineau, C. Gadolinium dose enhancement determination by unlaminated EBT3 films irradiated with ^{192}Ir brachytherapy source. *Rad. Phys. Chem.* **2023**, *212*, 111103. [CrossRef]
48. Ma, C.M.; Coffey, C.W.; DeWerd, L.A.; Liu, C.; Nath, R.; Seltzer, S.M.; Seuntjens, J.P. AAPM protocol for 40–300 kV X-ray beam dosimetry in radiotherapy and radiobiology. *Med. Phys.* **2001**, *28*, 868–893. [CrossRef]
49. Williams, M.; Metcalfe, P. Radiochromic film dosimetry and its applications in radiotherapy. In Proceedings of the AIP Conference, Wollongong, Australia, 15–18 September 2010; Volume 1345, pp. 75–99.
50. Das, I.J. 3. Physics and characteristic of radiochromic films: 3.6 Dose response. In *Radiochromic Film: Role and Applications in Radiation Dosimetry*; Das, I.J., Ed.; CRC Press: Boca Raton, FL, USA, 2017; pp. 41–44.

Disclaimer/Publisher's Note: The statements, opinions and data contained in all publications are solely those of the individual author(s) and contributor(s) and not of MDPI and/or the editor(s). MDPI and/or the editor(s) disclaim responsibility for any injury to people or property resulting from any ideas, methods, instructions or products referred to in the content.

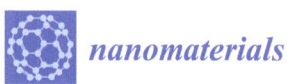

Article

MRI Detection and Therapeutic Enhancement of Ferumoxytol Internalization in Glioblastoma Cells

Michael S. Petronek [1,*], Nahom Teferi [2], Chu-Yu Lee [3], Vincent A. Magnotta [3] and Bryan G. Allen [1,*]

1. Department of Radiation Oncology, University of Iowa, Iowa City, IA 52242, USA
2. Department of Neurosurgery, University of Iowa, Iowa City, IA 52242, USA; nahom-teferi@uiowa.edu
3. Department of Radiology, University of Iowa, Iowa City, IA 52242, USA; vincent-magnotta@uiowa.edu (V.A.M.)
* Correspondence: michael-petronek@uiowa.edu (M.S.P.); bryan-allen@uiowa.edu (B.G.A.); Tel.: +1-319-356-8019 (M.S.P. & B.G.A.); Fax: +1-319-335-8039 (M.S.P. & B.G.A.)

Abstract: Recently, the FDA-approved iron oxide nanoparticle, ferumoxytol, has been found to enhance the efficacy of pharmacological ascorbate ($AscH^-$) in treating glioblastoma, as $AscH^-$ reduces the Fe^{3+} sites in the nanoparticle core. Given the iron oxidation state specificity of T_2* relaxation mapping, this study aims to investigate the ability of T_2* relaxation to monitor the reduction of ferumoxytol by $AscH^-$ with respect to its in vitro therapeutic enhancement. This study employed an in vitro glioblastoma MRI model system to investigate the chemical interaction of ferumoxytol with T_2* mapping. Lipofectamine was utilized to facilitate ferumoxytol internalization and assess intracellular versus extracellular chemistry. In vitro T_2* mapping successfully detected an $AscH^-$-mediated reduction of ferumoxytol (25.6 ms versus 2.8 ms for FMX alone). The T_2* relaxation technique identified the release of Fe^{2+} from ferumoxytol by $AscH^-$ in glioblastoma cells. However, the high iron content of ferumoxytol limited T_2* ability to differentiate between the external and internal reduction of ferumoxytol by $AscH^-$ (ΔT_2* = +839% for external FMX and +1112% for internal FMX reduction). Notably, the internalization of ferumoxytol significantly enhances its ability to promote $AscH^-$ toxicity (dose enhancement ratio for extracellular FMX = 1.16 versus 1.54 for intracellular FMX). These data provide valuable insights into the MR-based nanotheranostic application of ferumoxytol and $AscH^-$ therapy for glioblastoma management. Future developmental efforts, such as FMX surface modifications, may be warranted to enhance this approach further.

Keywords: ferumoxytol; glioblastoma therapy; glioblastoma imaging; pha

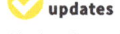

Citation: Petronek, M.S.; Teferi, N.; Lee, C.-Y.; Magnotta, V.A.; Allen, B.G. MRI Detection and Therapeutic Enhancement of Ferumoxytol Internalization in Glioblastoma Cells. *Nanomaterials* 2024, 14, 189. https://doi.org/10.3390/nano14020189

Academic Editor: James Chow

Received: 23 December 2023
Revised: 11 January 2024
Accepted: 12 January 2024
Published: 13 January 2024

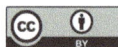

Copyright: © 2024 by the authors. Licensee MDPI, Basel, Switzerland. This article is an open access article distributed under the terms and conditions of the Creative Commons Attribution (CC BY) license (https://creativecommons.org/licenses/by/4.0/).

1. Introduction

Ferumoxytol (Feraheme®, FMX) is a clinically available, superparamagnetic iron oxide nanoparticle approved for treating iron deficiency anemia in patients with chronic kidney disease [1–4]. FMX can generate T1-contrast enhancement in tumor tissue in glioma imaging due to its ferromagnetic properties. FMX is a superparamagnetic iron oxide nanoparticle (SPION) with a Fe_3O_4 core that is about 30 nm in size, has a neutral charge, and resides within a carboxylated polymer coating [5]. Many units of the Fe_3O_4 core exist in one nanoparticle yielding a wide range of molecular weights with an average of about 730 kDa [6]. Because of the large iron content of one molecule of FMX (1 molecule has ≈ 5900 iron atoms or 1 nM FMX ≈ 5.9 μM iron), it can function as a T_1/T_2* MRI contrast agent [7,8]. Ferumoxytol's iron content and ferromagnetic properties also allow its use as a T_2*-contrast agent because T_2* relaxation times are largely influenced by paramagnetic and ferromagnetic materials (e.g., iron). FMX's superparamagnetic properties alter T_2* relaxation times [9,10]. FMX is an attractive MR contrast agent because it has a significantly longer intravascular half-life ($t_{1/2} \approx$ 14–21 h) than gadolinium-based compounds ($t_{1/2} \approx$ 1 h) [7,11].

Beyond its utility as an MRI contrast agent, FMX has shown potential as an anti-cancer therapy [12,13]. The anti-cancer mechanism of FMX has been suggested to be due to its redox activity. It has previously been shown that the Fe_3O_4 core can be oxidized by ionizing radiation, showing that FMX can serve as a reserve of redox-active iron [14]. FMX also reacts with H_2O_2 stimulating the release of iron from the nanoparticle. Thus, FMX may undergo redox reactions with a wide array of species. Ascorbate ($AscH^-$) is a one-electron reductant that can readily reduce some complexes of ferric (Fe^{3+}) to ferrous (Fe^{2+}) iron [15]. $AscH^-$ can reduce and release Fe^{2+} from ferritin, a Fe^{3+}-containing biological macromolecule that is the primary mechanism for intracellular iron storage [16–18]. Recently, it has been reported that $AscH^-$ catalyzes the decomposition of the FMX Fe_3O_4 core [19]. The chemical interaction between FMX and $AscH^-$ can be characterized by a significant reduction in FMX size (≈66% reduction in 24 h), a release of redox-active Fe^{2+} that follows Michaelis–Menton kinetics, and a significant increase in H_2O_2 generation. The decomposition of FMX by $AscH^-$ was reported to enhance glioblastoma cell killing and importantly, the enhanced toxicity of FMX and $AscH^-$ was glioblastoma specific, as no significant in vitro toxicity was observed in normal human astrocytes [19]. Thus, the chemical pairing of FMX and $AscH^-$ represents a novel therapeutic strategy. However, the utility of FMX as an MRI contrast agent suggests that FMX and $AscH^-$ may have nanotheranostic potential.

T_2^* relaxation mapping is a quantitative MRI technique used primarily to indicate total iron content [20]. This technique is widely applicable clinically for cardiac and hepatic iron overload [21–26]. Recent studies have shown that beyond total iron content, T_2^* can provide information on the oxidation state of iron, specificity differentiating between Fe^{3+} and Fe^{2+} [27,28]. This effect is theorized to result from proton– electron dipole–dipole interactions associated with the number of unpaired electrons (i.e., electron spin magnetic moment) of transition metals [29]. Moreover, a recent phase 2 clinical trial testing $AscH^-$ therapy in combination with radiation and temozolomide showed that patients with short T_2^* relaxation times (i.e., high iron content) had significantly greater therapy responses [30]. Because T_2^* relaxation appears to be largely dependent on the paramagnetic properties of metals and can detect alterations in these electronic spin properties (e.g., reduction/oxidation of iron), T_2^* mapping may serve as a useful tool in the evaluation of FMX redox chemistry. Therefore, changes in T_2^* relaxation may be reflective of the disruption of the FMX Fe_3O_4 core by $AscH^-$. This study aims to provide detailed proof-of-concept insights into the ability of T_2^* mapping to evaluate Fe_3O_4 disruptions by $AscH^-$ with respect to the in vitro toxicity of extracellular and intracellular FMX.

2. Materials and Methods

2.1. Cell Culture

Commercially available and validated U87, U251, and U118 glioblastoma cells were cultured in DMEM-F12 media (15% FBS, 1% penicillin-strep, 1% Na-pyruvate, 1.5% HEPES, 0.1% insulin, and 0.02% fibroblast growth factor) and grown to 70–80% confluence at 21% O_2 before experimentation. Cells were treated for 1 h with $AscH^-$ (20 pmol cell^{-1}; ≈8–10 mM), diluted from a 1 M stock of $AscH^-$ in H_2O with pH = 7, in complete cell culture media without FBS or Na-pyruvate to prevent scavenging of H_2O_2. Cells were treated with 100 µM deferoxamine mesylate salt (DFO; Sigma, St. Louis, MO, USA; D9533) from a 110 mM stock in H_2O. FMX was used from the commercially available Feraheme® (30 mg mL^{-1} stock in saline).

2.2. In Vitro MRI Studies

Glioblastoma cells were treated with 20 pmol cell^{-1} $AscH^-$ for 1 h with 20 µg mL^{-1} FMX or pre-incubated for 24 h with 20 µg mL^{-1} FMX-L prior to the 1 h $AscH^{-1}$ treatment. Following treatment, cells were trypsinized, re-suspended in sterile PBS, and transferred to PCR wells embedded in a 1% agarose gel phantom. Cells were allowed to collect at the bottom of the PCR well to form a pellet to be imaged. Cell pellets were then imaged on a 7T GE MR901 small animal scanner, a part of the small animal imaging core at the

University of Iowa. T_2^* weighted images were collected using a gradient-echo sequence (TR = 10 ms, TE = 2.2, 8.2, 14.2, and 20.2 ms, matrix = 256 × 256, FOV = 25 × 20 mm, 2 signal averages). A B_0 shimming routine was performed to limit the effect of macroscopic field inhomogeneities. T_2^* maps were generated using a combination of 4 echo times collected and fitting each voxel to a mono-exponential curve using in-house Python code. Images were imported to 3D Slicer software (V5.0.3) where regions of interest (ROIs) were delineated as a 1 mm diameter cylinder in the center of the tube and mean T_2^* values were calculated using the label statistics tool within 3D Slicer [31].

2.3. FMX Internalization with Lipofectamine

Lipofectamine FMX (FMX-L) was generated using the commercially available lipofectamine 3000 reagents (Thermofisher Scientific, Waltham, MA, USA; L3000015). Functionalization was completed by diluting FMX at 1:16 in 1% FBS containing DMEM-F12 media (1 mL) with 10 μL P3000 reagent, vortexing vigorously for 5 s, and then diluting the FMX/P3000 stock at 1:1 with lipofectamine 3000. The samples were incubated at room temperature for 15 min prior to utilization. FMX-L was generated new for every experiment. The cells were then treated with FMX-L for 24 h in 1% FBS containing DMEM-F12 medium. The cells were washed with 1X D-PBS prior to additional studies to remove extracellular FMX.

2.4. Quantitation of Intracellular Iron

Intracellular iron concentrations were validated colorimetrically following a 24 h treatment with either 20 μg mL^{-1} FMX or FMX-L using a ferrozine-based assay [32,33]. Following treatment, cells were washed with sterile PBS, trypsinized, and centrifuged at 1200 rpm for 5 min. The cell pellets were resuspended in 1X RIPA buffer (Sigma-Aldrich, St. Louis, MO, USA; R0278) and sonicated 3 × 10 s to lyse the cells. Cell lysis solution was then diluted 1:1 in 2.5 M glacial acetic acid pH = 4.5 with 5 mM ferrozine and 10 mM AscH$^-$. The sample and buffer mixture were centrifuged at maximum speed (14,000× g) for 10 min to remove protein aggregates. The supernatant (200 μL) was placed in a 96-well dish [33]. Ultraviolet-visible light (UV-Vis) spectroscopic measurements were performed using a 96-well plate reader. Fe^{2+} (ferrozine)$_3$ complex formation was monitored by analyzing absorbance at 562 nm. Fe^{2+} concentrations were determined using Beer's Law for absorbance at 562 nm (ε_{562} = 27,900 M^{-1} cm^{-1}) with a path length, of L = 0.55 cm (200 μL sample).

2.5. Cellular Iron Staining

To visualize the iron deposition following FMX treatment, cells were stained using a Prussian Blue technique using an iron staining kit (Abcam, Cambridge, U.K.; ab150674) using the manufacturer's protocol. Following treatment, cells were washed with 1X D-PBS and fixed with formalin for 5 min. The cells were then washed with distilled H$_2$O and incubated for 15 min with a 1:1 mixture of potassium ferrocyanide and 2% hydrochloric acid. After staining, cells were washed with distilled H$_2$O and stained for 5 min with a nuclear-fast red counterstain. Finally, cells were washed with distilled H$_2$O and allowed to dry. The cells were then imaged using a phase contrast microscope with a 40× objective lens.

2.6. Electron Paramagnetic Resonance Evaluation of FMX Concentrations in Cell Culture Media

The FMX concentrations were determined by measuring the peak-to-peak signal intensity of the EPR spectrum of the low-spin Fe$_3$O$_4$ complex at $g \approx 2$ as previously described [14]. Using a Bruker EMX spectrometer, the following scan parameters were used to collect spectra: center field = 3508.97 G, sweep width = 2000 G, frequency = 9.85 GHz, power attenuation = 18 dB, modulation frequency = 100 kHz, modulation amplitude = 0.7 G, with spectra being generated from a signal average of 2 scans with 2048 resolution. U87 cells were incubated for 24 h with 20 μg mL^{-1} FMX or FMX-L.

3. Results

3.1. In Vitro Oxidation State Specificity of T_2^* Mapping

Before evaluating if T_2^* mapping can detect FMX and AscH$^-$ chemistry, the in vitro oxidation state specificity of T_2^* mapping was tested using a previously established MRI phantom model system [29]. It was observed that AscH$^-$ increased T_2^* relaxation times in U87, U251, and U118 GBM cell lines by 7 ms, 17 ms, and 10 ms, respectively (Figure 1). This is consistent with the previously observed increase in T_2^* relaxation times following a pharmacological ascorbate infusion in GBM subjects [27]. Moreover, the iron chelator deferoxamine (DFO) causes a decrease (U87 = −12 ms, U251 = −6 ms, and U118 = −18 ms) in T_2^* relaxation times indicative of a paramagnetic shift as a result of ferrioxamine (DFO-Fe^{3+}) complex formation. This is consistent with the ability of DFO to bind and maintain Fe in the +3 oxidation state (Fe^{3+}) [34]. Thus, T_2^* mapping can detect iron oxidation state changes associated with the oxidation when complexed by DFO or internally reduced by AscH$^-$.

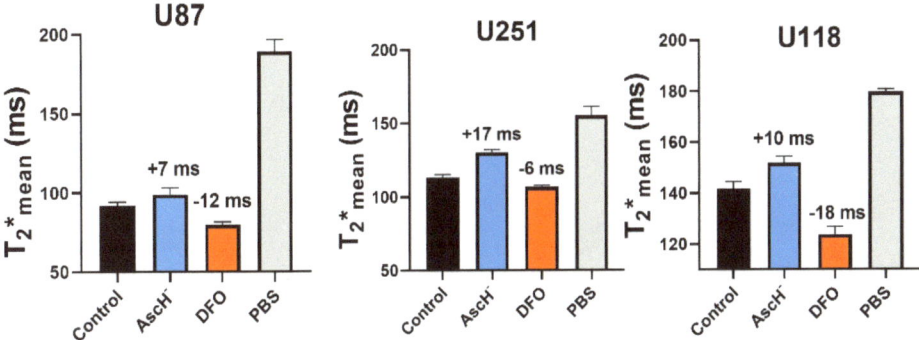

Figure 1. Pharmacological perturbations of intracellular iron can be detected in GBM cells using T_2^* mapping. Quantification of in vitro T_2^* maps of human GBM (U87, U251, U118) cells treated with P-AscH$^-$ (20 pmol cell^{-1}; range: 6–8 mM, 1 h) or DFO (200 µM, 24 h). Phosphate-buffered saline without cells was used as a positive control. Values represent the average magnitude of deflection in T_2^* relaxation from control (n = 3).

3.2. Lipofectamine Enhances FMX Internalization

A potential limitation of this approach is the extracellular nature of FMX [35]. Therefore, a proof-of-concept internalization model using lipofectamine was used to determine if T_2^* mapping can distinguish intracellular and extracellular FMX reduction by AscH$^-$. To validate this model system, U87 cells were incubated with 20 µg mL^{-1} FMX ± lipofectamine (FMX-L) for 24 h. The initial observation made using this approach was that cell pellets following treatment with FMX-L had a reddish hue that would be indicative of high iron content (Figure 2a). Quantitatively, there was a significant decrease in FMX concentrations in the cell culture media, evaluated using EPR spectroscopy (Figure 2b) [14]. This indicates a shift of FMX from the extracellular to the intracellular space. The cell pellets also showed a significant, ≥3-fold, increase in iron concentrations (Figure 2c). This was further validated using Prussian blue staining where intracellular iron was markedly increased following FMX-L treatment (Figure 2d). Interestingly, an increase in Prussian blue positive cells was visible following a 1 h FMX incubation. This effect was not as pronounced by 24 h. This suggests an initial extracellular accumulation of FMX that dissipates over time. Lipofectamine appears to be a valuable tool for facilitating FMX internalization and intracellular retention.

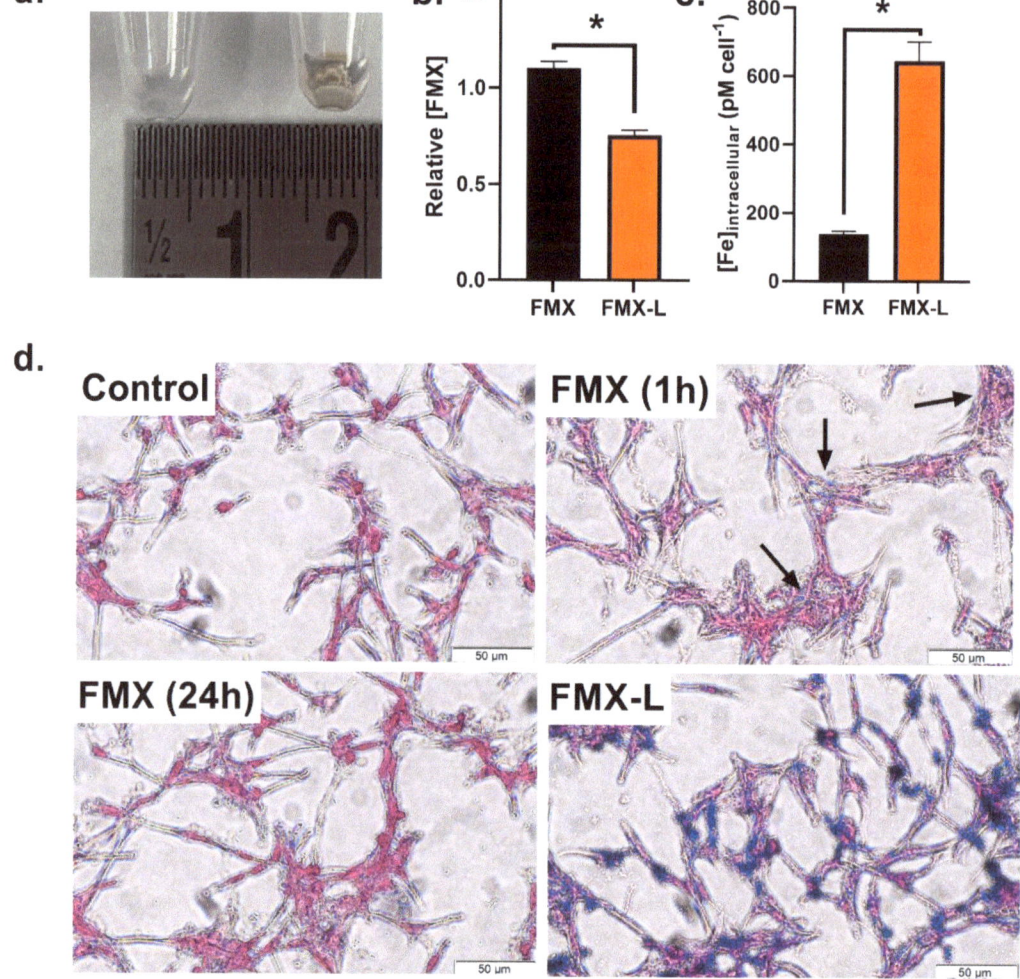

Figure 2. T_2^* **mapping detects FMX internalization and reduction in vitro.** (**a**) Cells were treated for 24 h followed by PBS washing and trypsinization. The large increase in intracellular iron content of FMX-L becomes apparent due to the reddish hue of the cell pellet. (**b**) Relative [FMX] concentrations in cell culture media following 24 h incubation. This was done by evaluating the EPR spectral peak of FMX at t = 0 and t = 24 h and normalizing both FMX and FMX-L peaks to FMX alone. (**c**) Intracellular, chelatable iron content in U87 cells following a 24 h incubation with FMX or FMX-L. Error bars represent mean ± SEM with * $p < 0.05$ using a Welch's *t*-test. (**d**) Representative phase contrast (40×) Prussian blue images for cellular iron content in U87 cells treated with FMX for 1 h and 24 h, or 24 h FMX-L. Black arrows indicate clusters of Prussian blue-positive cells.

3.3. FMX Internalization Enhances AscH⁻ Cytotoxicity

This FMX internalization model system was used to evaluate if changes in T_2^* relaxation times reflect the internal reduction of FMX by AscH⁻. U87 cells were either co-incubated for 1 h with 20 µg mL⁻¹ FMX ± 20 pmol cell⁻¹ AscH⁻ or pre-treated for 24 h FMX-L to load the cells with FMX prior to their 1 h AscH⁻ treatment. Following treatment, cells were pelleted for T_2^* map generation. From this experiment, it has been observed that following a 1 h treatment with FMX or a 24 h treatment with FMX-L caused a noticeable signal loss, likely due to the ferromagnetic properties of FMX (Figure 3a). In both FMX and FMX-L treated cells, there was an observable susceptibility artifact surrounding the cell pellet that was much larger in the FMX-L cells, indicative of the significant increases in intracellular iron content that were previously described. $AscH^-$-treated cells showed longer T_2* relaxation properties; however, this was difficult to qualitatively visualize in the FMX-L treated cells due to the large signal loss. Quantitatively, $AscH^-$ alone induced a 5 ms increase (control = 25.6 ms versus $AscH^-$ = 30.4 ms) in T_2 relaxation time, consistent with previous reports (Figure 3b) [27]. Both FMX and FMX-L cells caused a decrease in T_2* relaxation time to 2.8 and 1.9 ms, respectively. This is consistent with the observed FMX deposition with both treatments. In both cases (FMX and FMX-L), $AscH^-$ treated cells had significantly longer T_2* relaxation times (25.6 and 22.3 ms, respectively). The $T2*$ relaxation time change from baseline was significantly greater in those cells treated with FMX/FMX-L and $AscH^-$ than $AscH^-$ alone (Figure 3c). However, the internalization of FMX only partially increased the change in T_2* by $AscH^-$, suggesting that these doses of FMX for extracellular/intracellular differentiation were likely in the signal saturation range. Overall, these results further support the hypothesis that T_2* relaxation time can detect the reduction of FMX by $AscH^-$, but the high iron content of FMX may limit this effect.

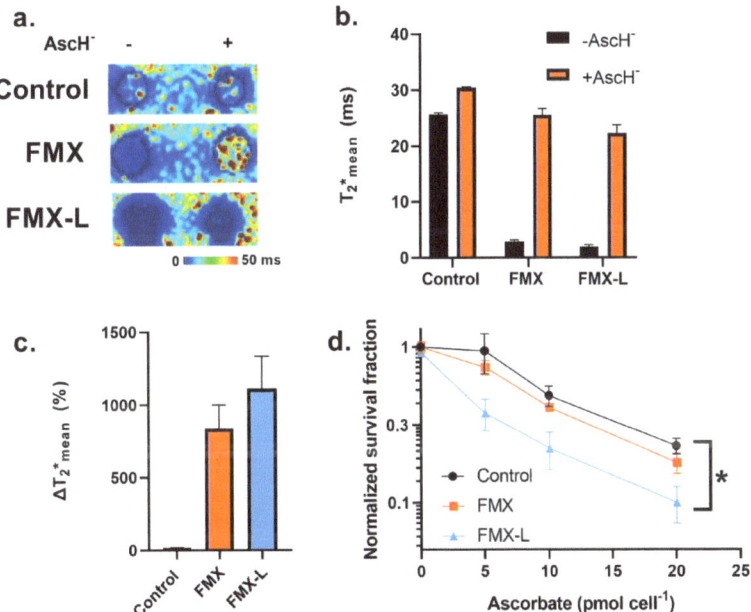

Figure 3. FMX internalization enhances $AscH^-$ cytotoxicity in glioblastoma cells. (**a**) Representative T_2* maps of U87 cell pellets treated with 20 pmol cell^{-1} $AscH^-$ ± standard 1 h co-incubation with 20 μg mL^{-1} FMX or 24 h pre-treatment with 20 μg mL^{-1} FMX-L. (**b**) Mean T_2* relaxation times in U87 cells treated with 20 pmol cell^{-1} $AscH^-$ ± standard 1 h co-incubation with 20 μg mL^{-1} FMX or 24 h pre-treatment with 20 μg mL^{-1} FMX-L. (**c**) Changes in T_2* relaxation time (% difference from untreated control) associated with 20 pmol cell^{-1} $AscH^-$ treatment standard 1 h co-incubation with 20 μg mL^{-1} FMX or 24 h pre-treatment with 20 μg mL^{-1} FMX-L. (**d**) Clonogenic dose–response curves for U87 cells treated with increasing concentrations of $AscH^-$ ± standard 1 h co-incubation with 20 μg mL^{-1} FMX or 24 h pre-treatment with 20 μg mL^{-1} FMX-L. Error bars represent mean ± SEM for three independent experiments with * $p < 0.05$ using a one-way ANOVA test with a post-hoc Tukey's test.

Moreover, it has recently been reported that the combination of FMX and AscH$^-$ exhibited enhanced cytotoxic effects in glioblastoma cells and significantly enhanced the standard of care therapy (radiation and temozolomide) in an in vivo animal model [19]. Thus, the therapeutic aspect of these imaging results was subsequently evaluated in glioblastoma cells. Based on the potential effects of FMX internalization on the ability of T_2^* to detect nanoparticle reduction, the effects on AscH$^-$ toxicity were evaluated. Consistent with these imaging results, FMX-L significantly enhanced the dose-dependent AscH$^-$ toxicity in U87 cells as FMX had a dose-enhancement ratio of 1.16 ($p = 0.09$) as compared to 1.54 for FMX-L ($p < 0.05$; Figure 3d). Thus, it appears that the internalization of FMX represents a novel strategy to enhance its utility in combination with AscH$^-$; however, this may be a context-dependent effect that warrants further consideration.

4. Discussion

This study describes the ability of T_2^* mapping to detect the release of ferrous iron from FMX by AscH$^-$. The primary utilization of FMX in the context of glioblastoma management is as an MR contrast agent [7,36,37]. FMX is also being investigated as a marker for glioblastoma progression [37]. Therefore, T_2^* may also be a valuable tool to identify regions of FMX accumulation. We demonstrate that FMX can decrease T_2^* relaxation times in vitro. This is consistent with previous data showing that FMX can decrease T_2^* relaxation times in humans 24 h following its administration likely owing to its 14–21 h intravascular half-life [7,38]. In this study, suprphysiological concentrations of AscH$^-$ (10 mM), which are typically achieved via intravenous injection during glioblastoma therapy, were used [39,40]. Thus, this chemical combination more closely replicates an interaction that may be observed during glioblastoma therapy. Adding a reducing agent (AscH$^-$) to FMX increases T_2^* relaxation times, which coincides with the release of Fe^{2+} from the nanoparticle core [19]. This is consistent with the iron oxidation state specificity of T_2^* mapping [29]. The oxidation state specificity of T_2^* mapping could be further validated in vitro in this study as AscH$^-$ induces an increase in T_2^* relaxation while DFO causes a decrease. Importantly, this chemistry effect was able to be replicated in the context of AscH$^-$ and FMX chemistry as the addition of AscH$^-$ can prolong FMX relaxation times. This indicates that AscH$^-$ can reduce the Fe^{3+} sites of FMX leading to an increase in the $Fe^{2+}:Fe^{3+}$ ratio, which can be detected with T_2^* mapping. These results are consistent with the increase in T_2^* associated with adding AscH$^-$ to FMX in an orthotopic glioblastoma model [19]. Thus, the present study provides further insights into the ability of T_2^* mapping to detect the catalyzed release of Fe^{2+} from the Fe_3O_4 core by AscH$^-$.

FMX and AscH$^-$ chemistry was detected in both the extracellular and intracellular space with FMX internalization facilitated by lipofectamine. In this cell culture model, adding FMX caused a significant decrease in T_2^* regardless of its localization. The internalization did appear to shorten T2* relaxation times further, consistent with the significant increase in cellular iron content; however, detectable differences were challenging due to potential signal saturation. In both cases, FMX and FMX-L, adding AscH$^-$ significantly increased T_2^* relaxation times. Following the internalization of FMX (FMX-L), the increase in T_2^* relaxation time induced by AscH$^-$ was slightly greater but was ultimately limited by the potential signal saturation caused by FMX. Thus, it is important to note that due to the large size ($\approx$30 nm) and high iron content of FMX, T_2^* relaxation appears to lose the ability to detect intracellular versus extracellular localization [19,41]. Therefore, the use of T_2^* may have an intrinsic technical limitation where the high iron concentrations of FMX limit the range of oxidation state specificity and impair the ability to evaluate FMX reduction by AscH$^-$. This can be overcome by using ultrashort echo time (UTE)-T_2^* and may warrant further investigation [42].

Furthering the nanotheranostic potential of FMX and AscH$^-$, the internalization of FMX significantly enhanced AscH$^-$ toxicity. Thus, the internalization of FMX may significantly enhance the therapeutic utility in combination with AscH$^-$ in GBM. Developmental efforts have been previously put forth to functionalize FMX and enhance tumor trafficking and internalization. For example, it has been shown that FMX functionalized with a Toll-like receptor 3 agonist enhanced melanoma tumor control [43]. Moreover, the trend towards a greater increase in T_2^* relaxation following internalization suggests that FMX reduction by $AscH^-$ is driving the enhanced toxicity. These results are also consistent with previous literature that demonstrates increases in intracellular iron content enhance $AscH^-$ toxicity [44]. This would support the hypothesis that cellular $AscH^-$ uptake by sodium vitamin C transporters (SVCTs) mediate $AscH^-$ toxicity in glioblastoma cells [45]. Therefore, it can be hypothesized that surface modifications of FMX to increase tumor trafficking and internalization can enhance the effectiveness of FMX and $AscH^-$ in the management of GBM and warrant further investigation.

5. Conclusions

In summary, this study provides important insights into the utility of T_2^* mapping as a tool for assessing FMX and $AscH^-$ chemistry in a biologically relevant model system. The large size of FMX can cause T_2^* signal saturation in GBM cells, limiting the ability to detect FMX internalization robustly. However, the oxidation state specificity of T_2^* mapping was partially retained. Moreover, the internalization of FMX significantly enhanced $AscH^-$ toxicity in glioblastoma cells. Thus, FMX internalization strategies (e.g., surface modifications) may warrant further investigation as a therapeutic approach. These data help contextualize the nanotheranostic application of FMX and $AscH^-$ therapy in glioblastoma to be considered in ongoing studies.

Author Contributions: Conception and design: M.S.P., V.A.M. and B.G.A.; Data collection and analysis: M.S.P., N.T. and C.-Y.L.; Data curation: M.S.P. and B.G.A.; Writing and editing: M.S.P., N.T., C.-Y.L., V.A.M. and B.G.A. All authors have read and agreed to the published version of the manuscript.

Funding: This work was supported by NIH grants P01 CA217797, R21CA270742, and the Gateway for Cancer Research grant, G-17-1500. Core facilities were supported in part by the Carver College of Medicine and the Holden Comprehensive Cancer Center, NIH P30 CA086862.

Data Availability Statement: Data is available upon request of the corresponding authors.

Acknowledgments: The content is solely the responsibility of the authors and does not represent the views of the National Institutes of Health.

Conflicts of Interest: The authors declare no conflicts of interest.

References

1. Macdougall, I.C.; Strauss, W.E.; Dahl, N.V.; Bernard, K.; Li, Z. Ferumoxytol for Iron Deficiency Anemia in Patients Undergoing Hemodialysis. The FACT Randomized Controlled Trial. *Clin. Nephrol.* **2019**, *91*, 237–245. [CrossRef] [PubMed]
2. Rosner, M.; Bolton, W. Ferumoxytol for the Treatment of Anemia in Chronic Kidney Disease. *Drugs Today* **2009**, *45*, 779–786. [CrossRef]
3. Rosner, M.H.; Auerbach, M. Ferumoxytol for the Treatment of Iron Deficiency. *Expert. Rev. Hematol.* **2011**, *4*, 399–406. [CrossRef] [PubMed]
4. Auerbach, M.; Chertow, G.M.; Rosner, M. Ferumoxytol for the Treatment of Iron Deficiency Anemia. *Expert Rev. Hematol.* **2018**, *11*, 829–834. [CrossRef]
5. Bullivant, J.P.; Zhao, S.; Willenberg, B.J.; Kozissnik, B.; Batich, C.D.; Dobson, J. Materials Characterization of Feraheme/Ferumoxytol and Preliminary Evaluation of Its Potential for Magnetic Fluid Hyperthermia. *Int. J. Mol. Sci.* **2013**, *14*, 17501–17510. [CrossRef]
6. Balakrishnan, V.S.; Rao, M.; Kausz, A.T.; Brenner, L.; Pereira, B.J.G.; Frigo, T.B.; Lewis, J.M. Physicochemical Properties of Ferumoxytol, a New Intravenous Iron Preparation. *Eur. J. Clin. Investig.* **2009**, *39*, 489–496. [CrossRef]
7. Toth, G.B.; Varallyay, C.G.; Horvath, A.; Bashir, M.R.; Choyke, P.L.; Daldrup-Link, H.E.; Dosa, E.; Finn, J.P.; Gahramanov, S.; Harisinghani, M.; et al. Current and Potential Imaging Applications of Ferumoxytol for Magnetic Resonance Imaging. *Kidney Int.* **2017**, *92*, 47–66. [CrossRef]
8. Manning, P.; Daghighi, S.; Rajaratnam, M.K.; Parthiban, S.; Bahrami, N.; Dale, A.M.; Bolar, D.; Piccioni, D.E.; McDonald, C.R.; Farid, N. Differentiation of Progressive Disease from Pseudoprogression Using 3D PCASL and DSC Perfusion MRI in Patients with Glioblastoma. *J. Neuro-Oncol.* **2020**, *147*, 681–690. [CrossRef]

9. Iv, M.; Samghabadi, P.; Holdsworth, S.; Gentles, A.; Rezaii, P.; Harsh, G.; Li, G.; Thomas, R.; Moseley, M.; Daldrup-Link, H.E.; et al. Quantification of Macrophages in High-Grade Gliomas by Using Ferumoxytol-Enhanced MRI: A Pilot Study. *Radiology* **2019**, *290*, 198–206. [CrossRef]
10. McCullough, B.J.; Kolokythas, O.; Maki, J.H.; Green, D.E. Ferumoxytol in Clinical Practice: Implications for MRI. *J. Magn. Reson. Imaging* **2013**, *37*, 1476–1479. [CrossRef]
11. Weinstein, J.S.; Varallyay, C.G.; Dosa, E.; Gahramanov, S.; Hamilton, B.; Rooney, W.D.; Muldoon, L.L.; Neuwelt, E.A. Superparamagnetic Iron Oxide Nanoparticles: Diagnostic Magnetic Resonance Imaging and Potential Therapeutic Applications in Neurooncology and Central Nervous System Inflammatory Pathologies, a Review. *J. Cereb. Blood Flow. Metab.* **2010**, *30*, 15–35. [CrossRef] [PubMed]
12. Trujillo-Alonso, V.; Pratt, E.C.; Zong, H.; Lara-Martinez, A.; Kaittanis, C.; Rabie, M.O.; Longo, V.; Becker, M.W.; Roboz, G.J.; Grimm, J.; et al. FDA-Approved Ferumoxytol Displays Anti-Leukaemia Efficacy against Cells with Low Ferroportin Levels. *Nat. Nanotechnol.* **2019**, *14*, 616–622. [CrossRef] [PubMed]
13. Zanganeh, S.; Hutter, G.; Spitler, R.; Lenkov, O.; Mahmoudi, M.; Shaw, A.; Pajarinen, J.S.; Nejadnik, H.; Goodman, S.; Moseley, M.; et al. Iron Oxide Nanoparticles Inhibit Tumour Growth by Inducing Pro-Inflammatory Macrophage Polarization in Tumour Tissues. *Nat. Nanotechnol.* **2016**, *11*, 986–994. [CrossRef] [PubMed]
14. Petronek, M.S.; Spitz, D.R.; Buettner, G.R.; Allen, B.G. Oxidation of Ferumoxytol by Ionizing Radiation Releases Iron. An Electron Paramagnetic Resonance Study. *J. Radiat. Res.* **2022**, *63*, 378–384. [CrossRef]
15. Buettner, G.; Anne Jurkiewicz, B. Catalytic Metals, Ascorbate and Free Radicals: Combinations to Avoid. *Radiat. Res.* **1996**, *145*, 532–541. [CrossRef] [PubMed]
16. Badu-Boateng, C.; Naftalin, R.J. Ascorbate and Ferritin Interactions: Consequences for Iron Release in Vitro and in Vivo and Implications for Inflammation. *Free. Radic. Biol. Med.* **2019**, *133*, 75–87. [CrossRef]
17. Badu-Boateng, C.; Pardalaki, S.; Wolf, C.; Lajnef, S.; Peyrot, F.; Naftalin, R.J. Labile Iron Potentiates Ascorbate-Dependent Reduction and Mobilization of Ferritin Iron. *Free. Radic. Biol. Med.* **2017**, *108*, 94–109. [CrossRef]
18. Harrison, P.M.; Arosio, P. The Ferritins: Molecular Properties, Iron Storage Function and Cellular Regulation. *Biochim. Biophys. Acta Bioenerg.* **1996**, *1275*, 161–203. [CrossRef]
19. Petronek, M.S.; Teferi, N.; Caster, J.M.; Stolwijk, J.M.; Zaher, A.; Buatti, J.M.; Hasan, D.; Wafa, E.I.; Salem, A.K.; Gillan, E.G.; et al. Magnetite Nanoparticles as a Kinetically Favorable Source of Iron to Enhance GBM Response to Chemoradiosensitization with Pharmacological Ascorbate. *Redox Biol.* **2023**, *62*, 102651. [CrossRef]
20. Chavhan, G.B.; Babyn, P.S.; Thomas, B.; Shroff, M.M.; Haacke, E.M. Principles, Techniques, and Applications of T_2^*-Based MR Imaging and Its Special Applications. *Radiographics* **2009**, *29*, 1433–1449. [CrossRef]
21. Anderson, L.; Holden, S.; Davis, B.; Prescott, E.; Charrier, C.; Bunce, N.; Firmin, D.; Wonke, B.; Porter, J.; Walker, J.; et al. Cardiovascular T2-Star (T2*) Magnetic Resonance for the Early Diagnosis of Myocardial Iron Overload. *Eur. Heart J. Cardiovasc. Imaging* **2001**, *22*, 2171–2179. [CrossRef] [PubMed]
22. Pepe, A.; Pistoia, L.; Martini, N.; De Marchi, D.; Barison, A.; Maggio, A.; Giovangrossi, P.; Bulgarelli, S.; Pasin, F.M.; Sarli, R.; et al. Detection of Myocardial Iron Overload with Magnetic Resonance By Native T1 and T2* Mapping Using a Segmental Approach. *Blood* **2018**, *132*, 2346. [CrossRef]
23. Henninger, B.; Kremser, C.; Rauch, S.; Eder, R.; Zoller, H.; Finkenstedt, A.; Michaely, H.J.; Schocke, M. Evaluation of MR Imaging with T1 and T2* Mapping for the Determination of Hepatic Iron Overload. *Eur. Radiol.* **2012**, *22*, 2478–2486. [CrossRef]
24. Wood, J.C. Magnetic Resonance Imaging Measurement of Iron Overload. *Curr. Opin. Hematol.* **2007**, *14*, 183–190. [CrossRef]
25. Wood, J.C.; Enriquez, C.; Ghugre, N.; Tyzka, J.M.; Carson, S.; Nelson, M.D.; Coates, T.D. MRI R2 and R2* Mapping Accurately Estimates Hepatic Iron Concentration in Transfusion-Dependent Thalassemia and Sickle Cell Disease Patients. *Blood* **2005**, *106*, 1460–1465. [CrossRef] [PubMed]
26. Ghugre, N.R.; Enriquez, C.M.; Gonzalez, I.; Nelson, M.D., Jr.; Coates, T.D.; Wood, J.C. MRI Detects Myocardial Iron in the Human Heart. *Magn. Reson. Med.* **2006**, *56*, 681–686. [CrossRef] [PubMed]
27. Cushing, C.M.; Petronek, M.S.; Bodeker, K.L.; Vollstedt, S.; Brown, H.A.; Opat, E.; Hollenbeck, N.J.; Shanks, T.; Berg, D.J.; Smith, B.J.; et al. Magnetic Resonance Imaging (MRI) of Pharmacological Ascorbate-Induced Iron Redox State as a Biomarker in Subjects Undergoing Radio-Chemotherapy. *Redox Biol.* **2021**, *38*, 101804. [CrossRef]
28. Birkl, C.; Birkl-Toeglhofer, A.M.; Kames, C.; Goessler, W.; Haybaeck, J.; Fazekas, F.; Ropele, S.; Rauscher, A. The Influence of Iron Oxidation State on Quantitative MRI Parameters in Post Mortem Human Brain. *NeuroImage* **2020**, *220*, 117080. [CrossRef]
29. Petronek, M.S.; St-Aubin, J.J.; Lee, C.Y.; Spitz, D.R.; Gillan, E.G.; Allen, B.G.; Magnotta, V.A. Quantum Chemical Insight into the Effects of the Local Electron Environment on T2*-Based MRI. *Sci. Rep.* **2021**, *11*, 20817. [CrossRef]
30. Petronek, M.S.; Monga, V.; Bodeker, K.L.; Kwofie, M.; Lee, C.-Y.; Mapuskar, K.A.; Stolwijk, J.M.; Zaher, A.; Wagner, B.A.; Smith, M.C.; et al. Magnetic Resonance Imaging of Iron Metabolism with T_2^* Mapping Predicts an Enhanced Clinical Response to Pharmacological Ascorbate in Patients with GBM. *Clin. Cancer Res.* **2023**. [CrossRef]
31. Fedorov, A.; Beichel, R.; Kalpathy-Cramer, J.; Finet, J.; Fillion-Robin, J.-C.; Pujol, S.; Bauer, C.; Jennings, D.; Fennessy, F.; Sonka, M.; et al. 3D Slicer as an Image Computing Platform for the Quantitative Imaging Network. *Magn. Reson. Imaging* **2012**, *30*, 1323–1341. [CrossRef] [PubMed]
32. Stookey, L. Ferrozine-A New Spectrophotometric Reagent for Iron. *Anal. Chem.* **1970**, *42*, 779–781. [CrossRef]

33. Abbasi, U.; Abbina, S.; Gill, A.; Bhagat, V.; Kizhakkedathu, J.N. A Facile Colorimetric Method for the Quantification of Labile Iron Pool and Total Iron in Cells and Tissue Specimens. *Sci. Rep.* **2021**, *11*, 6008. [CrossRef] [PubMed]
34. Kiss, T.; Farkas, E. Metal-Binding Ability of Desferrioxamine B. *J. Incl. Phenom. Mol. Recognit. Chem.* **1998**, *32*, 385–403. [CrossRef]
35. McConnell, H.L.; Schwartz, D.L.; Richardson, B.E.; Woltjer, R.L.; Muldoon, L.L.; Neuwelt, E.A. Ferumoxytol Nanoparticle Uptake in Brain during Acute Neuroinflammation Is Cell-Specific. *Nanomedicine* **2016**, *12*, 1535–1542. [CrossRef]
36. Vasanawala, S.S.; Nguyen, K.-L.; Hope, M.D.; Bridges, M.D.; Hope, T.A.; Reeder, S.B.; Bashir, M.R. Safety and Technique of Ferumoxytol Administration for MRI. *Magn. Reson. Med.* **2016**, *75*, 2107–2111. [CrossRef] [PubMed]
37. Neuwelt, E.A.; Várallyay, C.G.; Manninger, S.; Solymosi, D.; Haluska, M.; Hunt, M.A.; Nesbit, G.; Stevens, A.; Jerosch-Herold, M.; Jacobs, P.M.; et al. The Potential of Ferumoxytol Nanoparticle Magnetic Resonance Imaging, Perfusion, and Angiography in Central Nervous System Malignancy: A Pilot Study. *Neurosurgery* **2007**, *60*, 601–611, discussion 611–612. [CrossRef]
38. Stirrat, C.G.; Alam, S.R.; MacGillivray, T.J.; Gray, C.D.; Forsythe, R.; Dweck, M.R.; Payne, J.R.; Prasad, S.K.; Petrie, M.C.; Gardner, R.S.; et al. Ferumoxytol-Enhanced Magnetic Resonance Imaging Methodology and Normal Values at 1.5 and 3T. *J. Cardiovasc. Magn. Reason.* **2016**, *18*, 46. [CrossRef]
39. Petronek, M.S.; Wagner, B.A.; Hollenbeck, N.J.; Caster, J.M.; Spitz, D.R.; Cullen, J.J.; Buettner, G.R.; Allen, B.G. Assessment of the Stability of Supraphysiological Ascorbate in Human Blood: Appropriate Handling of Samples from Clinical Trials for Measurements of Pharmacological Ascorbate. *Radiat. Res.* **2019**, *191*, 491–496. [CrossRef]
40. Allen, B.G.; Bodeker, K.L.; Smith, M.C.; Monga, V.; Sandhu, S.; Hohl, R.; Carlisle, T.; Brown, H.; Hollenbeck, N.; Vollstedt, S.; et al. First-in-Human Phase I Clinical Trial of Pharmacologic Ascorbate Combined with Radiation and Temozolomide for Newly Diagnosed Glioblastoma. *Clin. Cancer Res.* **2019**, *25*, 6590–6597. [CrossRef]
41. Marashdeh, M.W.; Ababneh, B.; Lemine, O.M.; Alsadig, A.; Omri, K.; El Mir, L.; Sulieman, A.; Mattar, E. The Significant Effect of Size and Concentrations of Iron Oxide Nanoparticles on Magnetic Resonance Imaging Contrast Enhancement. *Results Phys.* **2019**, *15*, 102651. [CrossRef]
42. Hong, W.; He, Q.; Fan, S.; Carl, M.; Shao, H.; Chen, J.; Chang, E.Y.; Du, J. Imaging and Quantification of Iron-Oxide Nanoparticles (IONP) Using MP-RAGE and UTE Based Sequences. *Magn. Reson. Med.* **2017**, *78*, 226–232. [CrossRef] [PubMed]
43. Zhao, J.; Zhang, Z.; Xue, Y.; Wang, G.; Cheng, Y.; Pan, Y.; Zhao, S.; Hou, Y. Anti-Tumor Macrophages Activated by Ferumoxytol Combined or Surface-Functionalized with the TLR3 Agonist Poly (I:C) Promote Melanoma Regression. *Theranostics* **2018**, *8*, 6307–6321. [CrossRef] [PubMed]
44. Brandt, K.E.; Falls, K.C.; Schoenfeld, J.D.; Rodman, S.N.; Gu, Z.; Zhan, F.; Cullen, J.J.; Wagner, B.A.; Buettner, G.R.; Allen, B.G.; et al. Augmentation of Intracellular Iron Using Iron Sucrose Enhances the Toxicity of Pharmacological Ascorbate in Colon Cancer Cells. *Redox Biol.* **2018**, *14*, 82–87. [CrossRef]
45. Burgess, E.R.; Crake, R.L.I.; Phillips, E.; Morrin, H.R.; Royds, J.A.; Slatter, T.L.; Wiggins, G.A.R.; Vissers, M.C.M.; Robinson, B.A.; Dachs, G.U. Increased Ascorbate Content of Glioblastoma Is Associated With a Suppressed Hypoxic Response and Improved Patient Survival. *Front. Oncol.* **2022**, *12*, 829524. [CrossRef]

Disclaimer/Publisher's Note: The statements, opinions and data contained in all publications are solely those of the individual author(s) and contributor(s) and not of MDPI and/or the editor(s). MDPI and/or the editor(s) disclaim responsibility for any injury to people or property resulting from any ideas, methods, instructions or products referred to in the content.

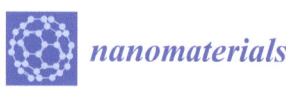

Article

Radiofluorination of an Anionic, Azide-Functionalized Teroligomer by Copper-Catalyzed Azide-Alkyne Cycloaddition

Barbara Wenzel [1,*], Maximilian Schmid [2,3], Rodrigo Teodoro [1], Rareș-Petru Moldovan [1], Thu Hang Lai [1], Franziska Mitrach [2], Klaus Kopka [1,4], Björn Fischer [3], Michaela Schulz-Siegmund [2], Peter Brust [1] and Michael C. Hacker [2,3,*]

[1] Department of Neuroradiopharmaceuticals, Institute of Radiopharmaceutical Cancer Research, Helmholtz-Zentrum Dresden-Rossendorf, 04318 Leipzig, Germany; r.teodoro@life-mi.com (R.T.); r.moldovan@hzdr.de (R.-P.M.); t.lai@hzdr.de (T.H.L.); k.kopka@hzdr.de (K.K.); peterbrustdeu@aol.com (P.B.)
[2] Institute of Pharmacy, Pharmaceutical Technology, Leipzig University, 04317 Leipzig, Germany; maximilian.schmid@uni-leipzig.de (M.S.); franziska.mitrach@uni-leipzig.de (F.M.); schulz@uni-leipzig.de (M.S.-S.)
[3] Institute of Pharmaceutics and Biopharmaceutics, Heinrich Heine University Düsseldorf, 40225 Düsseldorf, Germany; bjoern.fischer@hhu.de
[4] Faculty of Chemistry and Food Chemistry, School of Science, Technical University Dresden, 01069 Dresden, Germany
* Correspondence: b.wenzel@hzdr.de (B.W.); mch@mchlab.de (M.C.H.)

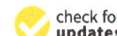

Citation: Wenzel, B.; Schmid, M.; Teodoro, R.; Moldovan, R.-P.; Lai, T.H.; Mitrach, F.; Kopka, K.; Fischer, B.; Schulz-Siegmund, M.; Brust, P.; et al. Radiofluorination of an Anionic, Azide-Functionalized Teroligomer by Copper-Catalyzed Azide-Alkyne Cycloaddition. *Nanomaterials* **2023**, *13*, 2095. https://doi.org/10.3390/nano13142095

Academic Editors: Alexey Pestryakov and Placido Mineo

Received: 16 May 2023
Revised: 6 July 2023
Accepted: 14 July 2023
Published: 18 July 2023

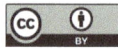

Copyright: © 2023 by the authors. Licensee MDPI, Basel, Switzerland. This article is an open access article distributed under the terms and conditions of the Creative Commons Attribution (CC BY) license (https://creativecommons.org/licenses/by/4.0/).

Abstract: This study describes the synthesis, radiofluorination and purification of an anionic amphiphilic teroligomer developed as a stabilizer for siRNA-loaded calcium phosphate nanoparticles (CaP-NPs). As the stabilizing amphiphile accumulates on nanoparticle surfaces, the fluorine-18-labeled polymer should enable to track the distribution of the CaP-NPs in brain tumors by positron emission tomography after application by convection-enhanced delivery. At first, an unmodified teroligomer was synthesized with a number average molecular weight of 4550 ± 20 Da by free radical polymerization of a defined composition of methoxy-PEG-monomethacrylate, tetradecyl acrylate and maleic anhydride. Subsequent derivatization of anhydrides with azido-TEG-amine provided an azido-functionalized polymer precursor (**o14PEGMA-N$_3$**) for radiofluorination. The ^{18}F-labeling was accomplished through the copper-catalyzed cycloaddition of **o14PEGMA-N$_3$** with diethylene glycol–alkyne-substituted heteroaromatic prosthetic group [^{18}F]2, which was synthesized with a radiochemical yield (RCY) of about 38% within 60 min using a radiosynthesis module. The ^{18}F-labeled polymer [^{18}F]**fluoro-o14PEGMA** was obtained after a short reaction time of 2–3 min by using CuSO$_4$/sodium ascorbate at 90 °C. Purification was performed by solid-phase extraction on an anion-exchange cartridge followed by size-exclusion chromatography to obtain [^{18}F]**fluoro-o14PEGMA** with a high radiochemical purity and an RCY of about 15%.

Keywords: teroligomer; fluorine-18; ^{18}F-polymer; click reaction; CuAAC; PEG-[^{18}F]FPyKYNE

1. Introduction

Amphiphilic polymers and nanomaterials have emerged as promising platforms for cancer therapy due to their unique properties, such as tunable size and shape, high surface-area-to-volume ratio and ability to target tumor cells. Therapeutic effects are associated with the observation that larger molecular systems can passively accumulate in tumors due to the *enhanced permeability and retention* (*EPR*) effect first described by Maeda et al. [1]. Synthetic polymers of the organic type can be effectively controlled in their composition and appearance and offer the advantage of convenient structural modifications. This motivates the intense investigation into polymeric nanosystems for the targeted delivery of drugs or imaging probes [2–7].

The topic of this research collaboration is the development of calcium phosphate nanoparticles (CaP-NPs) stabilized by suitable polymers and loaded with small interfering

RNA (siRNA) in order to investigate their potential for a targeted localized tumor therapy via convection-enhanced delivery (CED). CED is a technique to deliver therapeutics directly to the tumor using one or more stereotactically placed catheters [8]. For the pharmacotherapy of brain tumors this method bears particular advantages, such as bypassing the blood–brain barrier with consequently increasing drug doses at the therapeutic side and less systemic side effects compared to conventional application forms. In a first step, we have recently developed CaP-NPs stabilized with polymeric amphiphiles as a suitable siRNA carrier material [9]. One future intention of this research project is to investigate the distribution of these loaded CaP-NPs after delivery to the desired brain region in rats using positron emission tomography (PET). PET is a non-invasive imaging technique that allows the visualization of the distribution of radioactive substances in vitro and in vivo. The PET radionuclide fluorine-18 was selected for our purpose because of its reasonable half-life (109.7 min) and chemical properties that allow for covalent incorporation in molecules, which often ensures a higher stability of the radiolabel as compared to complexed radiometals. Therefore, the development and synthesis of an ^{18}F-radiolabeled polymer was needed as it fulfilled the requirements with respect to stabilizing as well as imaging of the nanoparticles.

To date, only a few ^{18}F-labeled polymers have been described in the literature. In 2009, Herth et al. [10] reported on the synthesis of *N*-(2-hydroxypropyl)-methylacrylamide (HPMA)-based polymeric structures, which were radiolabeled by coupling the phenolic tyramine functionalities of the polymer with 2-[^{18}F]fluoroethyl-1-tosylate ([^{18}F]FETos). This procedure was used for development and preclinical PET studies of HPMA-based polymeric conjugates [10–12]. In an approach to generate ^{18}F-labeled polyester-based nanoparticles, Di Mauro and co-workers [13] used 4-[^{18}F]fluorobenzyl-2-bromoacetamide ([^{18}F]FBBA) for condensation with a thiol-functionalized polyethylenglycolic ester and subsequently prepared nanoparticles from the radiofluorinated polymer. Highly efficient cycloaddition reactions, so called click reactions, which are well established for ^{18}F-labeling of sensitive biomolecules, have also been used for the generation of radiolabeled polymers by instant conjugation to functionalized polymers. As one example, the copper-catalyzed azide-alkyne cycloaddition (CuAAC) of 1-azido-2-(2-(2-[^{18}F]-fluoroethoxy)ethoxy)ethane to different alkyne-functionalized polymers has been described [14,15]. Moreover, one example for a copper-free strain-promoted azide-alkyne cycloaddition (SPAAC) of [^{18}F]fluoroethylazide with a cyclooctyne-functionalized hydrophilic polymer (ethyl poly(2-ethyl-2-oxazoline)) was published [16].

Copper-catalyzed click reactions are known for their mild conditions, the use of aqueous reaction media and a fast conversion rate. In particular, the latter is of importance for our purpose due to the relatively short half-life of the fluorine-18 radionuclide, which limits the synthesis time. We therefore focused on this reaction type, in which the polymer provides the azide functionalities for coupling with a suitable alkyne bearing and radiolabeled group. Because of its relatively hydrophilic character suitable for the desired reaction conditions, [^{18}F]2-fluoro-3-(2-(2-(prop-2-ynyloxy)ethoxy)ethoxy)pyridine ([^{18}F]2, in the literature is named as PEG-[^{18}F]FPyKYNE) [17,18] was selected as the alkyne-bearing group. The concept of the entire study is illustrated in Scheme 1.

Here, we describe the two-step ^{18}F-radiolabeling procedure and purification of an anionic amphiphilic teroligomer accomplished by the copper-catalyzed cycloaddition of the alkyne-substituted aromatic group [^{18}F]2 to an azide-functionalized amphiphilic oligomer.

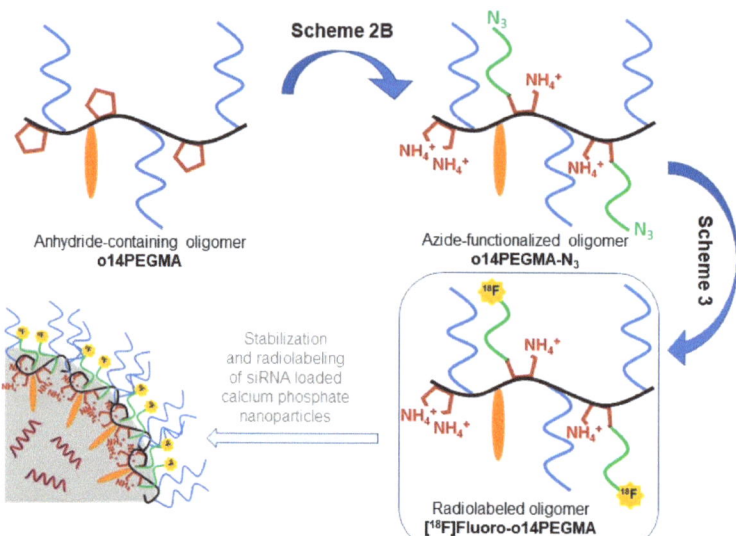

Scheme 1. Schematic illustration of the material concept investigated in this study. An amphiphilic anhydride group-containing oligomer (**o14PEGMA**) is synthesized from tetradecyl acrylate (orange), mPEG-MAc (blue) and maleic anhydride (red) [9]. The anhydride groups are derivatized, and unreacted anhydrides are hydrolyzed, yielding the azide-functionalized (green) teroligomer **o14PEGMA-N$_3$** (see also Scheme 2B). The water-soluble oligomer is then conjugated with a suitable alkyne-bearing and radiolabeled group in a copper-catalyzed azide-alkyne cycloaddition, yielding [^{18}F]fluoro-o14PEGMA (see also Scheme 3). The radiofluorinated oligomer would then be available as a stabilizer for the fabrication of siRNA-loaded CaP-NPs in analogy to our previous study [9].

2. Materials and Methods

2.1. Oligomer Synthesis

2.1.1. Materials

Tetrahydrofuran (THF) and diethyl ether were HPLC-grade and obtained from VWR International GmbH (Darmstadt, Germany). For polymer synthesis, THF was dried by refluxing over potassium and sodium and subsequently distilled. Maleic anhydride (MA) and aniline were purchased from Thermo Fisher Scientific and VWR International GmbH, respectively. Tetradecyl acrylate (TDA) and poly(ethylene glycol) methyl ether methacrylate (methoxy-PEG-monomethacrylate, mPEG-MAc) with an average Mn of 950 were obtained from TCI Deutschland GmbH (Eschborn, Germany) and used as received. 2,2′-Azobis(2-methylpropionitril) (AIBN), 2-(2-(2-(2-azidoethoxy)ethoxy)ethoxy)ethan-1-amine (azido-TEG-amine) and triethylamine (TEA) were from Sigma-Aldrich Chemie GmbH (Taufkirchen, Germany). Acetone was purchased from Carl Roth GmbH + Co. KG (Karlsruhe, Germany), and aqueous ammonia (25% m/V) was obtained from Grüssing GmbH (Filsum, Germany). Deuterated solvents, CDCl$_3$, DMSO-D6, both with tetramethyl silane, and D$_2$O were purchased from ARMAR GmbH (Leipzig, Germany). Float-A-Lyzer® dialysis devices from Repligen Europe B.V. (Dreda, The Netherlands), with a cellulose ester membrane and a molecular weight cut off of 0.1–0.5 kDa were used.

2.1.2. Synthesis of Pristine Teroligomer **o14PEGMA** (1:1:2.5)

The synthesis of the pristine teroligomer oligo(TDA-co-mPEG-MAc-co-MA) (**o14PEGMA**) composed of TDA (14 in oligomer code), mPEG-MAc (PEG in oligomer code) and MA was performed as recently described [9]. In brief, the three comonomers were mixed in a molar ratio of 1:1:2.5 (TDA/mPEG-MAc/MA) in quantities of 4.1 mL (13.3 mmol) of TDA, 11.5 mL

(13.3 mmol) of mPEG-MAc and 3.27 g (33.3 mmol) of MA. The comonomers were dissolved or diluted in an appropriate amount of THF and added to the flask at 60 °C. The final reaction volume was 300 mL (total comonomer concentration: 0.2 mol/L). After addition of 0.2 g of AIBN, the reaction mixture was stirred for 18 h and concentrated by rotary evaporation. The crude product was three times precipitated in diethyl ether, isolated and vacuum dried over several days. The resulting purified o14PEGMA was analyzed by gel permeation chromatography (GPC) and ^{1}H NMR as described before [9]. The amount of incorporated anhydride groups and the chemical intactness were determined before and after hydrolysis using conductometric titration and by a titration method according to Brown and Fujimorij after anhydride aminolysis [19].

2.1.3. Synthesis of Azide-Modified Teroligomer and Isolation as Ammonium Salt (o14PEGMA-N$_3$)

Based on the results of the anhydride quantification by titration and molecular size determination by GPC, the pristine teroligomer **o14PEGMA** was derivatized with azido-TEG-amine in a molar ratio that was set to 25% of intact anhydrides (8.4 µmol). TEA was added in an amount equal to 5% of chemically intact anhydrides. In a typical batch, azido-TEG-amine (0.471 µL, 2.1 µmol) and base (0.060 µL, 427 nmol) were added to 100 mg (22 µmol) of **o14PEGMA** dissolved in acetone and magnetically stirred at room temperature for 4 h. After removal of the volatile components by vacuum drying, the raw product was dissolved in aqueous ammonia (1 M) and maintained at 40 °C for 12 h [20] to hydrolyze any remaining anhydride and to form the ammonium salt **o14PEGMA-N$_3$**. Then, the reaction mixture was concentrated by rotary evaporation and subjected to dialysis against water for 10 h with four changes of the outer phase to obtain purified **o14PEGMA-N$_3$** as a sticky white hygroscopic solid. Proton NMR analysis of the linker modified oligomer **o14PEGMA-N$_3$** was inconclusive, because it was impossible to distinguish between TEG-azide and the mPEG-MAc chains, which are chemically identical, an observation which has already been described in the literature [21].

2.1.4. Fourier Transform Infrared Spectroscopy (FT-IR) and Confocal Raman Spectroscopy

FT-IR and confocal Raman spectroscopy were applied to visualize the amidation of **o14PEGMA** with azido-TEG-amine. FT-IR analysis of samples was performed on a Nicolet iS™ 50-FT-IR with a Smart Performer Sample Unit (Thermo Scientific) equipped with the Omnic Spectra Software 2.2.4.3 provided with the instrument.

Samples of the dry polymer were also investigated using the confocal Raman microscope alpha-300 R (WITec, Ulm, Germany). A single mode laser with a wavelength of 532 nm was applied for excitation. Using a Zeiss EC Epiplan-Neofluar Dic 50x/0.8 microscope objective, the laser power on the samples was set to 20 mW. The Raman microscope was equipped with a WITec UHTS 300 spectrometer and an Andor iDus Deep Depletion CCD camera, which was cooled down to -60 °C. By using a reflection grating with 600 lines/mm, an average spectral resolution of 3.8 cm^{-1}/pixel was achieved. Raman spectra were recorded using an exposure time of 20 s by accumulating 10×2 s. For the data interpretation, WITec FIVE 5.3.18.110 software was used. Samples were randomly measured at three positions, spectra were merged, baseline-corrected and -normalized.

2.2. Radiochemistry

2.2.1. Synthesis of Non-Radioactive Reference and Precursor

The compound 2-fluoro-3-(2-(2-(prop-2-ynyloxy)ethoxy)ethoxy)pyridine **2** and the corresponding trimethyl ammonium trifluoromethanesulfonate precursor **1** were synthesized as reported [17]. The identity of the compounds was controlled by NMR (spectra in Figure S1 in Supplementary Materials).

[3-(2-(Prop-2-ynyloxy)ethoxy)ethoxy)pyridine-2yl] trimethylammonium trifluoromethanesulfonate (**1**): ^{1}H NMR (300 MHz, CDCl$_3$) δ: 7.85 (dd, J = 4.9, 1.5 Hz, 1H), 7.01 (dd, J = 7.8,

1.5 Hz, 1H), 6.71 (dd, J = 7.8, 4.9 Hz, 1H), 4.21 (t, J = 2.2 Hz, 2H), 4.13 (dd, J = 5.6, 4.2 Hz, 2H), 3.89 (dd, J = 5.6, 4.3 Hz, 2H), 3.82–3.55 (m, 4H), 3.00 (s, 9H), 2.42 (t, J = 2.4 Hz, 1H).

2-Fluoro-3-(2-(2-(prop-2-yn-1-yloxy)ethoxy)ethoxy)pyridine (**2**): ^{1}H NMR (400 MHz, CDCl$_3$) δ: 7.75 (dt, J = 4.8, 1.6 Hz, 1H), 7.42–7.28 (m, 1H), 7.10 (ddd, J = 7.9, 4.9, 0.6 Hz, 1H), 4.41–4.12 (m, 4H), 4.01–3.84 (m, 2H), 3.83–3.73 (m, 2H), 3.73–3.57 (m, 2H), 2.44 (t, J = 2.4 Hz, 1H).

2.2.2. Analytics

Radio-thin-layer chromatography (radio-TLC) of the prosthetic group **[^{18}F]2** was performed on plates pre-coated with silica gel (Polygram® SIL G/UV254) and with ethyl acetate/n-hexane (3:1, v/v) as eluent. The plates were exposed to storage phosphor screens (BAS IP MS 2025 E, GE Healthcare Europe GmbH, Freiburg, Germany) and recorded using the Amersham Typhoon RGB Biomolecular Imager (GE Healthcare Life Sciences). Images were quantified using ImageQuant TL8.1 software (GE Healthcare Life Sciences).

Analytical radio-HPLC separations were performed on either (i) a JASCO LC-2000 system, incorporating a PU-2080Plus pump, AS-2055Plus auto injector (100 µL sample loop), and a UV-2070Plus (JASCO Deutschland GmbH, Pfungstadt, Germany) detector coupled with a radioactivity HPLC flow monitor (Gabi Star, raytest Isotopenmessgeräte GmbH, Straubenhardt, Germany) or (ii) a JASCO LC-4000 system, incorporating a PU-4180-LPG pump, AS-4050 auto injector (100 µL sample loop) and a UV-diode array detector MD-4015 coupled with a radio flow monitor (Gabi Nova, Elysia-raytest GmbH, Straubenhardt, Germany). Data analysis was performed either using Galaxy chromatography (Agilent Technologies) or ChromNAV 2.3C (JASCO Deutschland GmbH, Pfungstadt, Germany) software. For **[^{18}F]2**, a Reprosil-Pur C18-AQ column (250 × 4.6 mm; 5 µm; Dr. Maisch HPLC GmbH; Ammerbuch-Entringen, Germany) with ACN/aq. 20 mM NH$_4$OAc (pH 6.8) as eluent mixture and a flow of 1.0 mL/min was used (gradient: eluent A 10% ACN/aq. 20 mM NH$_4$OAc; eluent B 90% ACN/aq. 20 mM NH$_4$OAc; 0–5 min 100% A, 5–25 min up to 100% B, 25–29 min 100% B, 29–30 min up to 100% A, 30–35 min 100% A). For the radiolabeled polymer **[^{18}F]o14PEGMA** the following systems were used: (1) A HiTrap^{TM} Desalting 5 mL column (GE Healthcare Europe GmbH, Freiburg, Germany) with ethanol/aq. 25 mM sodium phosphate buffer (pH 7.0) as eluent mixture and a flow of 1.0 mL/min (either in gradient mode with eluent A of 100% ethanol and eluent B of 100% aq. 25 mM sodium phosphate pH 7; 0–10 min 10% A, 10–11 min up to 25% A, 11–17 min 25% A, 17–18 min up to 10% A, 18–25 min 10% A; or in isocratic mode with 10% A and 90% B) and (2) a Reprosil-Pur C18-AQ column (250 × 4.6 mm; 5 µm; Dr. Maisch HPLC GmbH; Ammerbuch-Entringen, Germany) with ACN/aq. 20 mM NH$_4$OAc (pH 6.8) as eluent mixture and a flow of 1.0 mL/min (gradient: eluent A 10% ACN/aq. 20 mM NH$_4$OAc; eluent B 90% ACN/aq. 20 mM NH$_4$OAc; 0–10 min 100% A, 10–25 min up to 100% B, 25–30 min 100% B, 30–31 min up to 100% A, 31–35 min 100% A).

The ammonium acetate and sodium phosphate concentration, stated as aq. 20 mM NH$_4$OAc and aq. 25 mM sodium phosphate, respectively, corresponds to the concentration in the aqueous component of an eluent mixture.

2.2.3. Radiosynthesis of **[^{18}F]2**

Remotely controlled radiosynthesis of **[^{18}F]2** (formerly named PEG-[^{18}F]PyKYNE) [17] was performed using a TRACERlab FX2 N synthesis module (GE Healthcare, Chicago, IL, USA) equipped with a Laboport vacuum pump N810.3FT.18 (KNF Neuburger GmbH, Freiburg, Germany), a BlueShadow UV detector 10D (KNAUER GmbH, Berlin, Germany) and TRACERlab FX software. No-carrier-added [^{18}F]fluoride was produced via the [^{18}O(p,n)^{18}F] nuclear reaction by irradiation of an [^{18}O]H$_2$O target (Hyox 18 enriched water, Rotem Industries Ltd., Mishor Yamin D.N AravaCity, Israel) on a Cyclone 18/9 (iba RadioPharma Solutions, Louvain-la-Neuve, Belgium) with a fixed energy proton beam using a Nirta [^{18}F]fluoride XL target.

As illustrated in the flow sheet of the synthesis module (Figure 1), [^{18}F]fluoride (4–6 GBq) was trapped on a Sep-Pak Accell Plus QMA Carbonate Plus light cartridge (Figure 1, entry 1; Waters GmbH, Eschborn, Germany) and eluted into the reactor with potassium carbonate (K_2CO_3, 1.8 mg, 13 µmol; entry 2) dissolved in 400 µL of water and 100 µL of ACN. After the addition of Kryptofix 2.2.2. in 1.5 mL ACN (11 mg, 29 µmol, entry 3), the mixture was dried by azeotropic distillation for 5 min at 65 °C and for 2 min at 85 °C. Thereafter, 1.0–1.5 mg of the trimethylammonium triflate precursor **1** dissolved in 800 µL of DMSO (entry 4) was added, and the reaction mixture was stirred at 120 °C for 8 min. After cooling, the reaction mixture was diluted with 3.5 mL of water and 0.5 mL of ACN and transferred into the injection vial (entry 6). Semi-preparative HPLC was performed using a Reprosil-Pur C18-AQ column (entry 7, 250 × 10 mm, Dr. Maisch HPLC GmbH, Ammerbuch-Entringen, Germany) with ACN/H_2O/TFA (35:75:0.05, $v/v/v$) as eluent at a flow of 4.5 mL/min. [^{18}F]**2** was collected into the dilution vessel (entry 8) previously loaded with 50 mL H_2O and 40 µL 1M aq. NaOH at retention times of 15–17 min. Final purification was performed by passing the solution through a Sep-Pak® C18 light cartridge (entry 9; Waters GmbH, Eschborn, Germany), followed by washing with 2 mL of water (entry 10). The cartridge was then removed from the automat and the trapped prosthetic group was manually eluted with 300–400 µL DMSO to prepare it for the subsequent click reaction. The quality control of the product was performed using radio-TLC and radio-HPLC.

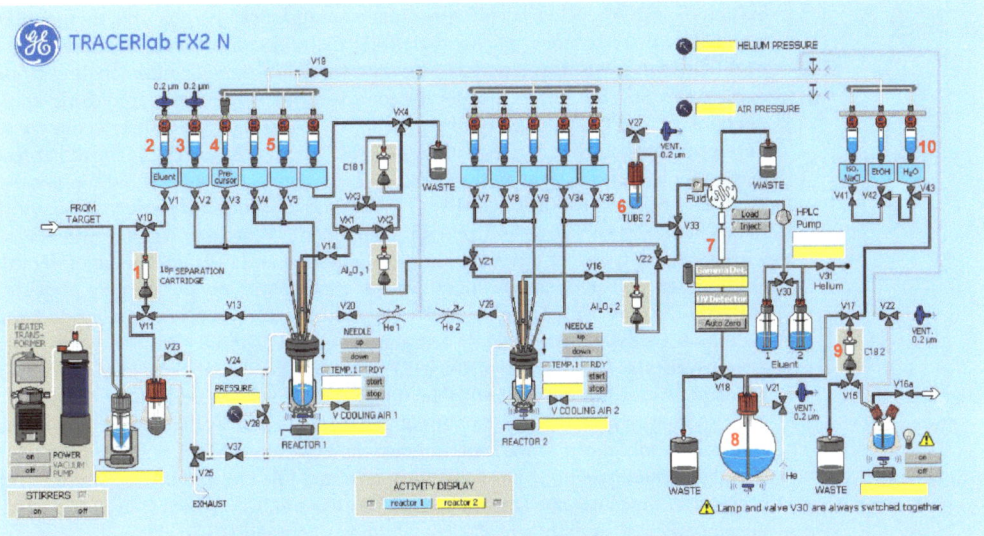

Figure 1. Flow sheet of the synthesis module TRACERlab FX2 N for the radiosynthesis of [^{18}F]**2**. (1) Sep-Pak Accell Plus QMA Carbonate Plus light cartridge, (2) K_2CO_3 (1.8 mg (13 µmol) in 400 µL water, 100 µL ACN), (3) $K_{2.2.2.}$ (11 mg (29 mmol) in 1.5 mL of ACN), (4) precursor **1** (1.0–1.5 mg (2.3–3.5 µmol) in 800 µL DMSO), (5) 3.5 mL of water + 0.5 mL of ACN, (6) injection vial, (7) Reprosil-Pur C18-AQ, 250 × 10 mm (ACN/H_2O/TFA (35:75:0.05, $v/v/v$), flow 4.0 mL/min), (8) 50 mL of water + 40 µL of 1M aq. NaOH, (9) Sep-Pak® C18 light, (10) 2 mL of water.

2.2.4. Radiosynthesis of the Teroligomer [^{18}F]**fluoro-o14PEGMA** by Click-Conjugation of [^{18}F]**2**

The CuAAC reactions of [^{18}F]**2** with azido-TEG-amine were initially performed to identify suitable reaction parameters and are described in the Supplementary Material.

For the generation of the radiolabeled polymer [^{18}F]**fluoro-o14PEGMA** a typical radiosynthesis procedure was performed as follows: The azide functionalized teroligomer **o14PEGMA-N$_3$** (2.0 mg, 0.44 µmol) was dissolved in 310 µL of water and mixed with

72 µL (36 µmol) of a freshly prepared aqueous 0.5 M sodium ascorbate solution and [^{18}F]2 (150–350 MBq) in 100 µL of DMSO. Thereafter, 18 µL (9 µmol) of an aqueous 0.5 M CuSO$_4$ solution was added under stirring, and the reaction mixture was heated up to 90 °C for 2–3 min. The reaction was performed under argon atmosphere, and all solvents were saturated with argon before usage. For the next step, the solution was cooled on ice, diluted with 20 mL of water and loaded on a Chromafix SB cartridge (size M, Macherey-Nagel GmbH & Co., KG, Düren, Germany), which was preconditioned with 10 mL of ethanol and 10 mL of water. The loaded cartridge was washed with 3 mL of water, and the product eluted with 1.7 mL of an aq. 1.0 M HCl solution. The obtained eluate was neutralized with about 0.3 mL of an aq. 5.0 M NaOH solution and directly injected in the semi-preparative size-exclusion chromatography (SEC) system (JASCO LC-2000 module with a PU-2080-20 pump and an UV/VIS-2075 detector; a radioactivity HPLC detector, whose measurement geometry was slightly modified (Gabi Star, Elysia-raytest GmbH); and a fraction collector (Advantec CHF-122SC)). Two in-line connected HiTrap^{TM} Desalting 5 mL columns (GE Healthcare Europe GmbH, Freiburg, Germany) were used with aq. 3.75 mM sodium phosphate buffer (pH 7) as eluent and a flow of 1.0 mL/min.

3. Results and Discussion

3.1. Polymer Synthesis and Characterization

With the aim to synthesize an ^{18}F-labeled amphiphilic polymer suitable for the generation of siRNA-loaded calcium phosphate nanoparticles as potential therapeutics for a targeted localized tumor application via CED, the azide-functionalized anionic teroligomer **o14PEGMA-N$_3$** was developed as precursor for a two-step ^{18}F-radiolabeling strategy, as depicted in Scheme 3. As a basis for the functionalization, the anhydride-containing teroligomer **o14PEGMA** was synthesized at first following a previously in our consortium developed free radical polymerization protocol (Scheme 2A) [9,22,23]. The molar feed used during the synthesis correlated to a mass percentage of the three building blocks of 18% TDA, 17% MA and 65% mPEG-MAc. TDA, a fatty alcohol acrylate derivative with a saturated chain, was chosen as hydrophobic component. A medium chain length was selected with regard to the respective membrane interaction and cellular uptake of the intended teroligomer-modified nanoparticles. Similar chain length can be found in phospholipids, such as 1,2-dimyristoyl-sn-glycero-3-phosphocholine, which has frequently been used for nanoscale drug delivery [24] or slightly altered as 1-monoethoxypolyethyleneglycol-2,3-dimyristylglycerol in the mRNA 1273 vaccine [25]. These examples indicate that the myristyl residue is compliant with the cellular uptake of nanostructures.

Another key factor is the amount of intact anhydrides, as their integrity influences the efficiency of modification and ionic interactions as well as exhibiting an appropriate balance to stabilize nanoparticles, as is currently reported [9]. The combination of two different titration methods revealed an anhydride intactness of 82%, which is in an expected range in comparison to similar anhydride-containing oligomers [23,26,27].

PEG is well known and widely used to prolong circulation time of submicron drug-delivery vehicles in the bloodstream and to reduce opsonization by immune cells [28,29]. However, it is important to balance the PEG content of the teroligomer. While PEG structures contribute to physical stabilization of the nanoparticles and prevent their aggregation, high contents should be avoided because they can reduce cellular uptake, binding efficiency and therefore the final efficacy of the therapeutic approach [30].

The number average molecular weight of the teroligomer was obtained by GPC as 4550 ± 20 Da ($Đ_M$ = 1.71 ± 0.0) [9]. The molecular weight is small enough to ensure for renal elimination but, at the same time, appropriate for interaction with a nanoparticle surface [31].

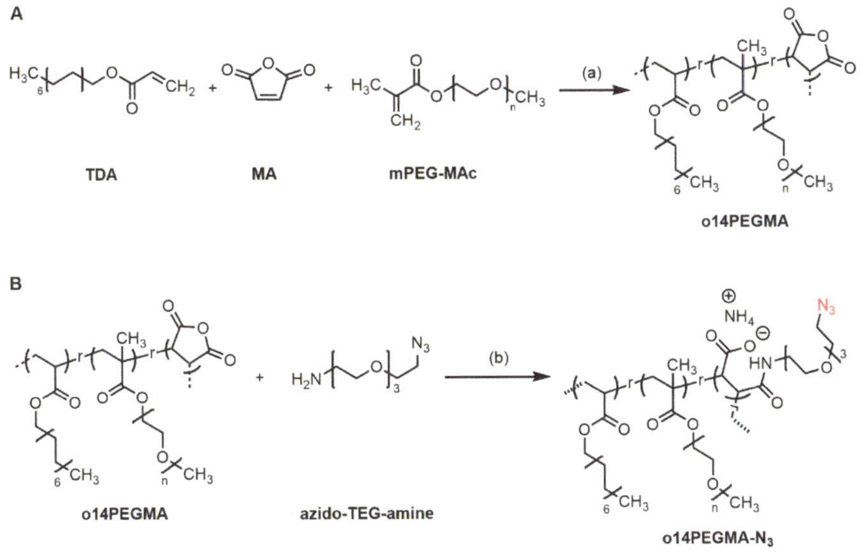

Scheme 2. Synthesis of (**A**) the pristine teroligomer **o14PEGMA** and (**B**) the azide-functionalized teroligomer **o14PEGMA-N$_3$**. Reagents and conditions: (a) free-radical polymerization with AIBN, 60 °C for 18 h under magnetic stirring; (b) (i) triethylamine in acetone, stirring at RT for 4 h, (ii) removal of acetone under vacuum; (iii) 1M aqueous ammonia, magnetic stirring at 40 °C for 12 h.

3.2. Linker Modification

In order to render the teroligomer accessible for ^{18}F-radiolabeling with the prosthetic group [^{18}F]2 via copper-catalyzed click reaction, **o14PEGMA** was derivatized with azido-TEG-amine and isolated as the corresponding ammonium salt (**o14PEGMA-N$_3$**, Scheme 2B). The composition was determined by combining ^{1}H NMR results (mPEG-MAc and TDA content) with the MA content from the conductometric titration method. Based on these results, it can be concluded that the azido-TEG-amine linker group was successfully implemented into the teroligomer structure.

Further structural characterization of **o14PEGMA-N$_3$** was performed by FT-IR and confocal Raman spectroscopy. As shown in Figure 2A, the FT-IR spectra of azido-TEG-amine displayed a prominent peak at 2095 cm^{-1}, representing the asymmetric stretch modes of the delocalized azide–nitrogen double bond [32]. This signal of the azide group could not be clearly detected after attachment of the linker to the teroligomer and subsequent aminolysis. Nevertheless, we expect that a covalent derivatization was achieved, but the number of azide groups in the derivatized oligomer was below the detection limit of the FT-IR equipment. Despite the low number of azide groups, the ^{18}F-labeling could be achieved as will be shown in subsequent paragraphs. Beside the low concentration of the azido group, there is also a possibility that the signal has been shifted due to hydrogen bonding or interactions with the ammonium cations. Furthermore, the automatic atmospheric vapor compensation that affects this area of the spectrum could also have affected any small signal derived from the azide group. Nevertheless, an amide I symmetric stretch vibration of the amide carbonyl peak is clearly visible at 1635 cm^{-1} in the azide-modified oligomer **o14PEGMA-N$_3$**, which indicates a successful amidation with the linker molecule [33]. Clear evidence of ammonium salt formation can also be seen in the 3000 cm^{-1} region of the spectrum. At 1402 cm^{-1}, the amide III region is represented as an overlap of the symmetric stretch along the carbon nitrogen bond and the nitrogen hydrogen bond deformation in phase vibrations. Due to its deformation origin from the nitrogen hydrogen bond, this band also occurs in the ammonium salt of the unmodified oligomer [34]. At 1718 cm^{-1}, the symmetric stretching of the strong carbonyl bond originates from the acid form of the maleic anhydride. It is notable that, as described in the literature, there is a shoulder in the anhydride position at around 1780 cm^{-1} indicating that some chemically intact anhydrides can be found after hydrolysis due to chemical equilibrium [35]. As expected, the highest number of chemically intact anhydrides are found in the pristine oligomer. The band at 1637 cm^{-1} is indicative of carboxylate OH bending during interactions with bound water [36]. Taken together, indications of covalent attachment of the azide linker molecules to the oligomers have been seen with FT-IR. The analysis also shows that the anhydride moieties of the teroligomers were effectively hydrolyzed and transformed to their corresponding ammonium salts.

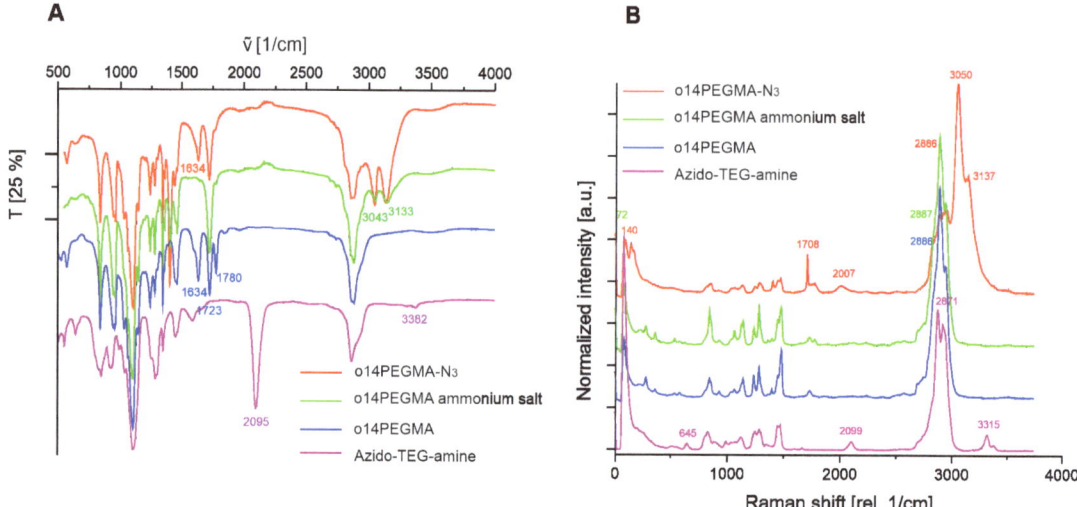

Figure 2. Spectra of **o14PEGMA-N$_3$**, **o14PEGMA**, the ammonium salt of **o14PEGMA** and azido-TEG-amine obtained by (**A**) FT-IR and (**B**) confocal Raman spectroscopy. Both methods complementarily indicate that azido-TEG-amine could be grafted on the **o14PEGMA** backbone by aminolysis. Additional peaks originating from azido-TEG-amine are visible in the reaction product **o14PEGMA-N$_3$** when compared to the non-derivatized ammonium salt of **o14PEGMA**.

Spectra recorded by confocal Raman spectroscopy (Figure 2B) also provided indications for successful azide modification. The azide group reveals signals at 645, 2099 and 3315 cm^{-1}, whereas a Raman transition was found around 2007 cm^{-1} for the azide-derivatized oligomer **o14PEGMA-N$_3$** [37]. The observation confirms interactions of the azide group with other functional moieties of the oligomer, which has already been suspected from the FT-IR data.

3.3. Radiochemistry

3.3.1. Radiosynthesis of the Alkyne-Substituted Heteroaromatic Group [^{18}F]2

Radiofluorination of [^{18}F]2, needed for coupling with the azide-modified oligomer **o14PEGMA-N$_3$**, was achieved by a nucleophilic heteroaromatic substitution reaction using a trimethylammonium triflate precursor (**1**) and the [^{18}F]F$^-$/K$_{2.2.2.}$/K$_2$CO$_3$ fluorination system according to the manual procedure described by Inkster et al. [17] (Scheme 3). The complete radiosynthesis was performed with an automated synthesis module. The setup of the module is described in the Materials and Methods section. Briefly, after trapping and elution of [^{18}F]fluoride from an anion exchange cartridge, the labeling reaction was performed in DMSO at 120 °C. For isolation of [^{18}F]2, the crude reaction mixture was diluted with water/acetonitrile and then directly applied to the implemented semi-preparative

HPLC system (for the chromatogram, see Figure S2 in Supplementary Materials). For the subsequent final purification by solid-phase extraction (SPE), the radiotracer fraction was collected in the collecting vial preloaded with water and a small amount of 1M NaOH to neutralize the acidic eluent containing 0.05% trifluoro acetic acid before loading on a C18 light cartridge. In contrast to the low sorption efficiencies (27–42%) described by Inkster et al. when using a light cartridge, with this procedure, 87 ± 1% (n = 5) of activity could be loaded. The Inkster group improved the SPE step by using two "full-size" C18 plus cartridges followed by elution of the activity with methanol and subsequent evaporation of the solvent. This process caused slight activity losses during evaporation and resulted in considerable longer total synthesis times (103 min) but reasonable radiochemical yields of 39 ± 9% could be achieved [17]. Nevertheless, this approach was less suitable for our purpose, because we aimed to generate the prosthetic group in a shorter time. In the next step, the activity loaded cartridge was removed from the synthesis module and [^{18}F]2 was manually eluted with a small volume of DMSO (300–400 µL) ready for subsequent click reactions. With this procedure, only 5 ± 1% (n = 8) of the activity remained on the cartridge resulting in total radiochemical yields (RCYs) of 38 ± 5 % (n = 10) and radiochemical purities of ≥99%. Thus, the results are comparable to the ones reported by Inkster et al. [17]. However, the entire process was reduced to about 60 min.

3.3.2. Radiosynthesis of the Teroligomer [^{18}F]fluoro-o14PEGMA by Conjugation of o14PEGMA-N$_3$ with [^{18}F]2

In order to find most suitable CuAAC reaction conditions for our purpose, an initial screening of different reaction parameters was performed using [^{18}F]2 and azido-TEG-amine as an easily available and broadly soluble coupling reagent (for details and Scheme S1, see Supplementary Materials). According to the literature, CuSO$_4$ and sodium ascorbate (NaAsc) as the reducing agent and a mixture of water/DMSO (4:1 (v/v)) as solvent were used. In a set of experiments, the following parameters were investigated: (i) the temperature (40, 70 and 90 °C), (ii) the concentration of the azide, (iii) the reaction time (5–60 min.) and (iv) the ratio of azide to CuSO$_4$. The molar ratio of CuSO$_4$ to NaAsc was kept constant at 1 to 4 to ensure effective reduction of Cu(II) to Cu(I). The formation of the radioactive triazole coupling product was monitored using radio-HPLC at different time points (for data, see Figure S3 in Supplementary Materials). In brief, the selected reaction system was shown to be suitable, and the formation of the coupling product could already be observed after short reaction times of 5 to 15 min. The conversion was mainly depending on the concentration of the azide and the reaction temperature. High yields and short reaction times could be achieved with high azide concentrations (25 µmol) already at low temperature (40 °C). However, the azide concentration is a parameter that is not very variable if the reaction conditions have to be transferred to the intended coupling reaction with the polymer, since the azide functionalities in the polymer only represent a small fraction of the molecular structure. Therefore, higher temperatures revealed to be necessary to achieve reasonable conversion yields for these reaction partners.

Based on the initial screening results, the first CuAAC reactions between the azide functionalized teroligomer o14PEGMA-N$_3$ and [^{18}F]2 (Scheme 3) were performed at 90 °C using (i) different polymer concentrations, (ii) a polymer to CuSO$_4$ ratio of 1:2 and (iii) water/DMSO as the solvent mixture (4:1 (v/v), 500 µL). The reaction mixtures were analyzed by radio-SEC and radio-RP-HPLC, taking samples at different time points. During the optimization of the reaction conditions, again a strong variation of the yields was observed depending on the amount of teroligomer. For example, using 2 mg of o14PEGMA-N$_3$ resulted in RCYs of about 60%, whereas 4 mg yielded approximately 80%. Moreover, it was found that already after 2–3 min of reaction time, the radioactive alkyne partner was quantitatively consumed and the coupling product formed. Longer reaction times lead to the decomposition of the radiolabeled product. In contrast to the initial screening with azido-TEG-amine as azide component, the ratio of polymer to CuSO$_4$ played an important role. A minimum molar ratio of 1:20 was necessary to achieve satisfying conversion yields (for comparison, the ratio azido-TEG-amine to CuSO₄ was 1:2). This excess of copper salt was probably needed due to a partial complexation of Cu ions by the carboxylate moieties of **o14PEGMA-N₃**.

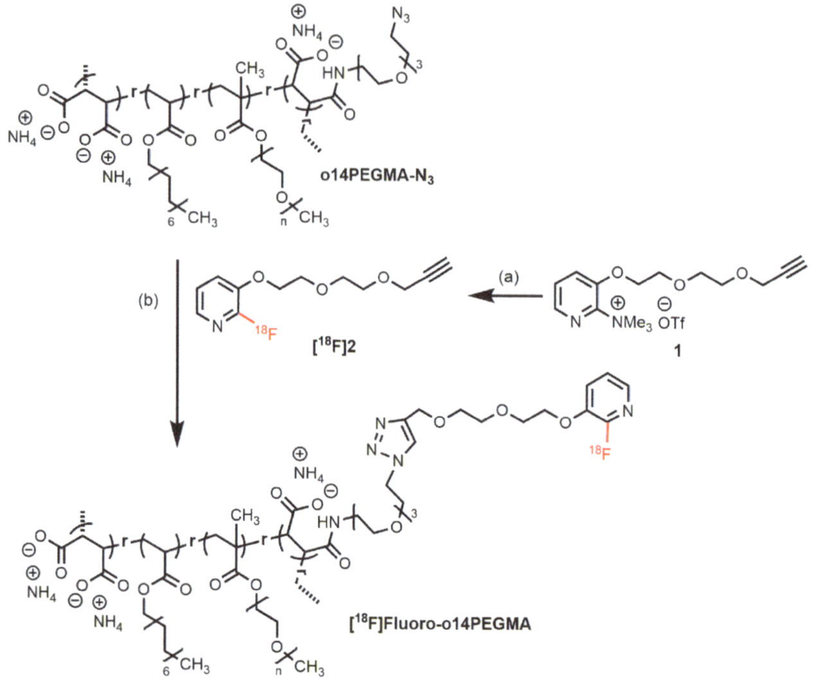

Scheme 3. Radiosynthesis of the teroligomer [^{18}F]**fluoro-o14PEGMA** by copper-catalyzed azide-alkyne cycloaddition of **o14PEGMA-N₃** and [^{18}F]**2**. Reaction conditions: (a) [^{18}F]F⁻/K$_{222}$/K$_2$CO$_3$, DMSO, 120 °C, 8 min; (b) NaAsc/CuSO₄ 4:1, DMSO/H₂O 1:4, 90 °C, 2–3 min.

For the purification of the radiolabeled teroligomer [^{18}F]**fluoro-o14PEGMA**, solid-phase extraction and subsequent isolation by size-exclusion chromatography was performed. The SPE step was found to be necessary to remove the excess of Cu ions. For this purpose, Sep-Pak® C18 and CHROMAFIX SB (anionic exchanger) cartridges of different size were tested. The best sorption efficiencies of the radiolabeled polymer could be obtained with the use of the CHROMAFIX SB cartridge, which correlates well with the anionic character of this amphiphilic polymer. The elution was tested under basic (100 mM PO$_4^{3-}$, 1.0 M NaOH) and acidic (0.1 and 1.0 M HCl) conditions, of which aqueous 1.0 M HCl was found to be most suitable as mainly the desired polymer was eluted with sufficient recovery. For final purification, the acidic eluate was neutralized and manually subjected to the SEC setup consisting of two in-line connected HiTrap™ columns with aqueous phosphate buffer as eluent (chromatogram see Figure 3). The final product was obtained by the collection of the radiolabeled polymer fraction without the need for further manipulation. All manual steps of the polymer radiolabeling and purification process occurred over about 40 min, and an RCY of about 15% (n = 3) was achieved (calculated on the basis of applied [^{18}F]**2**). A rather high loss of activity has been observed during the SEC purification, with almost 30% of activity remaining on the columns. Overall, formulation of the pure [^{18}F]**fluoro-o14PEGMA** could be obtained with a total synthesis time of about 120 min.

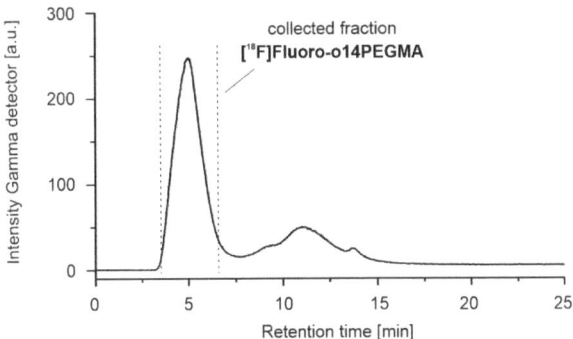

Figure 3. Exemplary radio-chromatogram of the semi-preparative SEC purification of the radiolabeled teroligomer [^{18}F]fluoro-o14PEGMA (conditions: 2 HiTrap^{TM} desalting 5 mL columns in line, 3.75 mM aq. phosphate pH 7, flow 1.0 mL/min).

The analyses of the radiolabeled teroligomer [^{18}F]fluoro-o14PEGMA fraction was performed using radio-SEC and radio-RP-HPLC. Figure 4A,B shows representative examples of the corresponding analytical radio-chromatograms obtained with the purified ^{18}F-labeled polymer. As expected, [^{18}F]fluoro-o14PEGMA eluted in the SEC system at short retention times close to the void volume due to its macromolecular structure (Figure 4A). A rather pronounced tailing was observed over the entire elution process indicating undesired adsorption processes of [^{18}F]fluoro-o14PEGMA on the phase material, a phenomenon which is well known [38]. This observation in the analytical scale corresponds to the observed activity loss on the HiTrap^{TM} columns during semi-preparative SEC purification. In the RP system with gradient mode (Figure 4B), adsorption is the main determinant for retention. As a consequence, the terpolymer does not elute before a certain concentration of the organic modifier is reached during the gradient run, which allows the desorption [38].

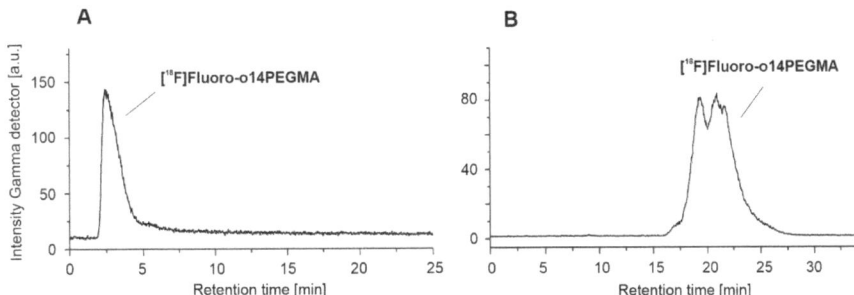

Figure 4. Exemplary radio-chromatograms of the analytical quality control of [^{18}F]fluoro-o14PEGMA using (**A**) radio-SEC (HiTrap^{TM} desalting 5 mL column, 10% ethanol/25 mM aq. phosphate pH 7, flow 1.0) and (**B**) radio-RP-HPLC (Reprosil Pur C18 AQ 250 × 4.6 mm, gradient ACN/20 mM aq. NH$_4$OAc, flow 1.0).

4. Conclusions

This study presents a procedure for the generation and analysis of modified amphiphilic polymers covalently labeled with fluorine-18. Applying a copper-catalyzed click-type cycloaddition reaction, the rather hydrophilic heteroaromatic prosthetic group [^{18}F]2 was coupled with an azide-functionalized teroligomer within 2–3 min. The partially anionic character of the radiolabeled product [^{18}F]fluoro-o14PEGMA allowed for its prepurification via SPE on an anion-exchange cartridge to remove the bulk of reaction additives. Final purification was performed by size-exclusion chromatography, and the radiolabeled teroligomer could be obtained as a phosphate-buffered solution that is ready for further use. The suitability of this new radiofluorinated polymer formulation for the generation of radiolabeled CaP-NPs is subject of current investigation.

Supplementary Materials: The following supporting information can be downloaded at: https://www.mdpi.com/article/10.3390/nano13142095/s1, Figure S1: ^{1}H NMR spectra of **1** and **2**; Figure S2: Semi-preparative HPLC of [^{18}F]2; Figure S3: Formation of the triazole coupling product [^{18}F]3, which is dependent on reaction time, temperature and concentration; Scheme S1: Click-coupling reaction of [^{18}F]2 with azido-TEG-amine.

Author Contributions: Conceptualization, P.B., M.S.-S., M.C.H., B.W. and R.T.; methodology, M.C.H., B.W., M.S., R.T., R.-P.M., F.M. and B.F.; validation, B.W., M.S., M.C.H. and B.F.; investigation, M.S., B.W., R.T., T.H.L., B.F. and R.-P.M.; writing—original draft preparation, B.W., M.C.H. and M.S.; writing—review and editing, R.T., R.-P.M., T.H.L., F.M., K.K., B.F., M.S.-S. and P.B.; project administration, P.B., M.S.-S., M.C.H. and K.K.; funding acquisition, P.B. and M.S.-S. All authors have read and agreed to the published version of the manuscript.

Funding: This research was funded by the Europäischer Fonds für regionale Entwicklung (EFRE) and the Sächsische Aufbaubank (SAB, Saxony, Germany, Grant-ID: 100344836).

Data Availability Statement: All data are contained within the article and Supplementary Materials.

Acknowledgments: We are very thankful to K. Franke and S. Fischer for providing [^{18}F]fluoride.

Conflicts of Interest: The authors declare no conflict of interest.

References

1. Maeda, H. The enhanced permeability and retention (EPR) effect in tumor vasculature: The key role of tumor-selective macromolecular drug targeting. *Adv. Enzym. Regul.* **2001**, *41*, 189–207. [CrossRef]
2. Duncan, R. Polymer conjugates as anticancer nanomedicines. *Nat. Rev. Cancer* **2006**, *6*, 688–701. [CrossRef] [PubMed]
3. Duncan, R.; Vicent, M.J. Polymer therapeutics-prospects for 21st century: The end of the beginning. *Adv. Drug Deliv. Rev.* **2013**, *65*, 60–70. [CrossRef] [PubMed]
4. Pant, K.; Sedlacek, O.; Nadar, R.A.; Hruby, M.; Stephan, H. Radiolabelled Polymeric Materials for Imaging and Treatment of Cancer: Quo Vadis? *Adv. Healthc. Mater.* **2017**, *6*, 1601115. [CrossRef]
5. Stockhofe, K.; Postema, J.M.; Schieferstein, H.; Ross, T.L. Radiolabeling of Nanoparticles and Polymers for PET Imaging. *Pharmaceuticals* **2014**, *7*, 392–418. [CrossRef] [PubMed]
6. Delplace, V.; Couvreur, P.; Nicolas, J. Recent trends in the design of anticancer polymer prodrug nanocarriers. *Polym. Chem.* **2014**, *5*, 1529–1544. [CrossRef]
7. Parveen, S.; Arjmand, F.; Tabassum, S. Clinical developments of antitumor polymer therapeutics. *RSC Adv.* **2019**, *9*, 24699–24721. [CrossRef] [PubMed]
8. Bobo, R.H.; Laske, D.W.; Akbasak, A.; Morrison, P.F.; Dedrick, R.L.; Oldfield, E.H. Convection-enhanced delivery of macromolecules in the brain. *Proc. Natl. Acad. Sci. USA* **1994**, *91*, 2076–2080. [CrossRef]
9. Mitrach, F.; Schmid, M.; Toussaint, M.; Dukic-Stefanovic, S.; Deuther-Conrad, W.; Franke, H.; Ewe, A.; Aigner, A.; Wölk, C.; Brust, P.; et al. Amphiphilic Anionic Oligomer-Stabilized Calcium Phosphate Nanoparticles with Prospects in siRNA Delivery via Convection-Enhanced Delivery. *Pharmaceutics* **2022**, *14*, 326. [CrossRef]
10. Herth, M.M.; Barz, M.; Moderegger, D.; Allmeroth, M.; Jahn, M.; Thews, O.; Zentel, R.; Rösch, F. Radioactive Labeling of Defined HPMA-Based Polymeric Structures Using [^{18}F]FETos for In Vivo Imaging by Positron Emission Tomography. *Biomacromolecules* **2009**, *10*, 1697–1703. [CrossRef]
11. Allmeroth, M.; Moderegger, D.; Gündel, D.; Buchholz, H.G.; Mohr, N.; Koynov, K.; Rösch, F.; Thews, O.; Zentel, R. PEGylation of HPMA-based block copolymers enhances tumor accumulation in vivo: A quantitative study using radiolabeling and positron emission tomography. *J. Control Release* **2013**, *172*, 77–85. [CrossRef] [PubMed]
12. Schieferstein, H.; Kelsch, A.; Reibel, A.; Koynov, K.; Barz, M.; Buchholz, H.G.; Bausbacher, N.; Thews, O.; Zentel, R.; Ross, T.L. ^{18}F-Radiolabeling, Preliminary Evaluation of Folate-pHPMA Conjugates via PET. *Macromol. Biosci.* **2014**, *14*, 1396–1405. [CrossRef] [PubMed]
13. Di Mauro, P.P.; Gomez-Vallejo, V.; Maldonado, Z.B.; Roig, J.L.; Borros, S. Novel ^{18}F-Labeling Strategy for Polyester-Based NPs for In Vivo PET-CT Imaging. *Bioconjug. Chem.* **2015**, *26*, 582–592. [CrossRef] [PubMed]
14. Reibel, A.T.; Müller, S.S.; Pektor, S.; Bausbacher, N.; Miederer, M.; Frey, H.; Rösch, F. Fate of Linear and Branched Polyether-Lipids In Vivo in Comparison to Their Liposomal Formulations by ^{18}F-Radiolabeling and Positron Emission Tomography. *Biomacromolecules* **2015**, *16*, 842–851. [CrossRef] [PubMed]

15. Wagener, K.; Worm, M.; Pektor, S.; Schinnerer, M.; Thiermann, R.; Miederer, M.; Frey, H.; Rösch, F. Comparison of Linear and Hyperbranched Polyether Lipids for Liposome Shielding by ^{18}F-Radiolabeling and Positron Emission Tomography. *Biomacromolecules* **2018**, *19*, 2506–2516. [CrossRef]
16. Glassner, M.; Palmieri, L.; Monnery, B.D.; Verbrugghen, T.; Deleye, S.; Stroobants, S.; Staelens, S.; Wyffels, L.; Hoogenboom, R. The Label Matters: μPET Imaging of the Biodistribution of Low Molar Mass ^{89}Zr and ^{18}F-Labeled Poly(2-ethyl-2-oxazoline). *Biomacromolecules* **2017**, *18*, 96–102. [CrossRef]
17. Inkster, J.; Lin, K.S.; Ait-Mohand, S.; Gosselin, S.; Benard, F.; Guerin, B.; Pourghiasian, M.; Ruth, T.; Schaffer, P.; Storr, T. 2-Fluoropyridine prosthetic compounds for the ^{18}F-labeling of bombesin analogues. *Bioorganic Med. Chem. Lett.* **2013**, *23*, 3920–3926. [CrossRef]
18. Kuhnast, B.; Damont, A.; Hinnen, F.; Huss, C.; Dolle, F. PEG-[^{18}F] FPyZIDE and PEG-[^{18}F] FPyKYNE, Two New Fluoropyridine-Based Reagents for the Fluorine-18 Labeling of Macromolecules Using Click Chemistry. *J. Label. Compd. Radiopharm.* **2009**, *52*, S184.
19. Brown, A.; Fujimori, K. A Method for the Determination of Maleic-Anhydride Content in Copolymers. *Polym. Bull.* **1986**, *16*, 441–444. [CrossRef]
20. Endo, R.; Hinokuma, T.; Takeda, M. Studies of Solution Properties of Copolymers. 2. Copolymer of Maleic Anhydride and Styrene. *J. Polym. Sci. Part A-2 Polym. Phys.* **1968**, *6*, 665–673. [CrossRef]
21. Edward Semple, J.; Sullivan, B.; Vojkovsky, T.; Sill, K.N. Synthesis and facile end-group quantification of functionalized PEG azides. *J. Polym. Sci. Part A Polym. Chem.* **2016**, *54*, 2888–2895. [CrossRef] [PubMed]
22. Nawaz, H.A.; Schrock, K.; Schmid, M.; Krieghoff, J.; Maqsood, I.; Kascholke, C.; Kohn-Polster, C.; Schulz-Siegmund, M.; Hacker, M.C. Injectable oligomer-cross-linked gelatine hydrogels via anhydride-amine-conjugation. *J. Mater. Chem. B* **2021**, *9*, 2295–2307. [CrossRef] [PubMed]
23. Kascholke, C.; Loth, T.; Kohn-Polster, C.; Möller, S.; Bellstedt, P.; Schulz-Siegmund, M.; Schnabelrauch, M.; Hacker, M.C. Dual-Functional Hydrazide-Reactive and Anhydride-Containing Oligomeric Hydrogel Building Blocks. *Biomacromolecules* **2017**, *18*, 683–694. [CrossRef] [PubMed]
24. Wölk, C.; Janich, C.; Meister, A.; Drescher, S.; Langner, A.; Brezesinski, G.; Bakowsky, U. Investigation of Binary Lipid Mixtures of a Three-Chain Cationic Lipid with Phospholipids Suitable for Gene Delivery. *Bioconjug. Chem.* **2015**, *26*, 2461–2473. [CrossRef] [PubMed]
25. Olenick, L.L.; Troiano, J.M.; Vartanian, A.; Melby, E.S.; Mensch, A.C.; Zhang, L.L.; Hong, J.W.; Mesele, O.; Qiu, T.; Bozich, J.; et al. Lipid Corona Formation from Nanoparticle Interactions with Bilayers. *Chem* **2018**, *4*, 2709–2723. [CrossRef]
26. Loth, T.; Hennig, R.; Kascholke, C.; Hötzel, R.; Hacker, M.C. Reactive and stimuli-responsive maleic anhydride containing macromers—Multi-functional cross-linkers and building blocks for hydrogel fabrication. *React. Funct. Polym.* **2013**, *73*, 1480–1492. [CrossRef]
27. Li, H.; Nawaz, H.A.; Masieri, F.F.; Vogel, S.; Hempel, U.; Bartella, A.K.; Zimmerer, R.; Simon, J.C.; Schulz-Siegmund, M.; Hacker, M.C.; et al. Osteogenic Potential of Mesenchymal Stem Cells from Adipose Tissue, Bone Marrow and Hair Follicle Outer Root Sheath in a 3D Crosslinked Gelatin-Based Hydrogel. *Int. J. Mol. Sci.* **2021**, *22*, 5404. [CrossRef]
28. Seneca, S.; Simon, J.; Weber, C.; Ghazaryan, A.; Ethirajan, A.; Mailaender, V.; Morsbach, S.; Landfester, K. How Low Can You Go? Low Densities of Poly(ethylene glycol) Surfactants Attract Stealth Proteins. *Macromol. Biosci.* **2018**, *18*, e1800075. [CrossRef]
29. D'Souza, A.A.; Shegokar, R. Polyethylene glycol (PEG): A versatile polymer for pharmaceutical applications. *Expert. Opin. Drug Deliv.* **2016**, *13*, 1257–1275. [CrossRef]
30. Pozzi, D.; Colapicchioni, V.; Caracciolo, G.; Piovesana, S.; Capriotti, A.L.; Palchetti, S.; De Grossi, S.; Riccioli, A.; Amenitsch, H.; Lagana, A. Effect of polyethyleneglycol (PEG) chain length on the bio-nano-interactions between PEGylated lipid nanoparticles and biological fluids: From nanostructure to uptake in cancer cells. *Nanoscale* **2014**, *6*, 2782–2792. [CrossRef]
31. Dinari, A.; Moghadam, T.T.; Abdollahi, M.; Sadeghizadeh, M. Synthesis and Characterization of a Nano-Polyplex system of GNRs-PDMAEA-pDNA: An Inert Self-Catalyzed Degradable Carrier for Facile Gene Delivery. *Sci. Rep.* **2018**, *8*, 8112. [CrossRef] [PubMed]
32. Tao, P.; Li, Y.; Rungta, A.; Viswanath, A.; Gao, J.N.; Benicewicz, B.C.; Siegel, R.W.; Schadler, L.S. TiO_2 nanocomposites with high refractive index and transparency. *J. Mat. Chem.* **2011**, *21*, 18623–18629. [CrossRef]
33. Li, H.; Li, X.; Jain, P.; Peng, H.; Rahimi, K.; Singh, S.; Pich, A. Dual-Degradable Biohybrid Microgels by Direct Cross-Linking of Chitosan and Dextran Using Azide-Alkyne Cycloaddition. *Biomacromolecules* **2020**, *21*, 4933–4944. [CrossRef] [PubMed]
34. Mudunkotuwa, I.A.; Minshid, A.A.; Grassian, V.H. ATR-FTIR spectroscopy as a tool to probe surface adsorption on nanoparticles at the liquid-solid interface in environmentally and biologically relevant media. *Analyst* **2014**, *139*, 870–881. [CrossRef]
35. Kopf, A.H.; Koorengevel, M.C.; van Walree, C.A.; Dafforn, T.R.; Killian, J.A. A simple and convenient method for the hydrolysis of styrene-maleic anhydride copolymers to styrene-maleic acid copolymers. *Chem. Phys. Lipids* **2019**, *218*, 85–90. [CrossRef]
36. Oh, S.Y.; Yoo, D.I.; Shin, Y.; Seo, G. FTIR analysis of cellulose treated with sodium hydroxide and carbon dioxide. *Carbohydr. Res.* **2005**, *340*, 417–428. [CrossRef]

37. Jiang, J.R.; Zhu, P.F.; Li, D.M.; Chen, Y.M.; Li, M.R.; Wang, X.L.; Liu, B.B.; Cui, Q.L.; Zhu, H.Y. High pressure studies of trimethyltin azide by Raman scattering, IR absorption, and synchrotron X-ray diffraction. *RSC Adv.* **2016**, *6*, 98921–98926. [CrossRef]
38. Uliyanchenko, E.; van der Wal, S.; Schoenmakers, P.J. Challenges in polymer analysis by liquid chromatography. *Polym. Chem.* **2012**, *3*, 2313–2335. [CrossRef]

Disclaimer/Publisher's Note: The statements, opinions and data contained in all publications are solely those of the individual author(s) and contributor(s) and not of MDPI and/or the editor(s). MDPI and/or the editor(s) disclaim responsibility for any injury to people or property resulting from any ideas, methods, instructions or products referred to in the content.

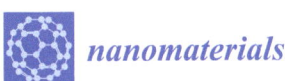

Article

Total Bio-Based Material for Drug Delivery and Iron Chelation to Fight Cancer through Antimicrobial Activity

Vincenzo Patamia [1], Chiara Zagni [1], Roberto Fiorenza [2], Virginia Fuochi [3,4], Sandro Dattilo [5], Paolo Maria Riccobene [5], Pio Maria Furneri [3,4], Giuseppe Floresta [1,*], and Antonio Rescifina [1,*]

1. Dipartimento di Scienze del Farmaco e della Salute, Università di Catania, Viale A. Doria 6, 95125 Catania, Italy; vincenzo.patamia@unict.it (V.P.); chiara.zagni@unict.it (C.Z.)
2. Dipartimento di Scienze Chimiche, Università di Catania, Viale A. Doria 6, 95125 Catania, Italy; roberto.fiorenza@unict.it
3. Department of Biomedical and Biotechnological Sciences (Biometec), University of Catania, 95125 Catania, Italy; vfuochi@unict.it (V.F.)
4. Center of Excellence for the Acceleration of Harm Reduction (Coehar), University of Catania, 95125 Catania, Italy
5. IPCB-CNR, Via Paolo Gaifami 18, Institute for Polymers, Composites, and Biomaterials, Via Paolo Gaifami 18, 95126 Catania, Italy; sandro.dattilo@cnr.it (S.D.); paolomaria.riccobene@cnr.it (P.M.R.)
* Correspondence: giuseppe.floresta@unict.it (G.F.); arescifina@unict.it (A.R.)

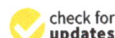

Citation: Patamia, V.; Zagni, C.; Fiorenza, R.; Fuochi, V.; Dattilo, S.; Riccobene, P.M.; Furneri, P.M.; Floresta, G.; Rescifina, A. Total Bio-Based Material for Drug Delivery and Iron Chelation to Fight Cancer through Antimicrobial Activity. *Nanomaterials* 2023, *13*, 2036. https://doi.org/10.3390/nano13142036

Academic Editor: James Chow

Received: 6 June 2023
Revised: 7 July 2023
Accepted: 8 July 2023
Published: 10 July 2023

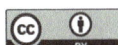

Copyright: © 2023 by the authors. Licensee MDPI, Basel, Switzerland. This article is an open access article distributed under the terms and conditions of the Creative Commons Attribution (CC BY) license (https://creativecommons.org/licenses/by/4.0/).

Abstract: Bacterial involvement in cancer's development, along with their impact on therapeutic interventions, has been increasingly recognized. This has prompted the development of novel strategies to disrupt essential biological processes in microbial cells. Among these approaches, metal-chelating agents have gained attention for their ability to hinder microbial metal metabolism and impede critical reactions. Nanotechnology has also contributed to the antibacterial field by offering various nanomaterials, including antimicrobial nanoparticles with potential therapeutic and drug-delivery applications. Halloysite nanotubes (HNTs) are naturally occurring tubular clay nanomaterials composed of aluminosilicate kaolin sheets rolled multiple times. The aluminum and siloxane groups on the surface of HNTs enable hydrogen bonding with biomaterials, making them versatile in various domains, such as environmental sciences, wastewater treatment, nanoelectronics, catalytic studies, and cosmetics. This study aimed to create an antibacterial material by combining the unique properties of halloysite nanotubes with the iron-chelating capability of kojic acid. A nucleophilic substitution reaction involving the hydroxyl groups on the nanotubes' surface was employed to functionalize the material using kojic acid. The resulting material was characterized using infrared spectroscopy (IR), thermogravimetric analysis (TGA), energy-dispersive X-ray spectroscopy (EDX), and scanning electron microscopy (SEM), and its iron-chelating ability was assessed. Furthermore, the potential for drug loading—specifically, with resveratrol and curcumin—was evaluated through ultraviolet (UV) analysis. The antibacterial assay was evaluated following CLSI guidelines. The results suggested that the HNTs–kojic acid formulation had great antibacterial activity against all tested pathogens. The outcome of this work yielded a novel bio-based material with dual functionality as a drug carrier and an antimicrobial agent. This innovative approach holds promise for addressing challenges related to bacterial infections, antibiotic resistance, and the development of advanced therapeutic interventions.

Keywords: resveratrol; curcumin; halloysite nanotubes; kojic acid; iron chelation; antibacterial

1. Introduction

Millions of people die from cancer yearly, making it the world's most prominent cause of death [1]. Researchers are dedicated to examining the origins of cancer and its progression, associated treatments, and postoperative interventions. Since growing evidence shows that bacteria can contribute to cancer's formation and interfere with therapy by mediating its carcinogenesis and related infections, bacteria, which initially appeared to be independent of cancer, have attracted substantial interest among all cancer-related variables [2]. By triggering inflammatory responses and secreting bacterial enzymes, toxins, and oncogenic peptides, bacteria can make tumor growth worse. As bacteria may survive in malignant tissues due to their bacteria-friendly microenvironment and the severely compromised immune function of patients, cancer patients are more likely to acquire bacterial infections after therapy, even if it has been shown that bacteria have the potential to be exploited as anticancer agents [3,4]. Clostridium and salmonella have been shown to infect and survive within the human body, including in tumors. In fact, patients with solid tumors had a 42% Gram-positive infection rate and a 27% Gram-negative infection rate, compared to 47% and 30% for patients with hematological malignancies, respectively [5]. Moreover, surgery is frequently performed to remove most solid tumors, leaving scars or grafts at risk of infection, leading to inflammation, slow wound healing, and other consequences [6].

For example, the malignant tissue must be removed to treat skin cancer, but preventing infection and ensuring wound healing is challenging following surgery. Once an infection has set in, the delicate tissue will bleed, exude abundantly, cause discomfort, and cause fever, which can be exceedingly harmful to cancer patients. The malignant bone is often replaced with an orthopedic implant in cases of bone tumor resection. The probable infection, however, may cause insufficient soft tissue coverage, difficulties with the incision, and implant failure [2,7].

The need for antibacterial medications with novel or better modes of action is a health challenge of the greatest relevance in the age of rising antimicrobial resistance [8]. One of the main methods to ensure progress seems to be to increase or enhance the chelating properties of already-existing medications, or to discover new, nature-inspired chelating agents [9]. Resistance-based infections frequently do not respond to standard treatments, prolonging sickness, raising expenditures, and increasing the chance of mortality. Because the current antimicrobial medications either have too many adverse effects or tend to lose their efficacy due to the selection of resistant strains, the creation of innovative antimicrobial treatments is becoming more and more challenging [10].

These facts have led to several new techniques for impeding crucial biological processes in microbial cells. One such technique centers on using metal-chelating agents, which can disrupt the metabolism of the metals vital to the microorganism, hindering the uptake and bioavailability of those metals for critical reactions [11].

The biological function of metal-dependent proteins, such as metalloproteases and transcription factors, can be inhibited by chelation activity, which disturbs the homeostasis of microbial cells and blocks microbial nutrition, growth, and development, cellular differentiation, adhesion to biotic (such as extracellular matrix components, cells, and/or tissues) and abiotic (such as plastic, silicone, and acrylic) structures, and in vivo infection. Curiously, chelating drugs also increase the effectiveness of traditional antibacterial substances [6,11,12].

Nanomaterials have all of the characteristics needed to address these problems and create new technologies that can effectively target bacterial infections [13,14]; they also have the potential to be used to treat cancer itself [15]. First, nanoscale particles' improved penetration and retention effects allow them to target tumor locations passively. Nanomaterials can be functionalized to actively target tumor tissues or cancer cells and accumulate at tumor sites through surface modification. For instance, cancer-targeting peptides can identify specific receptors [16–19], cationic elements can be added to nanomaterials' surfaces to improve their tumor-penetrating ability [20], and nanomaterials' shape or size can be altered to enhance tumor retention. Second, nanomaterials' distinctive hydrophobic and hydrophilic architectures enable the loading of various medications in relatively high quantities, improving their solubility and safeguarding them against deterioration [21–23].

Natural clay nanotubes, known as halloysite, are one such nanoscale delivery method. It was discovered that halloysite is a practical and affordable nanoscale container for the encapsulation of physiologically active compounds, such as medicines and biocides [24,25].

The nearby alumina and silica layers and their water hydration provide a packing disorder that causes the layers to roll up and bend, forming multilayer tubes [26]. Compared to other nanotubes, using halloysite has several advantages. Its production is neither laborious nor dangerous, since it occurs naturally. Compared to other nanotubes (such as carbon nanotubes and inorganic nanotubes composed of tungsten, titanium, etc.), it is less costly [27,28]. Large particle size, an abundance of hydrophilic hydroxyl groups for functionalization, high stability in biological fluids, and inexpensive cost are all benefits of HNTs for drug delivery carrier applications [29,30]. Halloysite nanotubes are harmless up to concentrations of 75 mg/mL, and parallel laser confocal observation of fluorescently labeled halloysite absorption of cells revealed the material's position inside the cells, close to the nucleus, demonstrating cellular uptake [30].

In this work, we modified HNTs with a derivative of kojic acid and then encapsulated them with resveratrol and curcumin—natural phenolic compounds with many beneficial effects on human health, such as antioxidant, anticancer, neuroprotective, and antiviral activities [31–33]. The successful preparation of this material was confirmed by various characterization methods. The novel material proved excellent drug-loading efficiency and chelating properties as proof of concept of a dual-acting antibacterial nanomaterial with resveratrol/curcumin and iron-depletion properties.

2. Materials and Methods

2.1. Materials

All of the required chemicals were purchased from Merck (Merck KGaA, Darmstadt, Germany) and used without further purification. The ^{1}H- and ^{13}C-NMR spectra were recorded at 300 K on a Varian UNITY Inova using DMSO-d_6 as the solvent at 500 MHz for ^{1}H-NMR and 125 MHz for ^{13}C-NMR.

2.2. Synthesis of HNTs

2.2.1. Synthesis of Chlorokojic Acid (2)

To a 100 mL round-bottomed reaction flask containing freshly distilled thionyl chloride (20 mL), kojic acid (**1**) (7.3 g) was added, and the mixture was magnetically stirred for 2 h. After one hour, a yellow-to-orange precipitate was formed. The product was collected by filtration, washed with petroleum ether, and then recrystallized from water to obtain colorless needles of chlorokojic acid (**2**) (5.2 g) at a 63% yield. The ^{1}H and ^{13}C NMR spectra of the compound were accordingly with the reported ones [34].

2.2.2. Synthesis of HNTs/Kojic Acid Derivative

To a 10 mL round-bottomed reaction flask containing DMF (2 mL), we added halloysite (400 mg, 1 eq, 1.36 mmol) and triethylamine (1.14 mL, 6 eq, 8.16 mmol), and the mixture was magnetically stirred at room temperature for 30 min. Subsequently, chlorokojic acid (437 mg, 2 eq, 2.72 mmol) was added, and the reaction mixture was left to stir overnight at 80 °C. Then, the precipitate was collected by filtration, washed with acetone several times (5 × 10 mL), and placed in an oven at 65 °C overnight to obtain the final product (470 mg) at a 60% yield.

2.3. IR and UV–vis

FTIR analyses in the 4000–400 cm^{-1} region were conducted using an FTIR System 2000 (PerkinElmer, Waltham, MA, USA) with KBr as the medium. UV–vis spectroscopy (JASCO V-730 spectrophotometer, Easton, MD, USA) was used to determine the encapsulation efficiency (EE) and the drug-loading capacity (DLC).

2.4. Resveratrol and Curcumin Uptake

The loading of resveratrol on the HNTs–kojic acid system was carried out as described in the literature [30,35], at different weight ratios: 1:1, 1:2.5, 1:5, and 1:10 (resveratrol:HNTs–kojic acid w/w, Figure S1). Briefly, a resveratrol solution in water was prepared (7.5 mg L^{-1}), and the correct amount of HNTs–kojic acid was suspended and kept under stirring for 1 h in the dark. Then, the suspension was centrifuged to separate the system from the uncharged drug. The loading capacities of curcumin were also evaluated, using different w/w ratios between the drug and the HNTs–kojic acid system. As described in the literature [36], a stock solution in ethanol was prepared (0.663 mg L^{-1}), and curcumin was loaded on the HNTs–kojic acid system employing different weight ratios: 1:10, 1:50, 1:100, and 1:1000 (curcumin:HNTs–kojic acid w/w, Figure S2).

2.5. ICP/MS

Quantitative determination of iron ions in solution was performed by inductively coupled plasma mass spectrometry (ICP/MS) with a Nexion 300X (PerkinElmer Inc. Waltham, Massachusetts, USA.) instrument, using kinetic energy discrimination (KED) for interference suppression. Each determination was performed three times. The accuracy of the analytical procedure was confirmed by measuring a standard reference material—Nist 1640a trace element in natural water—without observing an appreciable difference. Batch equilibrium tests were carried out to calculate the metal ions' removal percentage. In general, 10 mg of HNTs–kojic acid was immersed into iron(III) chloride (FeCl$_3$) solutions (5 mL and pH = 6) at different initial Fe concentrations of 1.50 and 10.00 mg L^{-1}. The vials were maintained under constant shaking at 25 °C and 180 rpm for 24 h, the suspension obtained was filtrated through a 0.22 nylon filter, and the solution was subjected to analysis by ICP-MS, as previously described.

2.6. SEM, EDX, and TGA

To study the morphology of the synthesized material, scanning electron microscopy (SEM) with a Phenomenex microscope was used. To increase conductivity before the test, the samples were pre-coated by gold sputter-coating. Images were then captured to examine the nanoclay morphology of the sample. The data were acquired and processed using Phenom Porometric 1.1.2.0 (Phenom-World BV, Eindhoven, the Netherlands). Energy-dispersive X-ray spectroscopy (EDX) was used to analyze the chemical elements in the material and determine its chemical composition. The material was subjected to thermogravimetric analysis (TGA) using a thermogravimetric apparatus (TA Instruments Q500) under a nitrogen atmosphere (flow rate: 60 mL/min) at a 10 °C/min heating rate, from 40 °C to 800 °C. The TGA sensitivity was 0.1 µg, with a weighting precision of ±0.01%.

2.7. Antibacterial Assay

The HNTs–kojic acid formulation was investigated for its antibacterial activity. *Escherichia coli* ATCC 25922, *Klebsiella pneumoniae* ATCC 700603, *Enterococcus faecalis* ATCC 29212, and *Staphylococcus aureus* ATCC 29213 strains were studied. The minimum inhibitory concentration (MIC) was determined through the broth microdilution technique, according to the recommendations stated in the Clinical and Laboratory Standards Institute (CLSI) document [37]. Briefly, a bacterial suspension of 0.5 McFarland was made for each strain under examination and, starting from the same suspension, the dilutions in broth were prepared to obtain a final concentration of 10^4 CFU/mL. The HNTs–kojic acid formulation was added at concentrations ranging from 1.5 mg to 24 mg. Each plate was prepared by including a positive control for bacterial growth (C+) and a negative control for sterility (C−). Each formulation was tested six times against each bacterial strain; the same experiment was repeated on a different day to ensure reproducibility.

3. Results and Discussion

3.1. Synthesis and Characterization

To produce a derivative able to react with the hydroxylic groups of the HNTs, a derivative of kojic acid (**1**) was produced, giving chlorokojic acid (**2**) through a simple reaction with thionyl chloride (Figure 1). Compound **2** was then reacted with the HNTs, as reported in Figure 2, giving the final product **3**, named HNTs–kojic acid. TGA of **2**,

HNTs, and **3** was performed, and the results are shown in Figures S3–S5. The maximal degradation rate of **2** is at 183 °C, while the highest-intensity peak of **3** is at 213 °C. In the DTG curve of **3**, a hump is visible at 194 °C, which is possibly due to chlorokojic acid, while the component of the peak at the higher temperature of 213 °C corresponds to the functionalized HNTs with chlorokojic acid. It is possible to infer that the percentage of functionalized HNTs with chlorokojic acid is higher than 10%.

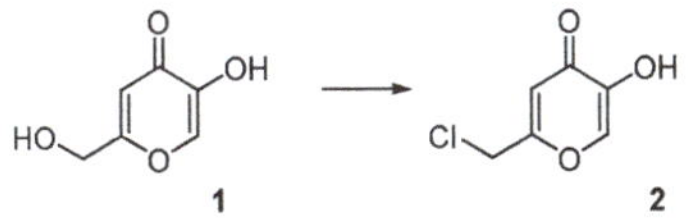

Figure 1. Synthesis of compound **2**.

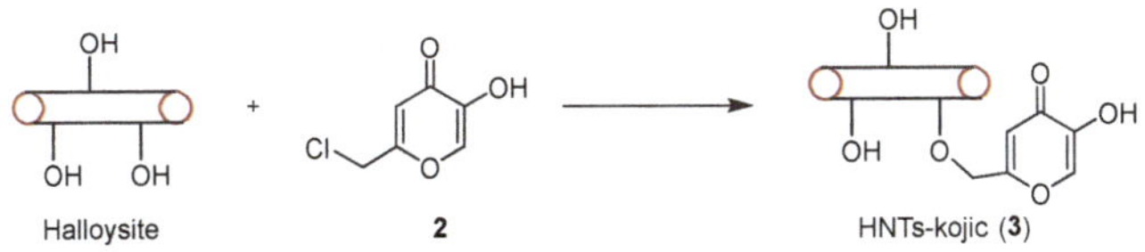

Figure 2. Synthesis of compound **3**.

Therefore, the material was characterized using IR, ICP/MS, SEM, and EDX, and the drug delivery capabilities were proven by drug-loading UV experiments with two natural molecules with antibacterial properties: resveratrol and curcumin [38–40].

The comparison of the IR spectra of HNTs and HNTs–kojic acid shows the successful functionalization of the halloysite nanotubes with kojic acid (Figure 3). In the spectrum of HNTs (red line), bands related to the OH groups are evident: the peak at 906 cm^{-1} is attributable to the Al-O-OH vibration, while the bands at 3695 and 3620 cm^{-1} can be attributed to the stretching vibration of the Al-OH groups. In addition, a strong peak related to O-Si-O is observed at around 1075 cm^{-1}, and the peaks at 793 and 752 cm^{-1} can be assigned to the stretching mode of apical Si-O [35].

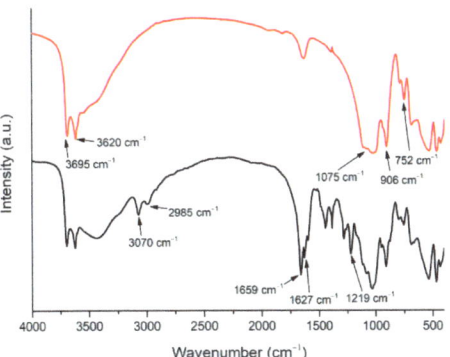

Figure 3. IR spectra of pristine halloysite (red line) and halloysite functionalized with kojic acid (black line).

From the spectrum related to the functionalized HNTs–kojic acid (black line), we can see the presence of signals related to halloysite nanotubes, along with typical kojic acid signals: at 2985 and 3070 cm^{-1}, the medium stretching of CH$_2$ [41]; at 1659 cm^{-1}, a strong signal related to conjugated ketone C=O; at 1627 cm^{-1}, the typical C=C stretching of an unsaturated ketone [42,43]; and finally, the stretching associated with C-O at 1219 cm^{-1}, which highlights the successful functionalization between the nanotubes and kojic acid.

ICP-MS spectra were recorded to verify the ability of the material to sequester iron(III) from the environment. The experiments revealed that HNTs–kojic acid chelates iron, i.e., eliminating gallium from solutions, with 65.33% retention of the ions when working with 1.50 mg/L of iron chloride, and 10.08% retention of the ions when working with 10.00 mg/L.

Figure 4 shows SEM images obtained of HNTs–kojic acid spread on a flat support. The presence of pure and functionalized HNTs was verified by SEM, as most of the sample consisted of cylindrical tubes [44]. The average particle size calculated from the SEM images was 400 nm.

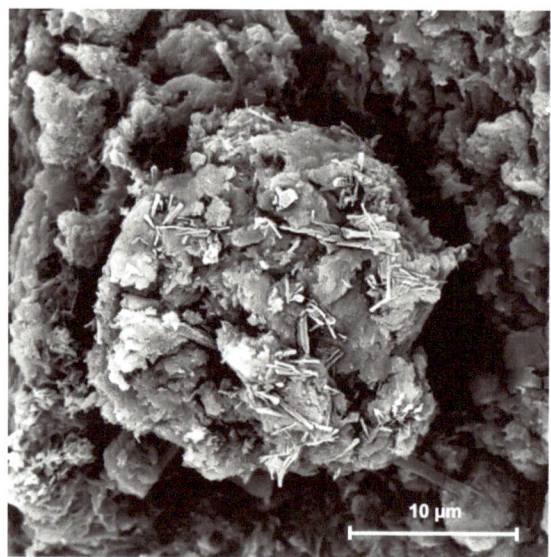

Figure 4. SEM image of HNTs–kojic acid.

The SEM-EDX elemental mapping of surface-modified HNTs–kojic acid is shown in Figure 5 and Table 1. The major constituents of HNTs are oxygen, aluminum, and silicon. The HNTs–kojic acid shows the presence of carbon, oxygen, silicon, and aluminum.

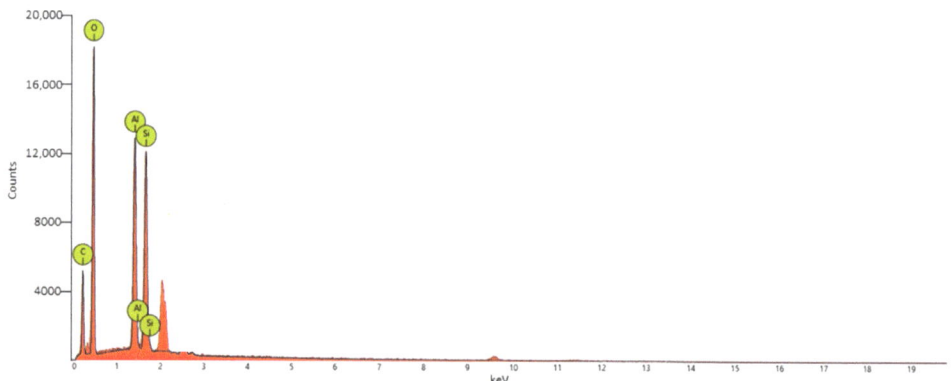

Figure 5. EDX spectrum of HNTs–kojic acid. The ordinate shows the counts, whereas the abscissa shows the keV. The unlabeled peaks at 2.1 and 9.6 keV correspond to gold, which is used to confer conductivity.

Table 1. Atomic and weight concentrations of HNTs–kojic acid obtained by EDX analysis.

Element Symbol	Atomic Conc. %	Weight Conc. %
O	45.27	45.06
C	40.70	30.41
Al	6.76	11.35
Si	6.22	10.87

3.2. Drug Loading and Release

Equations (1) and (2) describe the evaluation of drug-loading capacity (DLC) and encapsulation efficiency (EE) [35,45]:

$$DLC = \frac{loaded\ drug\ amount}{total\ HNTs - kojic\ amount} \quad (1)$$

$$EE = \frac{loaded\ drug\ amount}{total\ drug\ amount} \quad (2)$$

From Figure 6, it is clear that it is possible to obtain the highest EE with the highest amount of material. The results (DLC at a 1:1 loading ratio) are consistent with the literature concerning the release of resveratrol [35]. The same experiments were conducted with curcumin; once again, the DLC and EE values (Figure 7) detected by UV analysis were in excellent agreement with the literature [36,46,47].

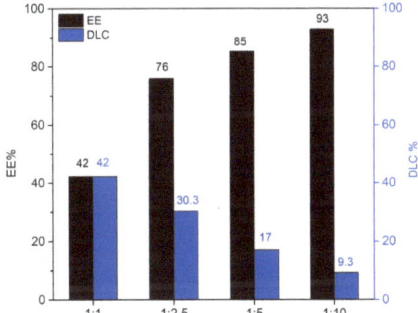

Figure 6. Encapsulation efficiency (EE) and drug-loading capacity (DLC) of resveratrol on the HNTs–kojic acid.

The difference between the loading capacity of resveratrol and curcumin with the HNTs–kojic acid system can be reasonably attributed, as reported in the literature, to the different solubility of the two drugs (resveratrol is weakly soluble in water, whereas curcumin is soluble in ethanol) [30,35,36,48]. However, the good interaction of the drugs with the peculiar nanotubular structure of the HNTs–kojic acid sample is promising for the possible application of this material in the field of drug carriers. The release kinetics of the drugs is reported in Figure 8. For these tests, we used the 1:1 resveratrol/HNTs–kojic acid and 1:100 curcumin/HNTs–kojic acid loading ratios to appreciate the drugs' release better. Consistent with the literature [30,35,49,50], up to 10 h, the release kinetics was relatively fast (about 40% for the resveratrol and 20% for the curcumin), after which the release became slower, with a waiver of 50% and about 30% in 20 h for the resveratrol and the curcumin, respectively, to reach 60% for the resveratrol and the 45% for the curcumin at 40 h. The latter drug was characterized by a slower kinetics compared to resveratrol. The quick drug release in the first hours was due to the rapid dissolution of the drugs adsorbed in the nanotubes of the halloysite, while the other drug molecules were gradually released from the sample surface, and this delivery was also affected by the diffusion phenomena.

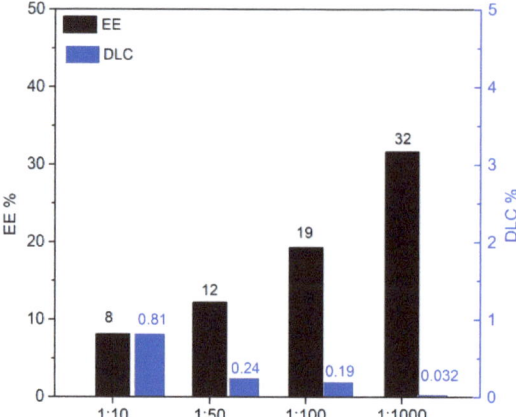

Figure 7. Encapsulation efficiency (EE) and drug-loading capacity (DLC) of curcumin on the HNTs–kojic acid.

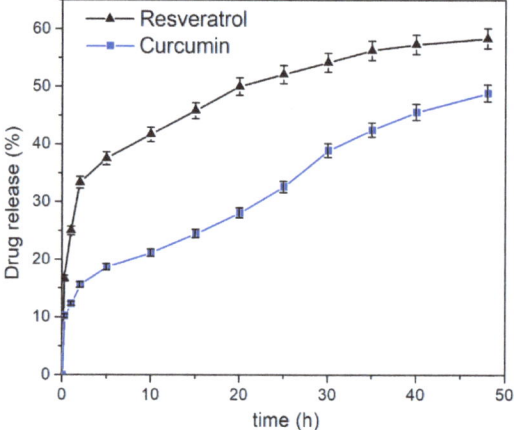

Figure 8. Release kinetics of resveratrol and curcumin from HNTs–kojic acid.

3.3. Microbiological Assays

The antibacterial assay was evaluated following CLSI guidelines. The results suggested that HNTs–kojic acid (**3**) had great antibacterial activity against all pathogens tested, with an MIC value equal to 3.0 mg, as shown in Figure 9. As evident from the bacterial growth curves, the new material demonstrated excellent antibacterial efficiency against both Gram-positive and Gram-negative strains.

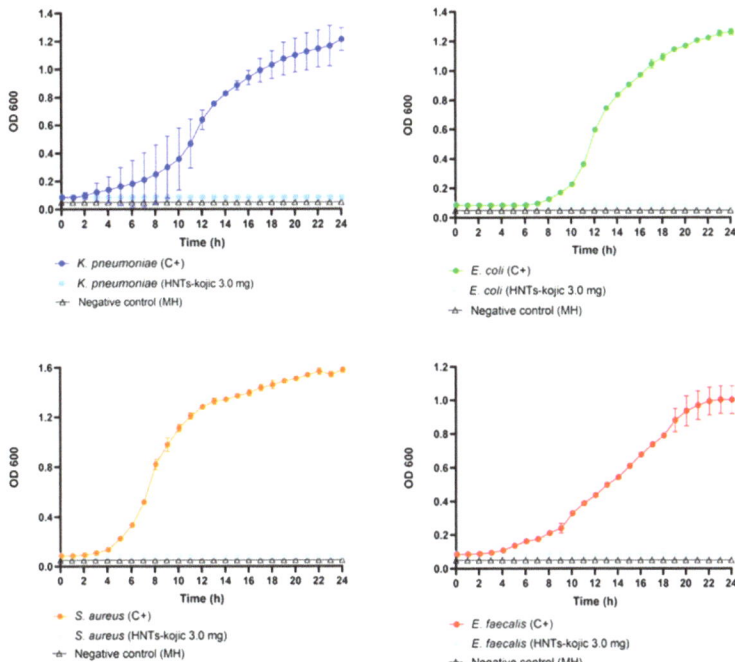

Figure 9. Growth curves (24 h) of the tested bacteria treated with the HNTs–kojic acid formulation.

4. Conclusions

The use of antibiotics in cancer therapy has advanced significantly, especially with the rapid development of nanomedicine. Significant efforts have been made to build nanosystems to improve the efficacy of medication delivery, adopt novel therapeutic agents or treatment modalities to reduce drug resistance, and implement local antimicrobial therapy. Nevertheless, there are always new difficulties associated with new approaches. Nanocarriers' size and surface charge are crucial, because they can affect the detection, adsorption, and removal of nanoparticles, influencing how widely distributed they are throughout the body. Even after they have reached the tumor site, smaller-scale nanoparticles in the circulatory system can be quickly cleared and leaked back into the circulation, whereas larger nanoparticles have strong retention but are unable to penetrate cells.

Antibacterial nanosystems have made impressive advances in cancer therapy overall, but there is still more work to be done before they can be used effectively and safely [51,52]. Because of their high biocompatibility and on-demand drug delivery, HNTs have received much interest recently in the biomedical area; by adding the appropriate chemotherapy or antibacterial medications, HNTs could be employed for antitumor or antibacterial treatments, as well as for the treatment of other diseases [29].

This work proposed the synthesis of a new nanomaterial based on HNTs and kojic acid (HNTs–kojic acid). HNTs–kojic acid was characterized by several techniques, and its iron chelation and drug delivery capabilities were well documented.

The system was developed to serve as a proof of concept of a dual-acting antibacterial nanomaterial with resveratrol/curcumin and iron-depletion properties for cancer and other infection-related applications. The chelating moiety of maltol was chemically bonded to the material, and the resveratrol/curcumin was incorporated into the HNTs cavity.

This new material proved that applying dual action due to the drug and the iron-chelating properties is possible with HNTs. Moreover, the results of the antibacterial evaluation conducted on this new formulation are auspicious. It was observed that, even at low concentrations, it exhibited antibacterial activity against both Gram-positive and Gram-negative bacteria. This suggests that the iron chelation action of the nanotubes is exceptionally efficient.

These findings open the way for further research and applications of the developed material in cancer treatment and other infection-related issues. Even if the use of HNTs in the treatment of tumors is still in the experimental stage, this new prototype material could have a wide range of applications in cancer and other fields, e.g., using HNTs–kojic acid with the already studied molecules, i.e., resveratrol or curcumin; using HNTs–kojic acid as a drug carrier for other molecules (antibacterial or others); reevaluation/potentiation of old antibiotics; or combined use of the aforementioned solutions.

Supplementary Materials: The following supporting information can be downloaded at: https://www.mdpi.com/article/10.3390/nano13142036/s1, Figure S1: UV spectra of the loading capacity of resveratrol on the HNTs–kojic acid system with different ratios. Figure S2: UV spectra of the loading capacity of curcumin on the HNTs–kojic acid system with different ratios. Figure S3: TGA of HNTs. Figure S4: TGA of **2**. Figure S5: TGA of **3**.

Author Contributions: Conceptualization, G.F. and V.P.; methodology, G.F., V.P., C.Z., R.F., V.F. and S.D.; validation, G.F., V.P., C.Z. and R.F.; investigation, G.F. and V.P.; resources, R.F., S.D., P.M.R., P.M.F. and A.R.; data curation, V.P., C.Z., R.F., P.M.R., V.F. and S.D.; writing—original draft preparation, G.F., V.P. and C.Z.; writing—review and editing, G.F. and A.R.; visualization, V.P. and C.Z.; supervision, V.P., P.M.F., G.F. and A.R.; project administration, G.F. and A.R., funding acquisition, A.R. All authors have read and agreed to the published version of the manuscript.

Funding: The research leading to these results received funding from the European Union—NextGenerationEU through the Italian Ministry of University and Research under PNRR—M4C2-I1.3 Project PE_00000019 "HEAL ITALIA" (Antonio Rescifina and Vincenzo Patamia), CUP E63C22002080006. The views and opinions expressed are those of the authors only and do not necessarily reflect those of the European Union or the European Commission. Neither the European Union nor the European Commission can be held responsible for them.

Data Availability Statement: Not applicable.

Conflicts of Interest: The authors declare no conflict of interest.

References

1. Siegel, R.L.; Miller, K.D.; Fuchs, H.E.; Jemal, A. Cancer statistics, 2022. *CA Cancer J. Clin.* **2022**, *72*, 7–33. [CrossRef] [PubMed]
2. Rao, J.; Yang, Y.; Pan Bei, H.; Tang, C.-Y.; Zhao, X. Antibacterial nanosystems for cancer therapy. *Biomater. Sci.* **2020**, *8*, 6814–6824. [CrossRef] [PubMed]
3. Xiao, L.; Zhang, Q.; Peng, Y.; Wang, D.; Liu, Y. The effect of periodontal bacteria infection on incidence and prognosis of cancer: A systematic review and meta-analysis. *Medicine* **2020**, *99*, e19698. [CrossRef] [PubMed]
4. Kalia, V.C.; Patel, S.K.S.; Cho, B.-K.; Wood, T.K.; Lee, J.-K. Emerging applications of bacteria as antitumor agents. *Semin. Cancer Biol.* **2022**, *86*, 1014–1025. [CrossRef]
5. Yadegarynia, D.; Tarrand, J.; Raad, I.; Rolston, K. Current spectrum of bacterial infections in patients with cancer. *Clin. Infect. Dis.* **2003**, *37*, 1144–1145. [CrossRef] [PubMed]
6. Simões, D.; Miguel, S.P.; Ribeiro, M.P.; Coutinho, P.; Mendonça, A.G.; Correia, I.J. Recent advances on antimicrobial wound dressing: A review. *Eur. J. Pharm. Biopharm.* **2018**, *127*, 130–141. [CrossRef]
7. Lascelles, B.D.; Dernell, W.S.; Correa, M.T.; Lafferty, M.; Devitt, C.M.; Kuntz, C.A.; Straw, R.C.; Withrow, S.J. Improved survival associated with postoperative wound infection in dogs treated with limb-salvage surgery for osteosarcoma. *Ann. Surg. Oncol.* **2005**, *12*, 1073–1083. [CrossRef]
8. Saha, M.; Sarkar, A. Review on Multiple Facets of Drug Resistance: A Rising Challenge in the 21st Century. *J. Xenobiot.* **2021**, *11*, 197–214. [CrossRef]
9. Repac Antić, D.; Parčina, M.; Gobin, I.; Petković Didović, M. Chelation in Antibacterial Drugs: From Nitroxoline to Cefiderocol and Beyond. *Antibiotics* **2022**, *11*, 1105. [CrossRef]
10. Boyd, N.K.; Teng, C.; Frei, C.R. Brief Overview of Approaches and Challenges in New Antibiotic Development: A Focus On Drug Repurposing. *Front. Cell. Infect. Microbiol.* **2021**, *11*, 684515. [CrossRef]
11. Santos, A.L.; Sodre, C.L.; Valle, R.S.; Silva, B.A.; Abi-Chacra, E.A.; Silva, L.V.; Souza-Goncalves, A.L.; Sangenito, L.S.; Goncalves, D.S.; Souza, L.O.; et al. Antimicrobial action of chelating agents: Repercussions on the microorganism development, virulence and pathogenesis. *Curr. Med. Chem.* **2012**, *19*, 2715–2737. [CrossRef] [PubMed]

12. Ghanem, S.; Kim, C.J.; Dutta, D.; Salifu, M.; Lim, S.H. Antimicrobial therapy during cancer treatment: Beyond antibacterial effects. *J. Intern. Med.* **2021**, *290*, 40–56. [CrossRef] [PubMed]
13. Ren, R.; Lim, C.; Li, S.; Wang, Y.; Song, J.; Lin, T.-W.; Muir, B.W.; Hsu, H.-Y.; Shen, H.-H. Recent Advances in the Development of Lipid-, Metal-, Carbon-, and Polymer-Based Nanomaterials for Antibacterial Applications. *Nanomaterials* **2022**, *12*, 3855. [CrossRef]
14. Yougbaré, S.; Mutalik, C.; Okoro, G.; Lin, I.H.; Krisnawati, D.I.; Jazidie, A.; Nuh, M.; Chang, C.C.; Kuo, T.R. Emerging Trends in Nanomaterials for Antibacterial Applications. *Int. J. Nanomed.* **2021**, *16*, 5831–5867. [CrossRef]
15. Shi, J.; Kantoff, P.W.; Wooster, R.; Farokhzad, O.C. Cancer nanomedicine: Progress, challenges and opportunities. *Nat. Rev. Cancer* **2017**, *17*, 20–37. [CrossRef]
16. Floresta, G.; Abbate, V. Recent progress in the imaging of c-Met aberrant cancers with positron emission tomography. *Med. Res. Rev.* **2022**, *42*, 1588–1606. [CrossRef] [PubMed]
17. Floresta, G.; Memdouh, S.; Pham, T.; Ma, M.T.; Blower, P.J.; Hider, R.C.; Abbate, V.; Cilibrizzi, A. Targeting integrin αvβ6 with gallium-68 tris (hydroxypyridinone) based PET probes. *Dalton Trans.* **2022**, *51*, 12796–12803. [CrossRef]
18. Failla, M.; Floresta, G.; Abbate, V. Peptide-based positron emission tomography probes: Current strategies for synthesis and radiolabelling. *RSC Med. Chem.* **2023**. [CrossRef]
19. Floresta, G.; Keeling, G.P.; Memdouh, S.; Meszaros, L.K.; de Rosales, R.T.M.; Abbate, V. NHS-Functionalized THP Derivative for Efficient Synthesis of Kit-Based Precursors for 68Ga Labeled PET Probes. *Biomedicines* **2021**, *9*, 367. [CrossRef]
20. Cilibrizzi, A.; Pourzand, C.; Abbate, V.; Reelfs, O.; Versari, L.; Floresta, G.; Hider, R. The synthesis and properties of mitochondrial targeted iron chelators. *Biometals* **2022**. [CrossRef]
21. Fang, X.; Wang, C.; Zhou, S.; Cui, P.; Hu, H.; Ni, X.; Jiang, P.; Wang, J. Hydrogels for Antitumor and Antibacterial Therapy. *Gels* **2022**, *8*, 315. [CrossRef] [PubMed]
22. Zagni, C.; Coco, A.; Patamia, V.; Floresta, G.; Curcuruto, G.; Mangano, K.; Mecca, T.; Rescifina, A.; Carroccio, S. Cyclodextrin-Based Cryogels for Controlled Drug Delivery. *Med. Sci. Forum* **2022**, *14*, 150. [CrossRef]
23. Zagni, C.; Dattilo, S.; Mecca, T.; Gugliuzzo, C.; Scamporrino, A.A.; Privitera, V.; Puglisi, R.; Carola Carroccio, S. Single and dual polymeric sponges for emerging pollutants removal. *Eur. Polym. J.* **2022**, *179*, 111556. [CrossRef]
24. Zagni, C.; Scamporrino, A.A.; Riccobene, P.M.; Floresta, G.; Patamia, V.; Rescifina, A.; Carroccio, S.C. Portable Nanocomposite System for Wound Healing in Space. *Nanomaterials* **2023**, *13*, 741. [CrossRef]
25. Price, R.R.; Gaber, B.P.; Lvov, Y. In-vitro release characteristics of tetracycline HCl, khellin and nicotinamide adenine dineculeotide from halloysite; a cylindrical mineral. *J. Microencapsul.* **2001**, *18*, 713–722. [CrossRef]
26. Lvov, Y.M.; Shchukin, D.G.; Möhwald, H.; Price, R.R. Halloysite clay nanotubes for controlled release of protective agents. *ACS Nano* **2008**, *2*, 814–820. [CrossRef]
27. Hasani, M.; Abdouss, M.; Shojaei, S. Nanocontainers for drug delivery systems: A review of Halloysite nanotubes and their properties. *Int. J. Artif. Organs.* **2021**, *44*, 426–433. [CrossRef]
28. Jha, R.; Singh, A.; Sharma, P.K.; Fuloria, N.K. Smart carbon nanotubes for drug delivery system: A comprehensive study. *J. Drug Deliv. Sci. Technol.* **2020**, *58*, 101811. [CrossRef]
29. Biddeci, G.; Spinelli, G.; Colomba, P.; Di Blasi, F. Nanomaterials: A Review about Halloysite Nanotubes, Properties, and Application in the Biological Field. *Int. J. Mol. Sci.* **2022**, *23*, 1518. [CrossRef]
30. Vergaro, V.; Lvov, Y.M.; Leporatti, S. Halloysite Clay Nanotubes for Resveratrol Delivery to Cancer Cells. *Macromol. Biosci.* **2012**, *12*, 1265–1271. [CrossRef]
31. Giordano, A.; Tommonaro, G. Curcumin and Cancer. *Nutrients* **2019**, *11*, 2376. [CrossRef] [PubMed]
32. Brisdelli, F.; D'Andrea, G.; Bozzi, A. Resveratrol: A natural polyphenol with multiple chemopreventive properties. *Curr. Drug Metab.* **2009**, *10*, 530–546. [CrossRef]
33. Gülçin, İ. Antioxidant properties of resveratrol: A structure–activity insight. *Innov. Food Sci. Emerg. Technol.* **2010**, *11*, 210–218. [CrossRef]
34. Ma, Y.; Luo, W.; Quinn, P.J.; Liu, Z.; Hider, R.C. Design, Synthesis, Physicochemical Properties, and Evaluation of Novel Iron Chelators with Fluorescent Sensors. *J. Med. Chem.* **2004**, *47*, 6349–6362. [CrossRef] [PubMed]
35. Patamia, V.; Fiorenza, R.; Brullo, I.; Zambito Marsala, M.; Balsamo, S.A.; Distefano, A.; Furneri, P.M.; Barbera, V.; Scirè, S.; Rescifina, A. A sustainable porous composite material based on loofah-halloysite for gas adsorption and drug delivery. *Mater. Chem. Front.* **2022**, *6*, 2233–2243. [CrossRef]
36. Dionisi, C.; Hanafy, N.; Nobile, C.; Giorgi, M.L.D.; Rinaldi, R.; Casciaro, S.; Lvov, Y.M.; Leporatti, S. Halloysite Clay Nanotubes as Carriers for Curcumin: Characterization and Application. *IEEE Trans. Nanotechnol.* **2016**, *15*, 720–724. [CrossRef]
37. CLSI. *M100: Performance Standards for Antimicrobial Susceptibility Testing*, 32nd. ed.; Clinical Laboratory Standards Institute: Wayne, PA, USA, 2022.
38. Vestergaard, M.; Ingmer, H. Antibacterial and antifungal properties of resveratrol. *Int. J. Antimicrob. Agents* **2019**, *53*, 716–723. [CrossRef]
39. Moghadamtousi, S.Z.; Kadir, H.A.; Hassandarvish, P.; Tajik, H.; Abubakar, S.; Zandi, K. A review on antibacterial, antiviral, and antifungal activity of curcumin. *Biomed. Res. Int.* **2014**, *2014*, 186864. [CrossRef]

40. Munir, Z.; Banche, G.; Cavallo, L.; Mandras, N.; Roana, J.; Pertusio, R.; Ficiarà, E.; Cavalli, R.; Guiot, C. Exploitation of the Antibacterial Properties of Photoactivated Curcumin as 'Green' Tool for Food Preservation. *Int. J. Mol. Sci.* **2022**, *23*, 2600. [CrossRef]
41. Patamia, V.; Tomarchio, R.; Fiorenza, R.; Zagni, C.; Scirè, S.; Floresta, G.; Rescifina, A. Carbamoyl-Decorated Cyclodextrins for Carbon Dioxide Adsorption. *Catalysts* **2023**, *13*, 41. [CrossRef]
42. Baharfar, R.; Alinezhad, H.; Azimi, R. Use of DABCO-functionalized mesoporous SBA-15 as catalyst for efficient synthesis of kojic acid derivatives, potential antioxidants. *Res. Chem. Intermed.* **2015**, *41*, 8637–8650. [CrossRef]
43. Andrade, G.F.; Lima, G.d.S.; Gastelois, P.L.; Assis Gomes, D.; Macedo, W.A.d.A.; de Sousa, E.M.B. Surface modification and biological evaluation of kojic acid/silica nanoparticles as platforms for biomedical systems. *Int. J. Appl. Ceram. Technol.* **2020**, *17*, 380–391. [CrossRef]
44. Murphy, Z.; Kent, M.; Freeman, C.; Landge, S.; Koricho, E. Halloysite nanotubes functionalized with epoxy and thiol organosilane groups to improve fracture toughness in nanocomposites. *SN Appl. Sci.* **2020**, *2*, 2130. [CrossRef]
45. Zhao, Y.; Cai, C.; Liu, M.; Zhao, Y.; Wu, Y.; Fan, Z.; Ding, Z.; Zhang, H.; Wang, Z.; Han, J. Drug-binding albumins forming stabilized nanoparticles for co-delivery of paclitaxel and resveratrol: In vitro/in vivo evaluation and binding properties investigation. *Int. J. Biol. Macromol.* **2020**, *153*, 873–882. [CrossRef] [PubMed]
46. Liu, M.; Chang, Y.; Yang, J.; You, Y.; He, R.; Chen, T.; Zhou, C. Functionalized halloysite nanotube by chitosan grafting for drug delivery of curcumin to achieve enhanced anticancer efficacy. *J. Mater. Chem. B* **2016**, *4*, 2253–2263. [CrossRef] [PubMed]
47. Rao, K.M.; Kumar, A.; Suneetha, M.; Han, S.S. pH and near-infrared active; chitosan-coated halloysite nanotubes loaded with curcumin-Au hybrid nanoparticles for cancer drug delivery. *Int. J. Biol. Macromol.* **2018**, *112*, 119–125. [CrossRef] [PubMed]
48. Chanphai, P.; Tajmir-Riahi, H.A. Encapsulation of micronutrients resveratrol, genistein, and curcumin by folic acid-PAMAM nanoparticles. *Mol. Cell. Biochem.* **2018**, *449*, 157–166. [CrossRef] [PubMed]
49. Farokh, A.; Pourmadadi, M.; Rashedi, H.; Yazdian, F.; Navaei-Nigjeh, M. Assessment of synthesized chitosan/halloysite nanocarrier modified by carbon nanotube for pH-sensitive delivery of curcumin to cancerous media. *Int. J. Biol. Macromol.* **2023**, *237*, 123937. [CrossRef] [PubMed]
50. Nyankson, E.; Awuzah, D.; Tiburu, E.K.; Efavi, J.K.; Agyei-Tuffour, B.; Paemka, L. Curcumin loaded Ag–TiO2-halloysite nanotubes platform for combined chemo-photodynamic therapy treatment of cancer cells. *RSC Adv.* **2022**, *12*, 33108–33123. [CrossRef]
51. Tiwari, S.; Juneja, S.; Ghosal, A.; Bandara, N.; Khan, R.; Wallen, S.L.; Ramakrishna, S.; Kaushik, A. Antibacterial and antiviral high-performance nanosystems to mitigate new SARS-CoV-2 variants of concern. *Curr. Opin. Biomed. Eng.* **2022**, *21*, 100363. [CrossRef]
52. Ermini, M.L.; Voliani, V. Antimicrobial Nano-Agents: The Copper Age. *ACS Nano* **2021**, *15*, 6008–6029. [CrossRef] [PubMed]

Disclaimer/Publisher's Note: The statements, opinions and data contained in all publications are solely those of the individual author(s) and contributor(s) and not of MDPI and/or the editor(s). MDPI and/or the editor(s) disclaim responsibility for any injury to people or property resulting from any ideas, methods, instructions or products referred to in the content.

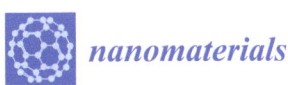

Article

Exploiting Blood Transport Proteins as Carborane Supramolecular Vehicles for Boron Neutron Capture Therapy

Tainah Dorina Marforio *, Edoardo Jun Mattioli, Francesco Zerbetto and Matteo Calvaresi *

Dipartimento di Chimica "Giacomo Ciamician", Alma Mater Studiorum-Università di Bologna, Via Francesco Selmi 2, 40126 Bologna, Italy; edoardojun.mattioli2@unibo.it (E.J.M.); francesco.zerbetto@unibo.it (F.Z.)
* Correspondence: tainah.marforio2@unibo.it (T.D.M.); matteo.calvaresi3@unibo.it (M.C.)

Abstract: Carboranes are promising agents for applications in boron neutron capture therapy (BNCT), but their hydrophobicity prevents their use in physiological environments. Here, by using reverse docking and molecular dynamics (MD) simulations, we identified blood transport proteins as candidate carriers of carboranes. Hemoglobin showed a higher binding affinity for carboranes than transthyretin and human serum albumin (HSA), which are well-known carborane-binding proteins. Myoglobin, ceruloplasmin, sex hormone-binding protein, lactoferrin, plasma retinol-binding protein, thyroxine-binding globulin, corticosteroid-binding globulin and afamin have a binding affinity comparable to transthyretin/HSA. The carborane@protein complexes are stable in water and characterized by favorable binding energy. The driving force in the carborane binding is represented by the formation of hydrophobic interactions with aliphatic amino acids and BH-π and CH-π interactions with aromatic amino acids. Dihydrogen bonds, classical hydrogen bonds and surfactant-like interactions also assist the binding. These results (i) identify the plasma proteins responsible for binding carborane upon their intravenous administration, and (ii) suggest an innovative formulation for carboranes based on the formation of a carborane@protein complex prior to the administration.

Keywords: carborane; boron neutron capture therapy (BNCT); virtual screening; docking; reverse docking; MD simulations; MM-GBSA; plasma proteins

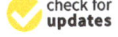

Citation: Marforio, T.D.; Mattioli, E.J.; Zerbetto, F.; Calvaresi, M. Exploiting Blood Transport Proteins as Carborane Supramolecular Vehicles for Boron Neutron Capture Therapy. *Nanomaterials* 2023, 13, 1770. https://doi.org/10.3390/nano13111770

Academic Editor: James Chow

Received: 21 April 2023
Revised: 26 May 2023
Accepted: 28 May 2023
Published: 31 May 2023

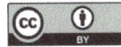

Copyright: © 2023 by the authors. Licensee MDPI, Basel, Switzerland. This article is an open access article distributed under the terms and conditions of the Creative Commons Attribution (CC BY) license (https://creativecommons.org/licenses/by/4.0/).

1. Introduction

Boron neutron capture therapy (BNCT) is a non-invasive binary approach for the treatment of difficult-to-cure tumors such as glioblastoma multiforme or head and neck cancers [1–6]. The effectiveness of BNCT is based on the adequate and selective accumulation of ^{10}B in the tumor tissue (approximately 10^9 atoms/cell), followed by irradiation with a thermal neutron beam. The fission reaction that occurs upon the neutron beam irradiation on the boron atom (^{10}B[n,α] ^{7}Li) produces a high linear energy transfer (LET) alpha particle (^{4}He), a recoiled lithium nucleus (^{7}Li) and γ radiation (0.48 MeV). The alpha particles, which have a LET in the range of 50–230 keV/μm, also possess a very short travel distance, causing their energy to be released within the diameter of the cell (Bragg's peak). Thus, BNCT is potentially highly selective, since only the cells that have accumulated enough boron are destroyed by the radiation. Low uptake and toxicity in healthy cells and persistence in the malignant tissues are the requirements for effective BNCT agents. The first boron-containing compounds employed in BNCT were based on boric acids and their derivatives (first-generation compounds). In the 1980s, concomitantly with the improvement of neutron beam sources, BPA (boronphenylalanine) and BSH (sodium borocaptate) were extensively employed in BNCT, and were authorized for clinical trials [7].

Nowadays, third-generation agents are emerging as potential drugs for BNCT clinical applications, such as boronated natural and non-natural amino acids [8,9], boronated drugs [10], nucleosides [11,12], porphyrines [13–15], antibodies [16] and carbohydrates [17].

Boron-based nanomaterials [18–21], such as polymers [22], liposomes [23–26], boron nitride [20,27] and other types of nanoparticles, were also developed [28–33].

Icosahedral carborane (1,2-C2B10H12) [4,34,35], which belongs to the family of closo-carboranes, promises to be a good boron agent candidate in BNCT because of (i) the presence of 10 boron atoms per molecule, (ii) its abiotic nature, which prevents metabolism and resistance by the living organism, and (iii) its chemical structure, which provides the cage with a strong hydrophobic character (3D aromaticity of the carborane cage) [36,37] facilitating the crossing of hydrophobic membranes, such as the cellular membrane [38–42]. On the other hand, the hydrophobicity of carboranes hampers their direct administration, being insoluble in blood; for their administration, organic solvents [43,44] or co-formulants [13,45–47] are usually used. The formation of complexes between the blood transport proteins and the carborane governs its cellular uptake and biodistribution. Human serum albumin (HSA) is one of the best biocompatible excipients for the solubilization and de-aggregation of cobalt bis(dicarbollide) derivatives in water [48]. Metallacarboranes bind to the surface of HSA [49] and hydrophobic interactions govern the binding because the binding affinity correlates with the lipophilicity of the metallacarborane derivatives [50].

The design of carriers able to transport carboranes in a physiological environment is a pressing task for BNCT's transition from an experimental modality to a widely accepted clinical approach.

The idea of employing proteins as hydrophilic carriers for hydrophobic drugs represents a novel and smart strategy to generate a biocompatible and water-soluble system for nanomedical and theranostic approaches [51–54]. Proteins are ideal supramolecular hosts for carrying and delivering carboranes since they meet the requirements of biocompatibility and water solubility and are naturally recognized by cells. Carborane has already demonstrated its ability to interact strongly with protein-binding sites; in fact, carborane derivatives have been used as inhibitors for many proteins such as HIV protease, human carbonic anhydrase, estrogen and androgen receptor, dihydrofolate reductase, translocator protein, retinoic acid receptor and retinoid X receptors, transthyretin, cyclooxygenase-2 and others [55,56].

Carboranes can generate a variety of intermolecular interactions (Scheme 1) with amino acids due to the presence of both acidic C-H and hydridic B-H groups, i.e., those bound to carbon and boron atoms, respectively: (i) "classical" hydrogen bonds (HB) between the acidic C-H groups of the carborane and a hydrogen bond acceptor (C–H···X), (ii) dihydrogen bonds (HH) between the hydridic B-H groups of the cage and a hydrogen bond donor (B–H···H–X), (iii) CH···π interactions between the acidic C-H groups of the carborane and aromatic residues, (iv) BH···π interactions between the hydridic B-H groups of the carborane and aromatic groups [37,57–61] and (vi) surfactant-like interactions where the non-polar portion of an amphiphilic molecule interacts with the hydrophobic cage of the carborane while the polar part protrudes in the solvent.

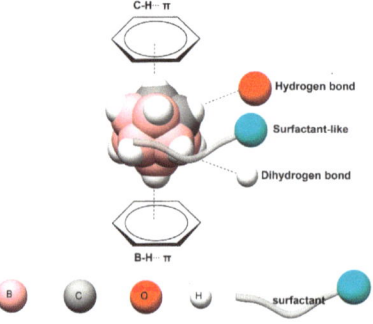

Scheme 1. Representation of the possible intermolecular interactions that can be generated between carborane and the protein-binding pockets.

Proteins, acting as Trojan horses [56,62,63], can also promote the accumulation of boron in the tumor tissue by taking advantage of the enhanced permeability and retention (EPR) effect and the tumor-targeting activity of some specific proteins [64–66].

Among the human proteome, blood transport proteins are the natural carriers of endogenous and exogenous hydrophobic molecules in the bloodstream [67]. Blood transport proteins have well-defined binding pockets for the transport of non-soluble compounds [67]. Human serum albumin (HSA), the most abundant protein in blood, and α-fetoprotein (AFP) and afamin are responsible for the binding of fatty acids, exogenous drugs and hormones [67]; vitamin D-binding protein (DBP), thyroxine-binding globulin (TBG), transthyretin (TTR), corticosteroid-binding globulin (CBG), sex hormone-binding globulin (SHBG) and plasma retinol-binding protein (RBP) carry hormones, steroids and vitamins in plasma [67]. Other proteins, such as hemoglobin (Hb), myoglobin (Mb), hemopexin (HPX) and haptoglobin (Hp), are heme-binding proteins and they are generally responsible for the transport of oxygen and carbon dioxide [67], while ceruloplasmin (CP), serotransferrin (TF), lactotransferrin (LF) and ferritin (FT) are involved in iron/copper transport and storage [67].

Carboranes are highly hydrophobic [36,37], and their transport in blood as pristine moieties is hardly possible. The notion of using plasma proteins as potential carriers of hydrophobic species is rather straightforward. In addition, the different chemical moieties present on the protein surface can be chemically functionalized with (i) targeting tags able to improve both the cell selectivity and promote the selective uptake of the carborane@protein hybrid in cancer therapy and (ii) imaging tags to create innovative, protein-based theranostic platforms [68].

Some of the blood transport plasma proteins can also be uptaken by cancer cells via active targeting: cancer cells can selectively accumulate human serum albumin and transferrin because of the high expression levels of albumin-binding proteins (gp60 and SPARC) and transferrin receptors. BNCT was clinically approved for head and neck cancers; it is well known that many head and neck cancers overexpress SPARC and transferrin receptors [69,70]. So, the use of HSA and transferrin as carborane carriers can be potentially exploited for the development of boron neutron capture targeted therapy.

HSA and transferrin are also effective carriers for delivery across the blood–brain barrier, and the dispersion of carborane by these proteins can be an opportunity for the application of BNCT to brain cancers [71].

Therefore, in this work, a reverse docking approach was used to investigate the interaction of blood plasma with carborane. Molecular dynamics (MD) simulations, followed by molecular mechanics/generalized Born surface area (MM-GBSA) analysis, quantitatively evaluated the affinity of carborane to blood transport proteins. This approach allows for (i) the identification of the most promising proteins to act as carriers for carborane in blood, (ii) the characterization of the carborane-binding pocket(s) and (iii) the determination of the nature of the non-covalent interactions between the amino acids of the protein and the ligand.

2. Materials and Methods

2.1. Blood Transport Protein Structural Database

Blood transport proteins were identified following the classification of Schaller [67]. When the 3D structures of the proteins are experimentally available, they were downloaded from the Protein Data Bank [72]. When multiple PDBs were available, a representative structure was identified, using as selecting criteria the completeness of the sequence, the absence of mutations and the highest resolution. These structures, reported in Table 1, were cleaned of their co-crystallized ligands, ions and water molecules. When the 3D structure was not experimentally available, as in the case of hemopexin, the computed structure model (CSM) was used [73].

Table 1. Structural database of blood transport protein structures used.

Protein	PDB/UNIPROT ID	Protein Concentration
Albumin	1N5U	42 mg/mL [74]
Afamin	6FAK	35 µg/mL [74]
α-fetoprotein	7YIM	20 ng/mL [75]
Cerulosplasmin	4ENZ	64.9 µg/mL [74]
Corticosteroid-binding globulin	2VDX	1.2 µg/mL [76]
Haptoglobulin	4X0L	1.1 mg/mL [74]
Hemoglobin	5HY8	41 µg/mL [74]
Hemopexin	P02790	257 µg/mL [74]
Lactotransferrin	1CB6	270 ng/mL [74]
Myoglobin	3RGK	210 ng/mL [76]
Plasma retinol-binding protein	5NU7	32 µg/mL [74]
Serotransferrin	6SOY	1.5 mg/mL [74]
Sex hormone-binding globulin	6PYF	260 µg/mL [76]
Thyroxine-binding globulin	2RIV	1.3 µg/mL [76]
Transthyretin	4QXV	109.6 µg/mL [74]
Vitamin D-binding protein	1KW2	62.36 µg/mL [74]

2.2. Docking and Refinement

The *ortho*-carborane structure was used as a representative of the closo-carboranes, due to its higher stability compared to meta- and para-carboranes. Docking calculations were carried out using the ortho-carborane structure and the blood transport proteins structural database, using the PatchDock algorithm [77], which is a valid tool for generating poses for rigid and spherical ligand molecules such as fullerenes [78–86], carbon nanotubes [87–90] and carboranes [55]. All the carborane@protein complexes obtained as poses of the docking procedure were then refined by minimization and MM-GBSA calculations. The first 50 poses, sorted by binding affinity, were further refined by 1 ns MD simulation followed by MM-GBSA calculations. For the complex of each blood transport protein, characterized by the highest affinity, 100 ns of MD simulations were carried out. In the case of human serum albumin (HSA), a refinement of 100 ns was carried out for all the possible binding pockets.

2.3. MD Simulations

The FF14SB force field [91], as implemented in Amber, was used to describe the proteins, while an ad hoc force field was used for the ortho-carborane, combining the GAFF force field with the parameters developed by Sarosi et al. [92]. In all simulations, the carborane@protein complexes were solvated by explicit water molecules (TIP3P model) and Na^+ and Cl^- counterions were added to neutralize the total charge of the system. Periodic boundary condition (PBC) and the particle mesh Ewald summations, with a cut-off radius of 10.0 Å, were used during all the simulations. RMSD values of carborane@protein complexes (see Figures S1–S15) were calculated using CPPTRAJ [93].

2.4. Molecular Mechanics/Generalized Born Surface Area (MM-GBSA) Calculations

From each MD trajectory, 1000 frames were extracted by CPPTRAJ [93] and employed as input for the MM-GBSA analysis [94]. The MM-GBSA analysis was carried out using the MM-PBSA.py module, considering an infinite cut-off in the calculation of the electrostatic and van der Waals (vdW) interactions. The generalized Born (GB) model developed by Hawkins and coworkers (GB^{HCT}) was used to compute the polar solvation term [95,96], whereas the non-polar solvation term was determined using solvent-accessible, surface-area-dependent terms. A fingerprint analysis, based on the decomposition of the total binding energy on a per-residue basis, offers the possibility to identify the protein residues more responsible for the binding of the ligand.

3. Results and Discussion

3.1. Identification of Blood Transport Proteins as Carriers for Carborane by Virtual Screening

A protocol of reverse docking was used to identify the propensity of the blood transport proteins to bind carborane. Figure 1 shows the strength of the interaction between blood transport proteins and carboranes, as calculated by the MD simulation followed by MM-GBSA analysis. The binding between carborane derivatives and HSA [18,49,97–100] and transthyretin [101] has already been experimentally demonstrated.

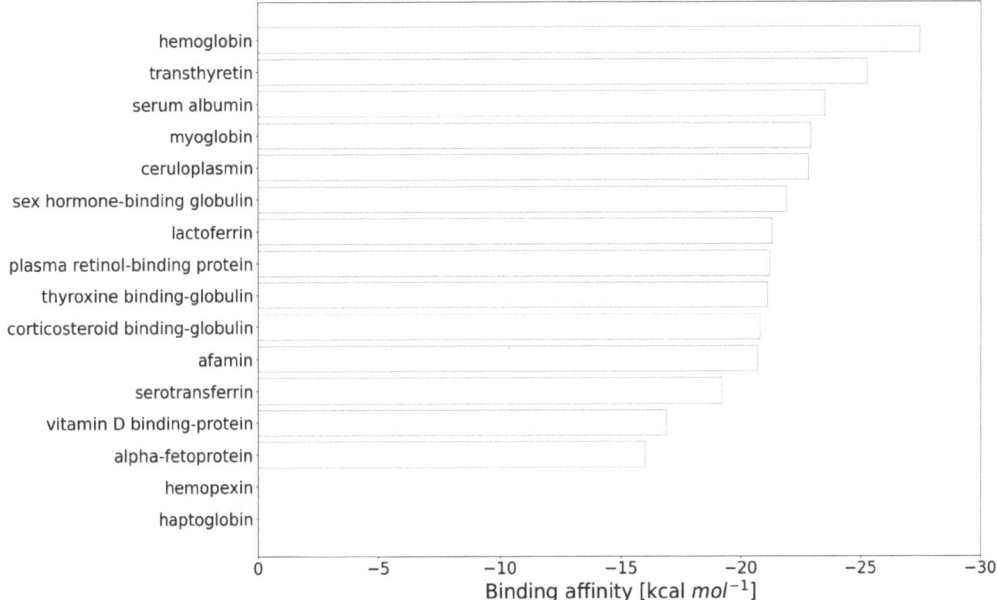

Figure 1. Binding affinity (kcal mol^{-1}) of the blood transport proteins for the carborane, sorted by the affinity for the ligand.

Hemoglobin has a stronger binding with carborane (-27.5 kcal mol^{-1}) with respect to transthyretin (-25.3 kcal mol^{-1}) and serum albumin (-23.5 kcal mol^{-1}). Eight other proteins, i.e., myoglobin (-22.9 kcal mol^{-1}), ceruloplasmin (-22.9 kcal mol^{-1}), sex hormone-binding protein (-22.5 kcal mol^{-1}), lactoferrin (-21.3 kcal mol^{-1}), plasma retinol-binding protein (-21.2 kcal mol^{-1}), thyroxine-binding globulin ($-21,1$ kcal mol^{-1}), corticosteroid-binding globulin (-20.8 kcal mol^{-1}) and afamin (-20.7 kcal mol^{-1}), show a binding affinity comparable (higher than 20 kcal mol^{-1}) to transthyretin and HSA, and can potentially bind carborane.

3.2. Carborane@HSA

Serum albumin (HSA) is the most abundant protein in the blood. HSA is responsible for the binding of fatty acids, exogenous drugs and hormones [67]. HSA has already demonstrated its ability to bind carborane derivatives [18,49,97–100].

The interactions of the carborane moieties with HSA were ascribed to the formation of hydrophobic interactions between the lipophilic cage of the carborane and the non-polar binding pockets of HSA.

Nevertheless, to our knowledge, the structural characterization of the carborane@HSA complex has never been reported. Following the proposed docking approach, we identified the most probable binding sites for carborane in HSA. The carborane occupies all the binding pockets that are specific for fatty acids (FA1–7), and the cleft site (Figure 2). The highly hydrophobic nature of the carborane explains its tendency to bind in the HSA pockets where hydrophobic molecules, such as warfarin (Sudlow's 1), ibuprofen (FA6), iodipamide (cleft), oxyphenbutazone (FA5) and diazepam (FA3,4), usually bind to HSA. Two additional binding pockets for the carborane were also identified. The binding affinity computed for the carborane in each of the nine pockets is reported in Figure 2B.

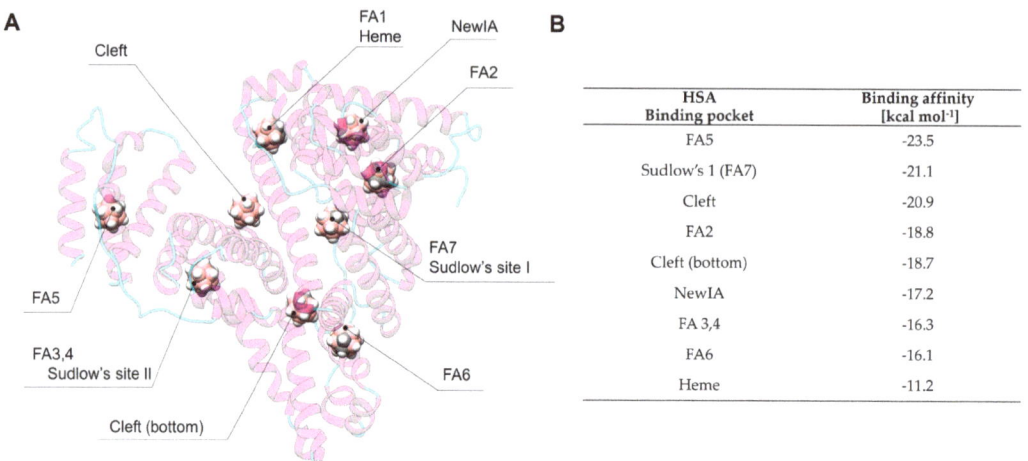

Figure 2. (**A**) The most probable carborane-binding sites in HSA; (**B**) the binding affinity of carborane for the HSA pockets computed by MM−GBSA approach after 100 ns of MD simulation in explicit water.

After 100 ns MD simulations, the three most favorable binding pockets were found to be FA5 (−23.5 kcal mol^{-1}), Sudlow's I (−21.1 kcal mol^{-1}) and the cleft region (−20.9 kcal mol^{-1}). Our results suggest that FA5, located in domain III of HSA, is the principal site for carborane binding in HSA. Carborane interacts with Phe554 (−1.3 kcal mol^{-1}) and Phe551 (−1.3 kcal mol^{-1}) by BH-π and CH-π interactions (Figure 3A). Leu529 (−0.9 kcal mol^{-1}) and Ala528 (−0.8 kcal mol^{-1}) give non-polar interactions with the carborane, while Lys525 (−0.8 kcal mol^{-1}) is characterized by a surfactant-like interaction: the aliphatic side-chain of Lys binds the hydrophobic surface of the carborane, while its hydrophilic head interacts with water.

At Sudlow's site I (Figure 3B), the carborane cage interacts by BH-π interactions with Trp214 (−2.0 kcal mol^{-1}) and with Phe212 (−1.1 kcal mol^{-1}). Leu198 (−1.0 kcal mol^{-1}) and Leu481 (−1.0 kcal mol^{-1}) are other residues responsible for the binding via hydrophobic interactions. Also in this binding pocket, similarly to Lys525 in FA5, Lys199 (−1.0 kcal mol^{-1}) gives surfactant-like interactions.

When carborane is located in the cleft (Figure 3C), only non-polar amino acids are responsible for the binding, specifically Val426 (−1.0 kcal mol^{-1}), Val455 (−1.0 kcal mol^{-1}), Leu430 (−0.9 kcal mol^{-1}), Ala191 (−0.9 kcal mol^{-1}) and Val456 (−0.8 kcal mol^{-1}).

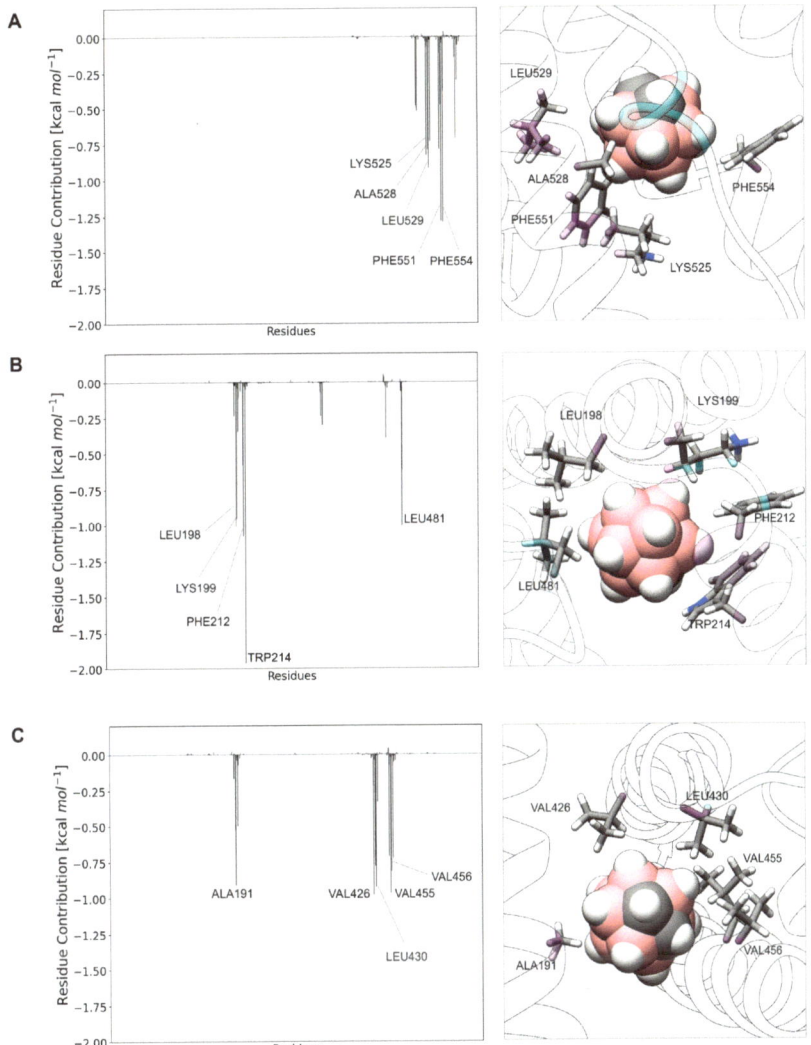

Figure 3. Fingerprint analysis and 3D representation of the interactions between carborane and HSA in the (**A**) FA5-binding pocket, (**B**) Sudlow's site I and (**C**) cleft region.

3.3. Carborane@transthyretin

Transthyretin (TTR) is a homotetramer, responsible for carrying the thyroid hormone thyroxine (T_4) [67]. TTR also acts as a carrier of retinol (vitamin A) through its association with retinol-binding protein (RBP) [67]. TTR is a 55 kDa protein and it comprises four subunits of 127 amino acids each [67]. The interface between two dimers creates the two binding pockets for T_4. Less than 1% of TTR's T_4-binding sites are occupied in blood. The docking and the MD simulations reveal that carborane occupies the T_4-binding site (Figure 4A), as also suggested by experimental studies [101]. In this binding pocket (Figure 4B,C), aliphatic amino acids such as the two Leu110 (-1.3 kcal mol^{-1}) and the two Ala108 (-0.9 kcal mol^{-1}) give strong hydrophobic interactions with the carborane. The hydroxyl side-chain of Thr119 (-0.9 kcal mol^{-1}) is involved in dihydrogen bonds with the hydridic B-H groups of the cage.

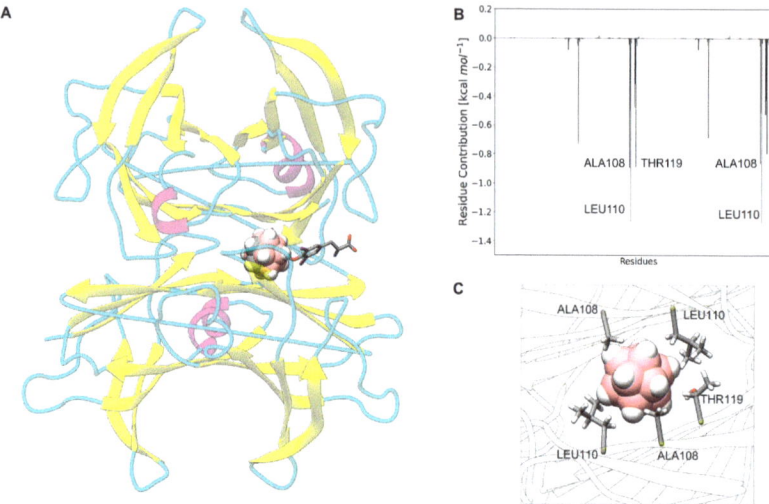

Figure 4. (**A**) A 3D representation of the carborane@transthyretin superimposed with T$_4$ (PDB ID 5CR1). (**B**) *Per*-residue decomposition energy. (**C**) Close-up of the most interacting protein residues with the ligand.

3.4. Carborane@hemoglobin

Hemoglobin (Hb) is a metalloprotein responsible for the transport of oxygen to the tissues. Hb (64 kDa) comprises four subunits, namely α and β chains of 141 and 146 residues, respectively, that pack into a tetramer α$_2$β$_2$ [67]. The four subunits interact via non-covalent interactions, and each chain contains a heme prosthetic group (i.e., iron protoporphyrin IX) which is responsible for the binding of molecular oxygen.

Carboranes occupy the heme-binding pockets of Hb (Figure 5A). This is not surprising since the heme-binding pockets in proteins are usually characterized by the presence of hydrophobic/aromatic residues responsible for the binding of the hydrophobic portions of the heme group.

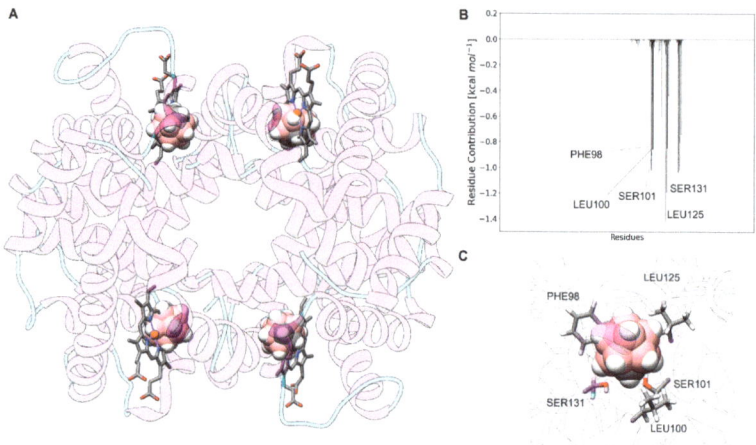

Figure 5. (**A**) A 3D representation of the carborane@hemoglobin superimposed with heme (PDB ID 5HY8). (**B**) *Per*-residue decomposition energy. (**C**) Close-up of the most interacting protein residues with the ligand.

The fingerprint analysis (Figure 5B,C) suggests that Phe98, Leu100 and Leu125 are the residues that mostly contribute to the stabilization of the carborane inside the heme-binding pocket: Phe98 (-1.4 kcal mol^{-1}) by BH-π interactions, and Leu100 (-1.2 kcal mol^{-1}) and Leu125 (-1.2 kcal mol^{-1}) by hydrophobic contacts. Two polar amino acids, i.e., Ser131 (-1.2 kcal mol^{-1}) and Ser101 (-1.1 kcal mol^{-1}), are also important for the binding, engaging dihydrogen bonds with the carborane cage.

3.5. Carborane@myoglobin

Myoglobin (Mb) is formed by a single polypeptide chain, folded into a globular shape. Mb shares almost identical secondary and tertiary structures with the α and β subunits of Hb and consequently binds only one heme group [67].

Mb is responsible for oxygen transport and storage in muscles [67]. In analogy to Hb, our in silico approach suggested that carborane occupies the binding pocket of the heme group of Mb (Figure 6A). His93 (-1.5 kcal mol^{-1}) and His97 (-0.9 kcal mol^{-1}) interact with the carborane cage by BH-π and CH-π interactions. Other three non-polar residues are responsible for the formation of the carborane@myoglobin complex via hydrophobic interactions, namely Ile99 (-1.1 kcal mol^{-1}), Leu104 (-1.0 kcal mol^{-1}) and Ile107 (-0.9 kcal mol^{-1}). The fingerprint analysis and the close-up of the most interacting residues are reported in Figure 6B,C, respectively.

Removing the heme group [50], it is possible to use myoglobin as a drug delivery system/supramolecular host for carborane.

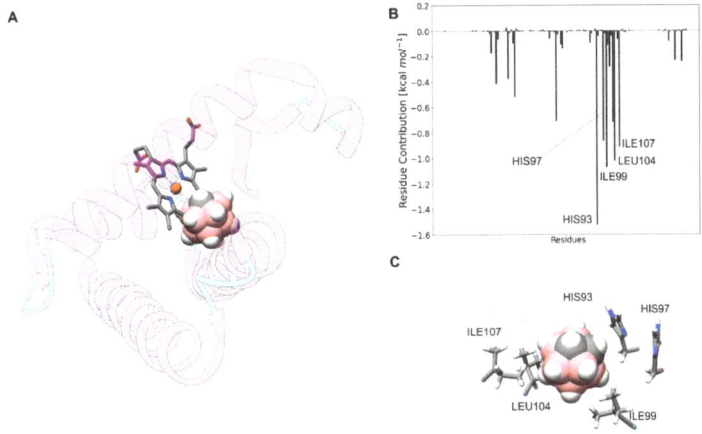

Figure 6. (**A**) A 3D representation of the carborane@myoglobin superimposed with the heme (PDB ID 3RGK). (**B**) Per-residue decomposition energy. (**C**) Close-up of the most interacting protein residues with the ligand.

3.6. Carborane@cerulosplamin

Ceruloplasmin (CP) is the most important copper-carrying protein in the blood and plays an important role in iron metabolism [67]. Ceruloplasmin is also able to prevent oxidative damage to biological systems (proteins, DNA and lipids) because of its antioxidant activity. CP has a molecular weight of ~132 kDa and is composed by a single peptide chain; in physiological conditions, it is a trimer [67]. Carborane binds CP at the interface of the three domains (Figure 7A), and the formation of the complex is stabilized by the formation of a set of BH-π and CH-π interactions with aromatic residues composing the binding pocket (Figure 7B,C), namely Phe303 (-1.5 kcal mol^{-1}), Tyr992 (-1.1 kcal mol^{-1}), Phe997 (-1.1 kcal mol^{-1}) and Tyr986 (-0.8 kcal mol^{-1}). The hydroxyl group of Thr301 (-0.7 kcal mol^{-1}), instead, generates a dihydrogen bond.

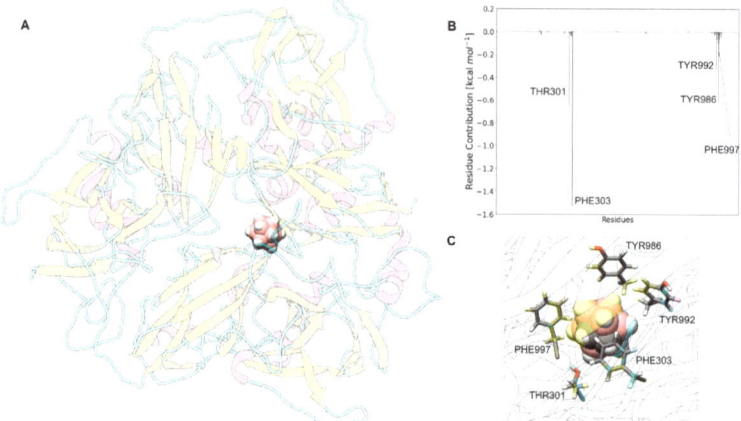

Figure 7. (**A**) A 3D representation of the ortho-carborane@cerulosplamin. (**B**) Per-residue decomposition energy. (**C**) Close-up of the most inter-acting protein residues with the ligand.

3.7. Carborane@sex Hormone-Binding Globulin

Sex hormone-binding globulin (SHBG) is a homodimeric glycoprotein responsible for carrying testosterone, dihydrotestosterone androgens and estradiol in the bloodstream [67]. It is produced by the liver. SHBG regulates the level of these hormones, keeping their concentration stable and preventing them from being broken down too quickly. Testosterone generally binds at the N-terminal domain and estrogen at the C-terminal portion of SHBG. The location of carborane in the protein is depicted in Figure 8A, indicating that the carborane is located in the binding pocket of dihydrosterone. At this binding site (Figure 8B,C), the carborane interacts with Phe67 (-1.8 kcal mol^{-1}) by BH-π and CH-π interactions and with the hydrophobic side-chains of Val105 (-0.9 kcal mol^{-1}), Met107 (-1.1 kcal mol^{-1}), Met139 (-0.8 kcal mol^{-1}) and Leu171 (-0.8 kcal mol^{-1}).

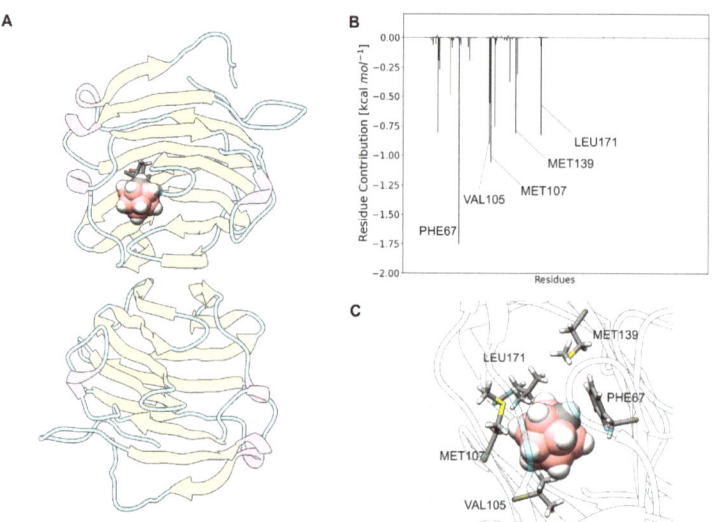

Figure 8. (**A**) A 3D representation of the carborane@sex hormone-binding globulin superimposed with dihydrosterone (PDB ID 1D2S) (**B**) *Per*-residue decomposition energy. (**C**) Close-up of the most interacting protein residues with the ligand.

3.8. Carborane@lactotransferrin

Transferrins (LT) are glycoproteins found in mammal fluids, such as blood (seotransferrin) and milk (lactotransferrin) [67]. Even if it is not a heme protein, transferrin is responsible for the binding of two iron atoms, their transport in the body and the regulation of the iron metabolism [67]. The residues involved in Fe(III) binding are also responsible for the recognition of the carborane cage (Figure 9A). In particular, as depicted in Figure 9B,C, the aromatic imidazole of Hie597 (-0.8 kcal mol^{-1}) and the phenol ring of Tyr528 (-0.8 kcal mol^{-1}) give BH-π and CH-π interactions with the aromatic cage of the carborane. Arg465 (-0.5 kcal mol^{-1}) interacts with its guanidinium group via cation-π and BH-π interactions, while two asparagine residues, Asn640 (-0.7 kcal mol^{-1}) and Asn644 (-0.6 kcal mol^{-1}), are involved in the dihydrogen bond with the carborane cage.

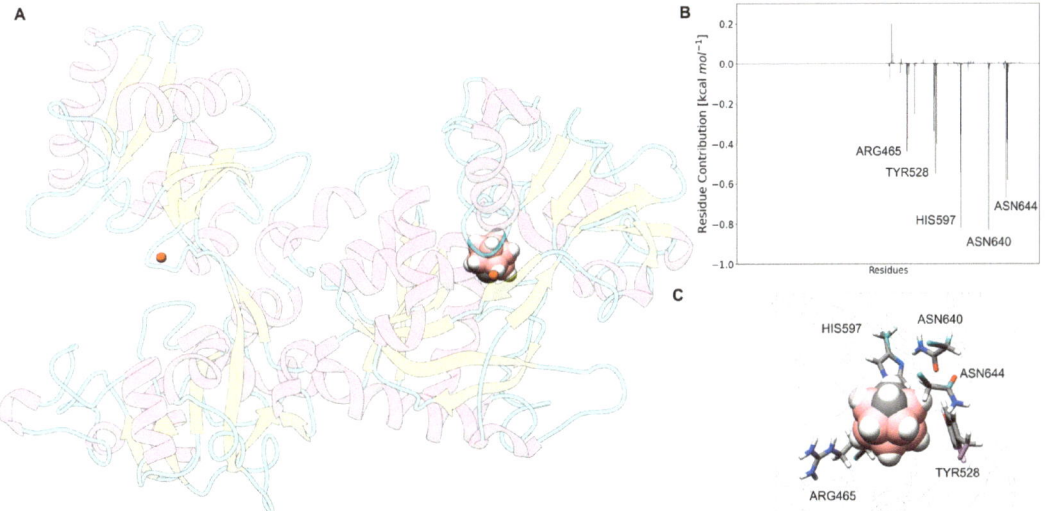

Figure 9. (**A**) A 3D representation of the carborane@lactotransferrin superimposed with the two Fe(III) (PDB ID 1B0L). (**B**) Per-residue decomposition energy. (**C**) Close-up of the most interacting protein residues with the ligand.

3.9. Carborane@plasma Retinol-Binding Protein

Plasma retinol-binding protein (RBP) is a single-chain protein of ~180 amino acids. RBP carries retinol (vitamin A) in blood, binding it in a hydrophobic pocket near the center of the protein [67]. Vitamin A is crucial for vision, immune function and cellular growth and differentiation; therefore, adequate levels of RBP are essential for the correct delivery of vitamin A in the body. Carborane occupies the retinol-binding pocket in RBP (Figure 10A); here, two methionine residues, Met88 (-1.1 kcal mol^{-1}) and Met73 (-0.9 kcal mol^{-1}), engage hydrophobic interactions with the carborane, while three aromatic amino acids, Tyr90 (-0.9 kcal mol^{-1}), Phe135 (-0.7 kcal mol^{-1}) and Phe36 (-0.7 kcal mol^{-1}), give BH-π and CH-π interactions with the aromatic cage of the carborane (Figure 10B,C).

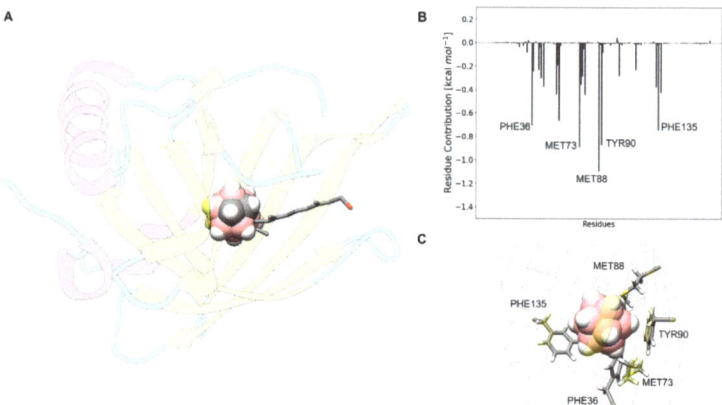

Figure 10. (**A**) A 3D representation of the carborane@plasma retinol-binding protein superimposed with retinol (PDB ID 5NU7). (**B**) Per-residue decomposition energy. (**C**) Close-up of the most interacting protein residues with the ligand.

3.10. Carborane@thyroxine-Binding Globulin

Thyroxine-binding globulin (TBG) regulates the binding of thyroxine (T_4) and tri-iodothyronine (T_3) [67], together with transthyretin and serum albumin. TBG has only one binding site for the thyroid hormones and has a molecular mass of ~54 kDa [67]. Carborane binds TBG in the T_4-binding pocket (Figure 11A) superimposing to one of the aromatic groups of the endogenous ligand. At this binding site (Figure 11B,C), Leu289 (-1.2 kcal mol^{-1}) gives hydrophobic interactions with the carborane. Two charged residues, Lys290 (-1.2 kcal mol^{-1}) and Arg401 (-1.0 kcal mol^{-1}), interact with the carborane cage with their aliphatic side chains via surfactant-like interactions. The aromatic Tyr40, instead, arranges its phenol group to give sandwich-like BH-π and CH-π interactions (-0.8 kcal mol^{-1}) with the carborane, while the hydroxyl portion of Ser43 (-0.7 kcal mol^{-1}) engages a dihydrogen bond with the hydridic B-H groups of the ligand.

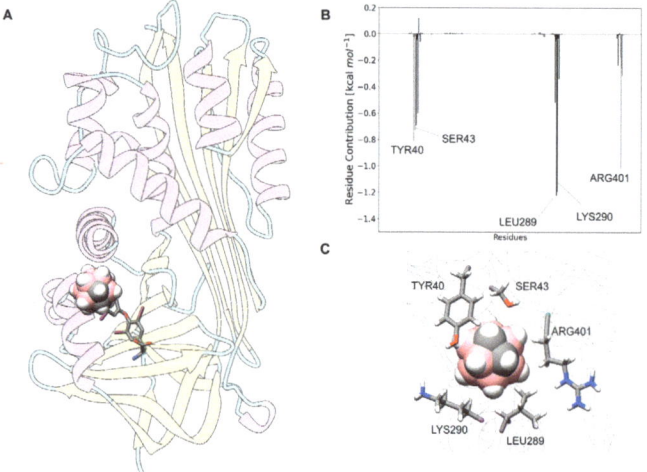

Figure 11. (**A**) A 3D representation of the ortho-carborane@thyroxine-binding protein superimposed with T_4 (PDB ID 2XN6). (**B**) Per-residue decomposition energy. (**C**) Close-up of the most interacting protein residues with the ligand.

3.11. Carborane@corticosteroid-Binding Globulin

Glucocorticoids and hormones, such as cortisol and progesterone, are mainly carried in the blood by corticosteroid-binding globulin (CBG), a member of the SERPIN (serine protease inhibitor) family [67]. CBG is a single-chain protein of 383 amino acids with a weight of ~52 kDa. The carborane binds in a pocket (Figure 12A–C) characterized by BH-π and CH-π interactions with Phe94 (-1.2 kcal mol^{-1}) and hydrophobic interactions with Leu93 and Leu374 (-0.9 kcal mol^{-1}). Very interestingly, here, a new type of interaction appears, i.e., a hydrogen bond with Asp367 (-0.9 kcal mol^{-1}). In fact, the negatively charged carboxylate group of Asp389 interacts with the acidic C-H groups of the carborane cage.

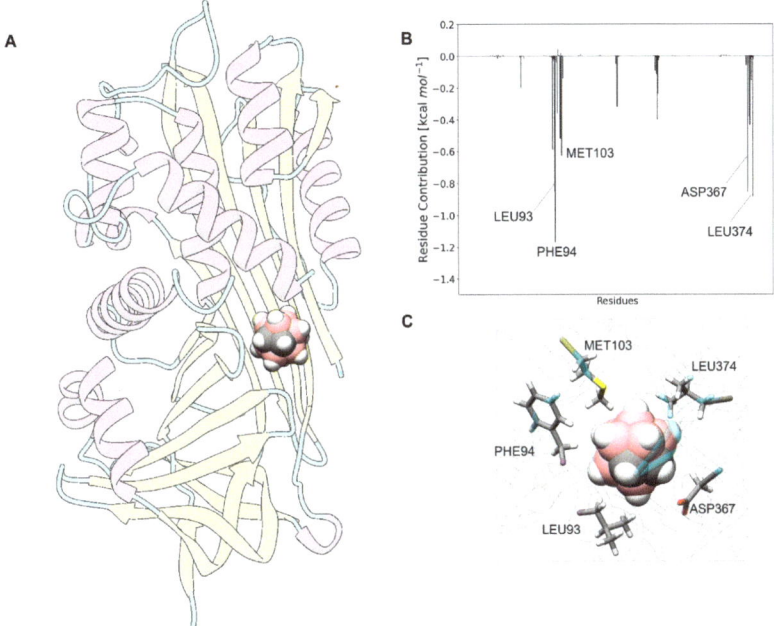

Figure 12. (**A**) A 3D representation of the ortho-carborane@corticosteroid-binding protein. (**B**) Per-residue decomposition energy. (**C**) Close-up of the most interacting protein residues with the ligand.

3.12. Carborane@afamin

Afamin belongs to the albumin gene family, and is mainly expressed in the liver; its role in humans is related to the metabolism syndrome, i.e., the regulation of glucose in blood, obesity and other parameters [67]. Afamin shares ~35% similarity with HSA, and it bears similar binding pockets such as Sudlow's site 1 and the deep cleft located in the center of the heart-shaped protein [67]. In these pockets, afamin is known to bind hydrophobic molecules, particularly vitamin E [67]. As represented in Figure 13A, carborane occupies Sudlow's site 1 of afamin, interacting with Ile293 (-1.2 kcal mol^{-1}), Ile294 (-0.9 kcal mol^{-1}), Val263 (-0.8 kcal mol^{-1}) and Val241 (-0.6 kcal mol^{-1}) with hydrophobic interactions, and with Phe145 (-0.8 kcal mol^{-1}) via BH-π interactions.

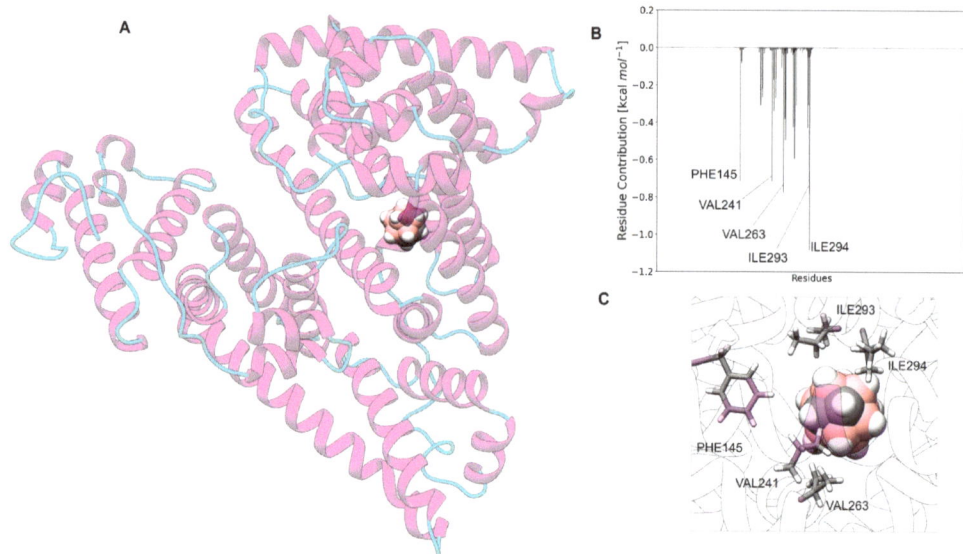

Figure 13. (**A**) A 3D representation of the carborane@afamin. (**B**) Per-residue decomposition energy. (**C**) Close-up of the most interacting protein residues with the ligand.

3.13. Analysis of the Nature of the Non-Covalent Interactions between the Amino Acids and the Carborane in the Protein-Binding Pockets

The analysis of the most interacting amino acids (the five most interacting amino acids were selected for every protein considered) allows the identification of the most recurrent amino acids, responsible for the interaction of a protein with the carborane cage (Figure 14).

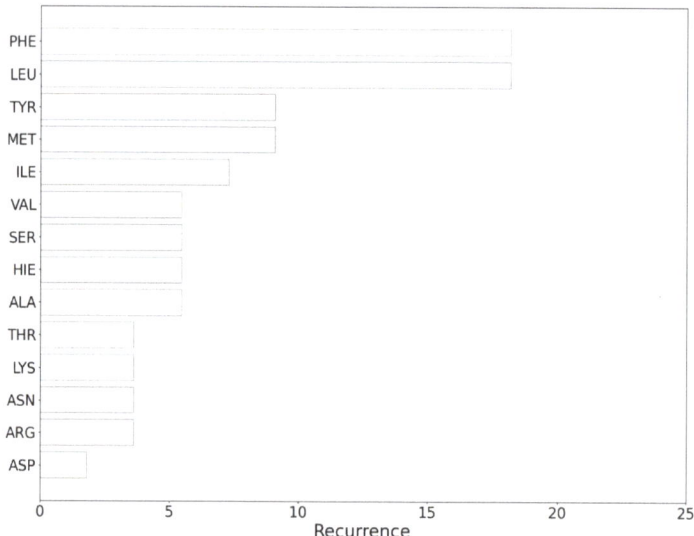

Figure 14. Recurrence (%) of amino acids in the binding pockets discussed in the present work.

The driving force in the recognition of the carborane in the protein-binding pockets is represented by:

(i) Hydrophobic interactions of the hydrophobic cage of the carborane with the aliphatic side chains of amino acids such as leucine (18%), methionine (9%), isoleucine (7%), valine (5%) and alanine (5%);

(ii) BH-π and CH-π interactions of the hydridic B-H groups and acidic C-H groups of the carborane with aromatic amino acids such as phenylalanine (18%), tyrosine (9%) and histidine (5%).

Other important contributions arise from the:

(iii) Formation of dihydrogen bonds with serine (5%), threonine (4%) and asparagine (4%), where serine and threonine use their hydroxylic moieties, while asparagine uses its amidic N-H to form the dihydrogen bonds with the hydridic B-H groups of the carborane;

(iv) Surfactant-like interactions with lysine (4%) and arginine (4%) which wrap the hydrophobic cage of the carborane with their aliphatic chains, while their hydrophilic moieties interact with water;

(v) Formation of classical hydrogen bonds with Asp (2.5%) where the carborane interacts with its acidic C-H groups with the carboxylate group of the amino acid.

4. Conclusions

A virtual screening approach allowed the identification of blood transport proteins as candidate carriers of carboranes. Human serum albumin (HSA) and transthyretin have already demonstrated their ability to bind carborane derivatives, but the structural characterization of their complexes has never been reported. Here, we identified the most probable binding sites for carborane in HSA, i.e., the FA5-binding pocket, Sudlow's I site and the cleft region. In transthyretin, as suggested also by experimental data, the carborane occupies the T4-binding site. Hemoglobin showed a higher binding affinity for carboranes than transthyretin and human serum albumin (HSA). Myoglobin, ceruloplasmin, sex hormone-binding protein, lactoferrin, plasma retinol-binding protein, thyroxine-binding globulin, corticosteroid-binding globulin and afamin have a binding affinity comparable to HSA/transthyretin. The "blind identification" of HSA and transthyretin as carborane-binding proteins (second and third position in the ranking) vouches for the accuracy of the model and validates its predictions.

Carborane shows the tendency to bind in the protein pockets where hydrophobic molecules, such as fatty acids, heme, thyroxine, androgens and retinol, are usually recognized. The driving force for the carborane binding is represented by the formation of hydrophobic interactions with aliphatic amino acids (i.e., leucine, methionine) and BH-π and CH-π interactions with aromatic amino acids (i.e., phenylalanine, tyrosine). Dihydrogen bonds, classical hydrogen bonds and surfactant-like interactions also assist the binding.

The blood transport proteins identified by the reverse docking protocol are potentially responsible to bind carborane upon their intravenous administration. These proteins can be also exploited, ex vivo, to develop boron neutron capture targeted therapy, following two different strategies: (i) the chemical conjugation of targeting (i.e., folate) and imaging (i.e., TRITC) tags on the surface of the protein to both improve the cell selectivity and promote the uptake of the carborane@protein hybrids in cancer cells, generating innovative protein-based theranostic platforms, and (ii) the selection of proteins that can be selectively uptaken by cancer cells via active targeting, such as albumin or transferrin, because their receptors are overexpressed in many cancer cells.

In addition, the dispersion of carboranes with specific proteins able to pass the BBB represents an opportunity for the development of a drug delivery system to target brain cancers with BNCT. Future works will be carried out to experimentally test the possibility to use the identified blood transport proteins as carborane carriers for BCNT.

Supplementary Materials: The following supporting information can be downloaded at: https://www.mdpi.com/article/10.3390/nano13111770/s1, Figures S1–S15: RMSD of carborane@protein complexes.

Author Contributions: Conceptualization, M.C.; investigation, data curation, formal analysis, methodology, T.D.M. and E.J.M.; writing—review and editing, all authors; supervision, F.Z. and M.C. All authors have read and agreed to the published version of the manuscript.

Funding: T.D.M. was supported by a FIRC-AIRC Fellowship for Italy (ID. 25554). E.J.M. was supported by Fondazione Umberto Veronesi.

Data Availability Statement: All data in this study can be requested from the corresponding authors (tainah.marforio2@unibo.it (T.D.M.); matteo.calvaresi3@unibo.it (M.C.)).

Acknowledgments: We acknowledge PRACE for awarding access to the Fenix Infrastructure resource at CINECA (IT), which is partially funded by the European Union's Horizon 2020 research and innovation program through the ICEI project under grant agreement no. 800858.

Conflicts of Interest: The authors declare no conflict of interest.

References

1. Malouff, T.D.; Seneviratne, D.S.; Ebner, D.K.; Stross, W.C.; Waddle, M.R.; Trifiletti, D.M.; Krishnan, S. Boron Neutron Capture Therapy: A Review of Clinical Applications. *Front. Oncol.* **2021**, *11*, 1820. [CrossRef] [PubMed]
2. Murphy, N.; McCarthy, E.; Dwyer, R.; Farràs, P. Boron Clusters as Breast Cancer Therapeutics. *J. Inorg. Biochem.* **2021**, *218*, 111412. [CrossRef]
3. Nuez-Martinez, M.; Pinto, C.I.G.; Guerreiro, J.F.; Mendes, F.; Marques, F.; Muñoz-Juan, A.; Xavier, J.A.M.; Laromaine, A.; Bitonto, V.; Protti, N.; et al. Cobaltabis(Dicarbollide) ([o-COSAN]−) as Multifunctional Chemotherapeutics: A Prospective Application in Boron Neutron Capture Therapy (BNCT) for Glioblastoma. *Cancers* **2021**, *13*, 6367. [CrossRef]
4. Messner, K.; Vuong, B.; Tranmer, G.K. The Boron Advantage: The Evolution and Diversification of Boron's Applications in Medicinal Chemistry. *Pharmaceuticals* **2022**, *15*, 264. [CrossRef] [PubMed]
5. Ali, F.; Hosmane, N.S.; Zhu, Y. Boron Chemistry for Medical Applications. *Molecules* **2020**, *25*, 828. [CrossRef]
6. Cheng, X.; Li, F.; Liang, L. Boron Neutron Capture Therapy: Clinical Application and Research Progress. *Curr. Oncol.* **2022**, *29*, 7868–7886. [CrossRef] [PubMed]
7. Lamba, M.; Goswami, A.; Bandyopadhyay, A. A Periodic Development of BPA and BSH Based Derivatives in Boron Neutron Capture Therapy (BNCT). *Chem. Commun.* **2021**, *57*, 827–839. [CrossRef] [PubMed]
8. Zharkov, D.O.; Yudkina, A.V.; Riesebeck, T.; Loshchenova, P.S.; Mostovich, E.A.; Dianov, G.L. Boron-Containing Nucleosides as Tools for Boron-Neutron Capture Therapy. *Am. J. Cancer Res.* **2021**, *11*, 4668–4682.
9. Gruzdev, D.A.; Levit, G.L.; Krasnov, V.P.; Charushin, V.N. Carborane-Containing Amino Acids and Peptides: Synthesis, Properties and Applications. *Coord. Chem. Rev.* **2021**, *433*, 213753. [CrossRef]
10. Alamón, C.; Dávila, B.; García, M.F.; Sánchez, C.; Kovacs, M.; Trias, E.; Barbeito, L.; Gabay, M.; Zeineh, N.; Gavish, M.; et al. Sunitinib-Containing Carborane Pharmacophore with the Ability to Inhibit Tyrosine Kinases Receptors FLT3, KIT and PDGFR-β, Exhibits Powerful In Vivo Anti-Glioblastoma Activity. *Cancers* **2020**, *12*, 3423. [CrossRef] [PubMed]
11. Barth, R.F.; Yang, W.; Al-Madhoun, A.S.; Johnsamuel, J.; Byun, Y.; Chandra, S.; Smith, D.R.; Tjarks, W.; Eriksson, S. Boron-Containing Nucleosides as Potential Delivery Agents for Neutron Capture Therapy of Brain Tumors. *Cancer Res.* **2004**, *64*, 6287–6295. [CrossRef] [PubMed]
12. Leśnikowski, Z.J.; Paradowska, E.; Olejniczak, A.B.; Studzińska, M.; Seekamp, P.; Schüßler, U.; Gabel, D.; Schinazi, R.F.; Plešek, J. Towards New Boron Carriers for Boron Neutron Capture Therapy: Metallacarboranes and Their Nucleoside Conjugates. *Bioorganic Med. Chem.* **2005**, *13*, 4168–4175. [CrossRef] [PubMed]
13. Smilowitz, H.M.; Slatkin, D.N.; Micca, P.L.; Miura, M. Microlocalization of Lipophilic Porphyrins: Non-Toxic Enhancers of Boron Neutron-Capture Therapy. *Int. J. Radiat. Biol.* **2013**, *89*, 611–617. [CrossRef]
14. Miura, M.; Morris, G.M.; Hopewell, J.W.; Micca, P.L.; Makar, M.S.; Nawrocky, M.M.; Renner, M.W. Enhancement of the Radiation Response of EMT-6 Tumours by a Copper Octabromotetracarboranylphenylporphyrin. *Br. J. Radiol.* **2014**, *85*, 443–450. [CrossRef]
15. Kawabata, S.; Yang, W.; Barth, R.F.; Wu, G.; Huo, T.; Binns, P.J.; Riley, K.J.; Ongayi, O.; Gottumukkala, V.; Vicente, M.G.H. Convection Enhanced Delivery of Carboranylporphyrins for Neutron Capture Therapy of Brain Tumors. *J. Neurooncol.* **2011**, *103*, 175–185. [CrossRef]
16. Hu, K.; Yang, Z.; Zhang, L.; Xie, L.; Wang, L.; Xu, H.; Josephson, L.; Liang, S.H.; Zhang, M.R. Boron Agents for Neutron Capture Therapy. *Coord. Chem. Rev.* **2020**, *405*, 213139. [CrossRef]
17. Imperio, D.; Panza, L. Sweet Boron: Boron-Containing Sugar Derivatives as Potential Agents for Boron Neutron Capture Therapy. *Symmetry* **2022**, *14*, 182. [CrossRef]
18. Schwarze, B.; Gozzi, M.; Zilberfain, C.; Rüdiger, J.; Birkemeyer, C.; Estrela-Lopis, I.; Hey-Hawkins, E. Nanoparticle-Based Formulation of Metallacarboranes with Bovine Serum Albumin for Application in Cell Cultures. *J. Nanoparticle Res.* **2020**, *22*, 24. [CrossRef]
19. Kawasaki, R.; Sasaki, Y.; Akiyoshi, K. Self-Assembled Nanogels of Carborane-Bearing Polysaccharides for Boron Neutron Capture Therapy. *Chem. Lett.* **2017**, *46*, 513–515. [CrossRef]

20. Silva, W.M.; Ribeiro, H.; Taha-Tijerina, J.J. Potential Production of Theranostic Boron Nitride Nanotubes (^{64}Cu-BNNTs) Radiolabeled by Neutron Capture. *Nanomaterials* **2021**, *11*, 2907. [CrossRef]
21. Chiang, C.W.; Chien, Y.C.; Yu, W.J.; Ho, C.Y.; Wang, C.Y.; Wang, T.W.; Chiang, C.S.; Keng, P.Y. Polymer-Coated Nanoparticles for Therapeutic and Diagnostic Non-^{10}B Enriched Polymer-Coated Boron Carbon Oxynitride (BCNO) Nanoparticles as Potent BNCT Drug. *Nanomaterials* **2021**, *11*, 2936. [CrossRef]
22. Pitto-Barry, A. Polymers and Boron Neutron Capture Therapy (BNCT): A Potent Combination. *Polym. Chem.* **2021**, *12*, 2035–2044. [CrossRef]
23. Takeuchi, I.; Kishi, N.; Shiokawa, K.; Uchiro, H.; Makino, K. Polyborane Encapsulated Liposomes Prepared Using PH Gradient and Reverse-Phase Evaporation for Boron Neutron Capture Therapy: Biodistribution in Tumor-Bearing Mice. *Colloid Polym. Sci.* **2018**, *296*, 1137–1144. [CrossRef]
24. Xiong, H.; Wei, X.; Zhou, D.; Qi, Y.; Xie, Z.; Chen, X.; Jing, X.; Huang, Y. Amphiphilic Polycarbonates from Carborane-Installed Cyclic Carbonates as Potential Agents for Boron Neutron Capture Therapy. *Bioconjugate Chem.* **2016**, *27*, 2214–2223. [CrossRef]
25. Lee, W.; Sarkar, S.; Ahn, H.; Kim, J.Y.; Lee, Y.J.; Chang, Y.; Yoo, J. PEGylated Liposome Encapsulating Nido-Carborane Showed Significant Tumor Suppression in Boron Neutron Capture Therapy (BNCT). *Biochem. Biophys. Res. Commun.* **2020**, *522*, 669–675. [CrossRef]
26. Tsygankova, A.R.; Gruzdev, D.A.; Kanygin, V.V.; Guselnikova, T.Y.; Telegina, A.A.; Kasatova, A.I.; Kichigin, A.I.; Levit, G.L.; Mechetina, L.V.; Mukhamadiyarov, R.A.; et al. Liposomes Loaded with Lipophilic Derivative of Closo-Carborane as a Potential Boron Delivery System for Boron Neutron Capture Therapy of Tumors. *Mendeleev. Commun.* **2021**, *31*, 659–661. [CrossRef]
27. Singh, B.; Kaur, G.; Singh, P.; Singh, K.; Kumar, B.; Vij, A.; Kumar, M.; Bala, R.; Meena, R.; Singh, A.; et al. Nanostructured Boron Nitride With High Water Dispersibility For Boron Neutron Capture Therapy. *Sci. Rep.* **2016**, *6*, 35535. [CrossRef]
28. Ailuno, G.; Balboni, A.; Caviglioli, G.; Lai, F.; Barbieri, F.; Dellacasagrande, I.; Florio, T.; Baldassari, S. Boron Vehiculating Nanosystems for Neutron Capture Therapy in Cancer Treatment. *Cells* **2022**, *11*, 4029. [CrossRef]
29. Sumitani, S.; Nagasaki, Y. Boron Neutron Capture Therapy Assisted by Boron-Conjugated Nanoparticles. *Polym. J.* **2012**, *44*, 522–530. [CrossRef]
30. Dukenbayev, K.; Korolkov, I.V.; Tishkevich, D.I.; Kozlovskiy, A.L.; Trukhanov, S.V.; Gorin, Y.G.; Shumskaya, E.E.; Kaniukov, E.Y.; Vinnik, D.A.; Zdorovets, M.V.; et al. Fe$_3$O$_4$ Nanoparticles for Complex Targeted Delivery and Boron Neutron Capture Therapy. *Nanomaterials* **2019**, *9*, 494. [CrossRef]
31. Ferreira, T.H.; Miranda, M.C.; Rocha, Z.; Leal, A.S.; Gomes, D.A.; Sousa, E.M.B. An Assessment of the Potential Use of BNNTs for Boron Neutron Capture Therapy. *Nanomaterials* **2017**, *7*, 82. [CrossRef]
32. Oleshkevich, E.; Morancho, A.; Saha, A.; Galenkamp, K.M.O.; Grayston, A.; Crich, S.G.; Alberti, D.; Protti, N.; Comella, J.X.; Teixidor, F.; et al. Combining Magnetic Nanoparticles and Icosahedral Boron Clusters in Biocompatible Inorganic Nanohybrids for Cancer Therapy. *Nanomedicine* **2019**, *20*, 101986. [CrossRef]
33. Ferrer-Ugalde, A.; Sandoval, S.; Pulagam, K.R.; Muñoz-Juan, A.; Laromaine, A.; Llop, J.; Tobias, G.; Núñez, R. Radiolabeled Cobaltabis(Dicarbollide) Anion-Graphene Oxide Nanocomposites for in Vivo Bioimaging and Boron Delivery. *ACS Appl. Nano Mater.* **2021**, *4*, 1613–1625. [CrossRef]
34. Yan, J.; Yang, W.; Zhang, Q.; Yan, Y. Introducing Borane Clusters into Polymeric Frameworks: Architecture, Synthesis, and Applications. *Chem. Commun.* **2020**, *56*, 11720–11734. [CrossRef]
35. Marfavi, A.; Kavianpour, P.; Rendina, L.M. Carboranes in Drug Discovery, Chemical Biology and Molecular Imaging. *Nat. Rev. Chem.* **2022**, *6*, 486–504. [CrossRef]
36. Poater, J.; Viñas, C.; Bennour, I.; Escayola, S.; Solà, M.; Teixidor, F. Too Persistent to Give Up: Aromaticity in Boron Clusters Survives Radical Structural Changes. *J. Am. Chem. Soc.* **2020**, *142*, 9396–9407. [CrossRef]
37. Farràs, P.; Juárez-Pérez, E.J.; Lepšík, M.; Luque, R.; Núñez, R. Metallacarboranes and Their Interactions: Theoretical Insights and Their Applicability. *Chem. Soc. Rev.* **2012**, *41*, 3445–3463. [CrossRef]
38. Issa, F.; Kassiou, M.; Rendina, L.M. Boron in Drug Discovery: Carboranes as Unique Pharmacophores in Biologically Active Compounds. *Chem. Rev.* **2011**, *111*, 5701–5722. [CrossRef]
39. Chen, Y.; Du, F.; Tang, L.; Xu, J.; Zhao, Y.; Wu, X.; Li, M.; Shen, J.; Wen, Q.; Cho, C.H.; et al. Carboranes as Unique Pharmacophores in Antitumor Medicinal Chemistry. *Mol. Ther. Oncolytics* **2022**, *24*, 400–416. [CrossRef]
40. Barry, N.P.E.; Sadler, P.J. Dicarba-Closo-Dodecarborane-Containing Half-Sandwich Complexes of Ruthenium, Osmium, Rhodium and Iridium: Biological Relevance and Synthetic Strategies. *Chem. Soc. Rev.* **2012**, *41*, 3264–3279. [CrossRef]
41. Fink, K.; Uchman, M. Boron Cluster Compounds as New Chemical Leads for Antimicrobial Therapy. *Coord. Chem. Rev.* **2021**, *431*, 213684. [CrossRef]
42. Stockmann, P.; Gozzi, M.; Kuhnert, R.; Sárosi, M.B.; Hey-Hawkins, E. New Keys for Old Locks: Carborane-Containing Drugs as Platforms for Mechanism-Based Therapies. *Chem. Soc. Rev.* **2019**, *48*, 3497. [CrossRef]
43. Fithroni, A.B.; Kobayashi, K.; Uji, H.; Ishimoto, M.; Akehi, M.; Ohtsuki, T.; Matsuura, E. Novel Self-Forming Nanosized DDS Particles for BNCT: Utilizing A Hydrophobic Boron Cluster and Its Molecular Glue Effect. *Cells* **2022**, *11*, 3307. [CrossRef]
44. Takeuchi, I.; Nomura, K.; Makino, K. Hydrophobic Boron Compound-Loaded Poly(l-Lactide-Co-Glycolide) Nanoparticles for Boron Neutron Capture Therapy. *Colloids Surf. B Biointerfaces* **2017**, *159*, 360–365. [CrossRef]

45. Alberti, D.; Protti, N.; Toppino, A.; Deagostino, A.; Lanzardo, S.; Bortolussi, S.; Altieri, S.; Voena, C.; Chiarle, R.; Crich, S.G.; et al. A Theranostic Approach Based on the Use of a Dual Boron/Gd Agent to Improve the Efficacy of Boron Neutron Capture Therapy in the Lung Cancer Treatment. *Nanomedicine* **2015**, *11*, 741–750. [CrossRef]
46. Heber, E.M.; Kueffer, P.J.; Lee, M.W.; Hawthorne, M.F.; Garabalino, M.A.; Molinari, A.J.; Nigg, D.W.; Bauer, W.; Hughes, A.M.; Pozzi, E.C.C.; et al. Boron Delivery with Liposomes for Boron Neutron Capture Therapy (BNCT): Biodistribution Studies in an Experimental Model of Oral Cancer Demonstrating Therapeutic Potential. *Radiat. Environ. Biophys.* **2012**, *51*, 195–204. [CrossRef]
47. Zhang, T.; Xu, D.; Yi, Y.; Wang, Y.; Cui, Z.; Chen, X.; Ma, Q.; Song, F.; Zhu, B.; Zhao, Z.; et al. Chitosan-Lactobionic Acid-Thioctic Acid-Modified Hollow Mesoporous Silica Composite Loaded with Carborane for Boron Neutron Capture Therapy of Hepatocellular Carcinoma. *Mater. Des.* **2022**, *223*, 111196. [CrossRef]
48. Rak, J.; Kaplánek, R.; Král, V. Solubilization and Deaggregation of Cobalt Bis(Dicarbollide) Derivatives in Water by Biocompatible Excipients. *Bioorganic Med. Chem. Lett.* **2010**, *20*, 1045–1048. [CrossRef]
49. Rak, J.; Jakubek, M.; Kaplánek, R.; Matějíček, P.; Král, V. Cobalt Bis(Dicarbollide) Derivatives: Solubilization and Self-Assembly Suppression. *Eur. J. Med. Chem.* **2011**, *46*, 1140–1146. [CrossRef]
50. Rak, J.; Dejlová, B.; Lampová, H.; Kaplánek, R.; Matějíček, P.; Cígler, P.; Král, V. On the Solubility and Lipophilicity of Metallacarborane Pharmacophores. *Mol. Pharm.* **2013**, *10*, 1751–1759. [CrossRef]
51. Marconi, A.; Giugliano, G.; Di Giosia, M.; Marforio, T.D.; Trivini, M.; Turrini, E.; Fimognari, C.; Zerbetto, F.; Mattioli, E.J.; Calvaresi, M. Identification of Blood Transport Proteins to Carry Temoporfin: A Domino Approach from Virtual Screening to Synthesis and In Vitro PDT Testing. *Pharmaceutics* **2023**, *15*, 919. [CrossRef]
52. Cantelli, A.; Malferrari, M.; Mattioli, E.J.; Marconi, A.; Mirra, G.; Soldà, A.; Marforio, T.D.; Zerbetto, F.; Rapino, S.; Di Giosia, M.; et al. Enhanced Uptake and Phototoxicity of C_{60}@albumin Hybrids by Folate Bioconjugation. *Nanomaterials* **2022**, *12*, 3501. [CrossRef]
53. Mattioli, E.J.; Ulfo, L.; Marconi, A.; Pellicioni, V.; Costantini, P.E.; Marforio, T.D.; Di Giosia, M.; Danielli, A.; Fimognari, C.; Turrini, E.; et al. Carrying Temoporfin with Human Serum Albumin: A New Perspective for Photodynamic Application in Head and Neck Cancer. *Biomolecules* **2023**, *13*, 68. [CrossRef]
54. Marconi, A.; Mattioli, E.J.; Ingargiola, F.; Giugliano, G.; Marforio, T.D.; Prodi, L.; Di Giosia, M.; Calvaresi, M. Dissecting the Interactions between Chlorin E6 and Human Serum Albumin. *Molecules* **2023**, *28*, 2348. [CrossRef]
55. Calvaresi, M.; Zerbetto, F. In Silico Carborane Docking to Proteins and Potential Drug Targets. *J. Chem. Inf. Model.* **2011**, *51*, 1882–1896. [CrossRef]
56. Di Giosia, M.; Zerbetto, F.; Calvaresi, M. Incorporation of Molecular Nanoparticles inside Proteins: The Trojan Horse Approach in Theranostics. *Acc. Mater. Res.* **2021**, *2*, 594–605. [CrossRef]
57. Frontera, A.; Bauzá, A. Closo-Carboranes as Dual CH···π and BH···π Donors: Theoretical Study and Biological Significance. *Phys. Chem. Chem. Phys.* **2019**, *21*, 19944–19950. [CrossRef]
58. Zou, W.; Zhang, X.; Dai, H.; Yan, H.; Cremer, D.; Kraka, E. Description of an Unusual Hydrogen Bond between Carborane and a Phenyl Group. *J. Organomet. Chem.* **2018**, *865*, 114–127. [CrossRef]
59. Saha, B.; Sharma, H.; Bhattacharyya, P.K. Nonclassical B-H_b···π Interaction in Diborane···localized-π Sandwiches: A DFT-D3 Study. *Int. J. Quantum. Chem.* **2019**, *119*, e25998. [CrossRef]
60. Fanfrlík, J.; Brynda, J.; Kugler, M.; Lepšík, M.; Pospísilová, K.; Holub, J.; Hnyk, D.; Nekvinda, J.; Gruner, B.; Rezacova, P. B-H···π and C-H···π Interactions in Protein-Ligand Complexes: Carbonic Anhydrase II Inhibition by Carborane Sulfonamides. *Phys. Chem. Chem. Phys.* **2023**, *25*, 1728. [CrossRef]
61. Zhang, X.; Dai, H.; Yan, H.; Zou, W.; Cremer, D. B−H···π Interaction: A New Type of Nonclassical Hydrogen Bonding. *J. Am. Chem. Soc.* **2016**, *138*, 4334–4337. [CrossRef]
62. Di Giosia, M.; Soldà, A.; Seeger, M.; Cantelli, A.; Arnesano, F.; Nardella, M.I.; Mangini, V.; Valle, F.; Montalti, M.; Zerbetto, F.; et al. A Bio-Conjugated Fullerene as a Subcellular-Targeted and Multifaceted Phototheranostic Agent. *Adv. Funct. Mater.* **2021**, *31*, 2101527. [CrossRef]
63. Cantelli, A.; Malferrari, M.; Solda, A.; Simonetti, G.; Forni, S.; Toscanella, E.; Mattioli, E.J.; Zerbetto, F.; Zanelli, A.; Di Giosia, M.; et al. Human Serum Albumin−oligothiophene Bioconjugate: A Phototheranostic Platform for Localized Killing of Cancer Cells by Precise Light Activation. *JACS Au* **2021**, *1*, 625–635. [CrossRef] [PubMed]
64. Zhang, N.; Mei, K.; Guan, P.; Hu, X.; Zhao, Y.; Zhang, N.; Mei, K.; Guan, P.; Hu, X.; Zhao, Y.L. Protein-Based Artificial Nanosystems in Cancer Therapy. *Small* **2020**, *16*, 1907256. [CrossRef] [PubMed]
65. Liang, K.; Chen, H. Protein-Based Nanoplatforms for Tumor Imaging and Therapy. *Wiley Interdiscip. Rev. Nanomed. Nanobiotechnol.* **2020**, *12*, e1616. [CrossRef]
66. Gou, Y.; Miao, D.; Zhou, M.; Wang, L.; Zhou, H.; Su, G. Bio-Inspired Protein-Based Nanoformulations for Cancer Theranostics. *Front. Pharmacol.* **2018**, *9*, 421. [CrossRef]
67. Schaller, J.; Gerber, S.; Kämpfer, U.; Lejon, S.; Trachsel, C. *Human Blood Plasma Proteins: Structure and Function*; John Wiley & Sons Ltd.: Hoboken, NJ, USA, 2008; pp. 1–526. [CrossRef]
68. Greco, G.; Ulfo, L.; Turrini, E.; Marconi, A.; Costantini, P.E.; Marforio, T.D.; Mattioli, E.J.; Di Giosia, M.; Danielli, A.; Fimognari, C.; et al. Light-Enhanced Cytotoxicity of Doxorubicin by Photoactivation. *Cells* **2023**, *12*, 392. [CrossRef]
69. Shan, L.; Hao, Y.; Wang, S.; Korotcov, A.; Zhang, R.; Wang, T.; Califano, J.; Gu, X.; Sridhar, R.; Bhujwalla, Z.M.; et al. Visualizing Head and Neck Tumors in Vivo Using Near-Infrared Fluorescent Transferrin Conjugate. *Mol. Imaging* **2008**, *7*, 42–49. [CrossRef]

70. Desai, N.; Trieu, V.; Damascelli, B.; Soon-Shiong, P. SPARC Expression Correlates with Tumor Response to Albumin-Bound Paclitaxel in Head and Neck Cancer Patients. *Transl. Oncol.* **2009**, *2*, 59–64. [CrossRef]
71. Calabrese, G.; Daou, A.; Barbu, E.; Tsibouklis, J. Towards Carborane-Functionalised Structures for the Treatment of Brain Cancer. *Drug Discov. Today* **2018**, *23*, 63–75. [CrossRef]
72. Berman, H.M.; Westbrook, J.; Feng, Z.; Gilliland, G.; Bhat, T.N.; Weissig, H.; Shindyalov, I.N.; Bourne, P.E. The Protein Data Bank. *Nucleic Acids Res.* **2000**, *28*, 235–242. [CrossRef]
73. Jumper, J.; Evans, R.; Pritzel, A.; Green, T.; Figurnov, M.; Ronneberger, O.; Tunyasuvunakool, K.; Bates, R.; Žídek, A.; Potapenko, A.; et al. Highly Accurate Protein Structure Prediction with AlphaFold. *Nature* **2021**, *596*, 583–589. [CrossRef]
74. Percy, A.J.; Chambers, A.G.; Smith, D.S.; Borchers, C.H. Standardized Protocols for Quality Control of MRM-Based Plasma Proteomic Workflows. *J. Proteome Res.* **2013**, *12*, 222–233. [CrossRef]
75. Polanski, M.; Anderson, N.L. A List of Candidate Cancer Biomarkers for Targeted Proteomics. *Biomark Insights* **2006**, *1*. [CrossRef]
76. Farrah, T.; Deutsch, E.W.; Omenn, G.S.; Campbell, D.S.; Sun, Z.; Bletz, J.A.; Mallick, P.; Katz, J.E.; Malmström, J.; Ossola, R.; et al. A High-Confidence Human Plasma Proteome Reference Set with Estimated Concentrations in PeptideAtlas. *Mol. Cell. Proteom.* **2011**, *10*, M110.006353. [CrossRef] [PubMed]
77. Schneidman-Duhovny, D.; Inbar, Y.; Polak, V.; Shatsky, M.; Halperin, I.; Benyamini, H.; Barzilai, A.; Dror, O.; Haspel, N.; Nussinov, R.; et al. Taking Geometry to Its Edge: Fast Unbound Rigid (and Hinge-Bent) Docking. *Proteins Struct. Funct. Genet.* **2003**, *52*, 107–112. [CrossRef] [PubMed]
78. Calvaresi, M.; Zerbetto, F. Baiting Proteins with C60. *ACS Nano* **2010**, *4*, 2283–2299. [CrossRef]
79. Calvaresi, M.; Zerbetto, F. Fullerene Sorting Proteins. *Nanoscale* **2011**, *3*, 2873–2881. [CrossRef]
80. Ahmed, L.; Rasulev, B.; Kar, S.; Krupa, P.; Mozolewska, M.A.; Leszczynski, J. Inhibitors or Toxins? Large Library Target-Specific Screening of Fullerene-Based Nanoparticles for Drug Design Purpose. *Nanoscale* **2017**, *9*, 10263–10276. [CrossRef]
81. di Giosia, M.; Valle, F.; Cantelli, A.; Bottoni, A.; Zerbetto, F.; Calvaresi, M. C60 Bioconjugation with Proteins: Towards a Palette of Carriers for All PH Ranges. *Materials* **2018**, *11*, 691. [CrossRef]
82. Calvaresi, M.; Furini, S.; Domene, C.; Bottoni, A.; Zerbetto, F. Blocking the Passage: C_{60} Geometrically Clogs K+ Channels. *ACS Nano* **2015**, *9*, 4827–4834. [CrossRef] [PubMed]
83. Calvaresi, M.; Arnesano, F.; Bonacchi, S.; Bottoni, A.; Calò, V.; Conte, S.; Falini, G.; Fermani, S.; Losacco, M.; Montalti, M.; et al. C_{60}@Lysozyme: Direct Observation by Nuclear Magnetic Resonance of a 1:1 Fullerene Protein Adduct. *ACS Nano* **2014**, *8*, 1871–1877. [CrossRef] [PubMed]
84. Calvaresi, M.; Bottoni, A.; Zerbetto, F. Thermodynamics of Binding between Proteins and Carbon Nanoparticles: The Case of C60@Lysozyme. *J. Phys. Chem. C* **2015**, *119*, 28077–28082. [CrossRef]
85. Marforio, T.D.; Mattioli, E.J.; Zerbetto, F.; Calvaresi, M. Fullerenes against COVID-19: Repurposing C_{60} and C_{70} to Clog the Active Site of SARS-CoV-2 Protease. *Molecules* **2022**, *27*, 1916. [CrossRef] [PubMed]
86. Malarz, K.; Korzuch, J.; Marforio, T.D.; Balin, K.; Calvaresi, M.; Mrozek-Wilczkiewicz, A.; Musiol, R.; Serda, M. Identification and Biological Evaluation of a Water-Soluble Fullerene Nanomaterial as BTK Kinase Inhibitor. *Int. J. Nanomed.* **2023**, *18*, 1709–1724. [CrossRef] [PubMed]
87. Di Giosia, M.; Valle, F.; Cantelli, A.; Bottoni, A.; Zerbetto, F.; Fasoli, E.; Calvaresi, M. Identification and Preparation of Stable Water Dispersions of Protein—Carbon Nanotube Hybrids and Efficient Design of New Functional Materials. *Carbon* **2019**, *147*, 70–82. [CrossRef]
88. Berto, M.; Di Giosia, M.; Giordani, M.; Sensi, M.; Valle, F.; Alessandrini, A.; Menozzi, C.; Cantelli, A.; Gazzadi, G.C.; Zerbetto, F.; et al. Green Fabrication of (6,5)Carbon Nanotube/Protein Transistor Endowed with Specific Recognition. *Adv. Electron. Mater.* **2021**, *7*, 2001114. [CrossRef]
89. Di Giosia, M.; Marforio, T.D.; Cantelli, A.; Valle, F.; Zerbetto, F.; Su, Q.; Wang, H.; Calvaresi, M. Inhibition of α-Chymotrypsin by Pristine Single-Wall Carbon Nanotubes: Clogging up the Active Site. *J. Colloid. Interface Sci.* **2020**, *571*, 174–184. [CrossRef]
90. Calvaresi, M.; Hoefinger, S.; Zerbetto, F. Probing the Structure of Lysozyme–Carbon-Nanotube Hybrids with Molecular Dynamics. *Chem. A Eur. J.* **2012**, *18*, 4308–4313. [CrossRef]
91. Wang, J.; Wolf, R.M.; Caldwell, J.W.; Kollman, P.A.; Case, D.A. Development and Testing of a General Amber Force Field. *J. Comput. Chem.* **2004**, *25*, 1157–1174. [CrossRef]
92. Sárosi, M.B.; Lybrand, T.P. Molecular Dynamics Simulation of Cyclooxygenase-2 Complexes with Indomethacin Closo-Carborane Analogs. *J. Chem. Inf. Model.* **2018**, *58*, 1990–1999. [CrossRef] [PubMed]
93. Roe, D.R.; Cheatham, T.E. PTRAJ and CPPTRAJ: Software for Processing and Analysis of Molecular Dynamics Trajectory Data. *J. Chem. Theory Comput.* **2013**, *9*, 3084–3095. [CrossRef]
94. Miller, B.R.; McGee, T.D.; Swails, J.M.; Homeyer, N.; Gohlke, H.; Roitberg, A.E. MMPBSA.Py: An Efficient Program for End-State Free Energy Calculations. *J. Chem. Theory Comput.* **2012**, *8*, 3314–3321. [CrossRef] [PubMed]
95. Hawkins, G.D.; Cramer, C.J.; Truhlar, D.G. Parametrized Models of Aqueous Free Energies of Solvation Based on Pairwise Descreening of Solute Atomic Charges from a Dielectric Medium. *J. Phys. Chem.* **1996**, *100*, 19824–19839. [CrossRef]
96. Hawkins, G.D.; Cramer, C.J.; Truhlar, D.G. Pairwise Solute Descreening of Solute Charges from a Dielectric Medium. *Chem. Phys. Lett.* **1995**, *246*, 122–129. [CrossRef]

97. Ol'shevskaya, V.A.; Nikitina, R.G.; Savchenko, A.N.; Malshakova, M.V.; Vinogradov, A.M.; Golovina, G.V.; Belykh, D.V.; Kutchin, A.V.; Kaplan, M.A.; Kalinin, V.N.; et al. Novel Boronated Chlorin E6-Based Photosensitizers: Synthesis, Binding to Albumin and Antitumour Efficacy. *Bioorganic Med. Chem.* **2009**, *17*, 1297–1306. [CrossRef]
98. Goszczyński, T.M.; Fink, K.; Kowalski, K.; Leśnikowski, Z.J.; Boratyński, J. Interactions of Boron Clusters and Their Derivatives with Serum Albumin. *Sci. Rep.* **2017**, *7*, 9800. [CrossRef]
99. Jena, B.B.; Satish, L.; Mahanta, C.S.; Swain, B.R.; Sahoo, H.; Dash, B.P.; Satapathy, R. Interaction of Carborane-Appended Trimer with Bovine Serum Albumin: A Spectroscopic Investigation. *Inorg. Chim. Acta* **2019**, *491*, 52–58. [CrossRef]
100. Fuentes, I.; Pujols, J.; Viñas, C.; Ventura, S.; Teixidor, F. Dual Binding Mode of Metallacarborane Produces a Robust Shield on Proteins. *Chem. A Eur. J.* **2019**, *25*, 12820–12829. [CrossRef]
101. Julius, R.L.; Farha, O.K.; Chiang, J.; Perry, L.J.; Hawthorne, M.F. Synthesis and Evaluation of Transthyretin Amyloidosis Inhibitors Containing Carborane Pharmacophores. *Proc. Natl. Acad. Sci. USA* **2007**, *104*, 4808–4813. [CrossRef]

Disclaimer/Publisher's Note: The statements, opinions and data contained in all publications are solely those of the individual author(s) and contributor(s) and not of MDPI and/or the editor(s). MDPI and/or the editor(s) disclaim responsibility for any injury to people or property resulting from any ideas, methods, instructions or products referred to in the content.

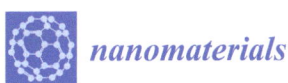

Article

Facile One-Pot Green Synthesis of Magneto-Luminescent Bimetallic Nanocomposites with Potential as Dual Imaging Agent

Radek Ostruszka [1], Denisa Půlpánová [2], Tomáš Pluháček [3], Ondřej Tomanec [4], Petr Novák [1], Daniel Jirák [2,5] and Karolína Šišková [1,*]

1. Department of Experimental Physics, Faculty of Science, Palacký University Olomouc, 77900 Olomouc, Czech Republic
2. Faculty of Health Studies, Technical University of Liberec, 46117 Liberec, Czech Republic
3. Department of Analytical Chemistry, Faculty of Science, Palacký University Olomouc, 77900 Olomouc, Czech Republic
4. Regional Centre of Advanced Technologies and Materials, Czech Advanced Technology and Research Institute, Palacký University Olomouc, 77900 Olomouc, Czech Republic
5. Radiodiagnostic and Interventional Radiology Department, Institute for Clinical and Experimental Medicine, 14021 Prague, Czech Republic
* Correspondence: karolina.siskova@upol.cz

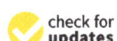

Citation: Ostruszka, R.; Půlpánová, D.; Pluháček, T.; Tomanec, O.; Novák, P.; Jirák, D.; Šišková, K. Facile One-Pot Green Synthesis of Magneto-Luminescent Bimetallic Nanocomposites with Potential as Dual Imaging Agent. *Nanomaterials* 2023, *13*, 1027. https://doi.org/10.3390/nano13061027

Academic Editor: James Chow

Received: 17 February 2023
Revised: 8 March 2023
Accepted: 9 March 2023
Published: 13 March 2023

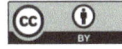

Copyright: © 2023 by the authors. Licensee MDPI, Basel, Switzerland. This article is an open access article distributed under the terms and conditions of the Creative Commons Attribution (CC BY) license (https://creativecommons.org/licenses/by/4.0/).

Abstract: Nanocomposites serving as dual (bimodal) probes have great potential in the field of bio-imaging. Here, we developed a simple one-pot synthesis for the reproducible generation of new luminescent and magnetically active bimetallic nanocomposites. The developed one-pot synthesis was performed in a sequential manner and obeys the principles of green chemistry. Briefly, bovine serum albumin (BSA) was exploited to uptake Au (III) and Fe (II)/Fe (III) ions simultaneously. Then, Au (III) ions were transformed to luminescent Au nanoclusters embedded in BSA (AuNCs-BSA) and majority of Fe ions were bio-embedded into superparamagnetic iron oxide nanoparticles (SPIONs) by the alkalization of the reaction medium. The resulting nanocomposites, AuNCs-BSA-SPIONs, represent a bimodal nanoprobe. Scanning transmission electron microscopy (STEM) imaging visualized nanostructures with sizes in units of nanometres that were arranged into aggregates. Mössbauer spectroscopy gave direct evidence regarding SPION presence. The potential applicability of these bimodal nanoprobes was verified by the measurement of their luminescent features as well as magnetic resonance (MR) imaging and relaxometry. It appears that these magneto-luminescent nanocomposites were able to compete with commercial MRI contrast agents as MR displays the beneficial property of bright luminescence of around 656 nm (fluorescence quantum yield of 6.2 ± 0.2%). The biocompatibility of the AuNCs-BSA-SPIONs nanocomposite has been tested and its long-term stability validated.

Keywords: nanocomposite material; imaging; gold nanocluster; luminescence material; MRI assessment; SPION; bovine serum albumin

1. Introduction

Today, nanocomposites that are simultaneously luminescent and magnetically active are the focus of many research groups due to their applications in nanomedicine (for instance, [1–5]). Several approaches can be used to combine luminescent and magnetic features within one nanocomposite: (i) luminescent nanostructures (NSs) (e.g., quantum dots and/or AuNSs) connected with magnetic NSs [6–12]; (ii) fluorescent (organic) dyes and magnetic NSs [13,14]; (iii) luminescent NSs and magnetic complexes (e.g., containing Gd^{3+}) [3,15,16]; and (iv) fluorescent dyes and magnetic complexes [17,18]. Here, we deal with the first approach (luminescent NSs and magnetic NSs) to achieve magneto-luminescent nanocomposites serving as dual (bimodal) probes.

Typical synthetic strategies for the fabrication of such magneto-luminescent nanocomposites can include: (a) complex multi-step synthesis via a series of sequential synthetic procedures with separately optimized steps (e.g., [6,7]); (b) one-pot method from as-prepared or commercially available structures (e.g., post-synthetic modifications) [13,14,16,17]; and/or (c) a one-pot method without the previous preparation of NSs components (e.g., [15,18]). Here, a straightforward synthesis of the (c) type with a high yield is presented.

Aside from the complexity of the preparation, the individual syntheses of NSs also differ in the total preparation time, ranging from a few minutes (in the case of microwave-assisted synthesis) [19–21] to tens of hours [7,15,18]. Today, simplicity, reproducibility, and green chemistry in NSs preparation are beneficial and highly recommended and are therefore applied in this work. Indeed, we have chosen a protein templated synthesis of luminescent Au nanoclusters based on our previous experience [19,22]. Bovine serum albumin (BSA), a transportation protein which is structurally analogous to human serum albumin, is successfully employed as a matrix for the formation of non-toxic luminescent Au nanoclusters embedded in BSA [19,22].

Furthermore, the same protein, BSA, has also been used by other authors in the generation of superparamagnetic iron oxide nanoparticles (SPIONs), which play a special role in the *in vivo* visualization of cells or biological tissues by ^{1}H MRI (magnetic resonance imaging) [23,24]. BSA in conjunction with SPIONs are exploited for two reasons: (i) achieving a better *in vivo* biocompatibility (e.g., [25–28]) and (ii) prolonging the blood circulation lifetime of SPIONs, representing MRI nanoprobes (e.g., [29–33]). Both properties are superior in SPIONs in comparison to, for instance, Gd (III) species, which are exhaustively reported in the literature, even in combination with AuNSs (e.g., [15,16]). Since Gd (III) species are toxic and represent potential risk to environment and human health [34], we instead decided to exploit SPIONs as MRI contrast agents in our nanocomposites. Wang Y. and co-authors [29] generated ultrasmall SPIONs directly in the presence of BSA under alkaline pH, i.e., using a one-step bio-mineralization method. In the works of other authors, BSA created only a part of the modification layers of SPIONs [30–33,35–37]. Nevertheless, none of these SPIONs-BSA nanocomposites manifested fluorescent properties in the visible region of the electromagnetic spectrum.

In the present study, a one-pot simultaneous bio-mineralization method of gold and iron ions in the presence of BSA under alkaline medium was developed to create new magneto-luminescent probes (further abbreviated as AuBSA-Fe). We demonstrate here that an easy, reproducible, highly efficient synthesis of new functional bimodal probes can be achieved by performing the one-pot sequential preparation procedure. Importantly, in comparison to most of the related literature [12], no abundant chemical agents are necessary and the use of organic solvents was totally avoided by us. Therefore, the synthesis can be regarded as a green one.

Several basic, as well as sophisticated experimental techniques, were exploited for the characterization of our bimodal AuBSA-Fe probes, such as steady-state fluorescence, dynamic light scattering (DLS), UV–Vis absorption measurements, scanning transmission electron microscopy (STEM), energy dispersive spectroscopy (EDS), Mössbauer spectroscopy, inductively coupled plasma mass spectrometry (ICP-MS), relaxation rates determination, and magnetic resonance imaging (MRI). Moreover, cell viability tests were performed by using Alamar blue assay (resazurin) and the long-term stability of AuBSA-Fe nanocomposites was verified by X-ray photoelectron spectroscopy (XPS), among others.

Our results clearly demonstrate that our AuBSA-Fe probes prepared by a simple one-pot sequential green synthetic procedure are superior to commercial MRI contrast agents owing to their bright luminescence at 656 nm when excited in the visible region (e.g., using 480 nm excitation wavelength).

2. Materials and Methods

2.1. Chemicals for Syntheses

Bovine serum albumin (BSA; >98%), gold(III) chloride trihydrate ($HAuCl_4 \cdot 3H_2O$, ≥99.9%), iron(II) chloride tetrahydrate ($FeCl_2 \cdot 4H_2O$; containing 93.4% of $FeCl_2$ and 6.6% of FeOOH according to Mössbauer spectroscopy), iron(III) chloride hexahydrate ($FeCl_3 \cdot 6H_2O$; ≥99%), and sodium hydroxide (NaOH; ≥98.0%) were purchased from Sigma-Aldrich (Saint Louis, MO, USA) and used as received (without any further purification) for all experiments. Nitric acid (69%, Analpure), hydrochloric acid (36%, Analpure), acid-certified reference materials of the calibration standard solution ASTASOL® of Au, Fe (1000 ± 2 mg·L^{-1}), and INT-MIX 1 (10.0 ± 0.1 mg·L^{-1}) were purchased from Analytika, Ltd., Prague, Czech Republic, and used only for ICP-MS analyses. Deionized (DI) water prepared by purging Milli-Q purified water (Millipore Corp., Bedford, MA, USA) was used in all experiments.

2.2. Chemicals for Alamar Blue Assay

Foetal bovine serum (FBS), L-glutamine, Penicillin-Streptomycin, sodium chloride (NaCl; ≥99.0%), potassium chloride (KCl; ≥99.0%), potassium dihydrogen phosphate (KH_2PO_4; ≥99.0%), disodium hydrogen phosphate (Na_2HPO_4; ≥99.0%), and trypsin (from the porcine pancreas) were purchased from Sigma-Aldrich (Saint Louis, MO, USA). Resazurin sodium salt (≥75%) was purchased from VWR International (Radnor, PA, USA). Dulbecco's modified Eagle's medium (DMEM, 11054) was purchased from Thermo Fisher Scientific (Waltham, MA, USA).

2.3. Syntheses of AuBSA and AuBSA-Fe—Their Purification, Concentrate Formation, and Storage

The synthetic procedure of AuBSA system follows the one used in our previous manuscript [22]. Briefly, DI water (0.2 mL) was added to an aqueous $HAuCl_4$ solution (0.8 mL, 12.5 mM) and, subsequently, BSA solution (1 mL, 1 mM) was introduced under vigorous stirring (600 rpm). After 90 s, NaOH solution (0.2 mL, 1 M) was added to obtain a basic environment (pH ≈ 12). Ninety seconds later, the mixed solution was heated up in a microwave oven for 10 s (power was set to 150 W). The preparation of the AuBSA-Fe system differs only in the gradual addition of DI water (0.05 mL), $FeCl_2$ (0.05 mL, 5 mM) and $FeCl_3$ (0.1 mL, 5 mM) to an aqueous $HAuCl_4$ solution instead of DI water volume (0.2 mL) alone.

After two hours of maturing at room temperature, the samples were dialyzed with a 14 kDa cut-off dialysis membrane (regenerated cellulose, Membra-Cel™) against DI water. Dialysis was performed at room temperature for 24 h, with DI water being changed twice: once after the first hour and then again after the second hour. Concentrated forms of samples were prepared using a centrifugal concentrator (30 kDa). The rotational speed was set to 5000 rpm and the centrifugation lasted for 5 min. This process was performed repeatedly until the desired concentration was reached. Dialyzed and concentrated samples were stored in the dark at 4 °C.

2.4. Characterization Techniques

2.4.1. Fluorescence Spectroscopy

The fluorescence measurements of AuBSA and AuBSA-Fe systems were performed on a JASCO F8500 (Jasco, Tokyo, Japan) spectrofluorometer using a 1 cm quartz cuvette. Excitation–emission 3D maps were measured in the excitation range of 250–850 nm with a data interval of 5 nm and in an emission range of 250–850 nm with a data interval of 1 nm and a scan speed of 5000 nm·min^{-1}. Emission spectra were measured in the range of 500–850 nm with a data interval of 1 nm and a scan speed of 100 nm·min^{-1}. The excitation wavelength was set to 480 nm. All spectra were corrected to avoid any deviations induced by instrumental components.

The quantum yield of fluorescence (Φ) was then calculated by Equation (1):

$$\Phi = \Phi_s \cdot \frac{F \cdot (1 - 10^{-A_s}) \cdot n^2}{F_s \cdot (1 - 10^{-A}) \cdot n_s^2}, \quad (1)$$

where F is the integrated fluorescence intensity, A is the absorbance, n is the index of refraction, and the subscript s indicates the standard. DCM, 4-(dicyanomethylene)-2-methyl-6-(4-dimethylaminostyryl)-4H-pyran, dissolved in ethanol (99.8%, Lach-Ner, Neratovice, Czech Republic) was used as a standard (Φ_s = 0.437 ± 0.024) [38].

Absorbance was measured on a Specord 250 Plus—223G1032 (Analytik Jena, Jena, Germany) with a double beam arrangement using a 1 cm quartz cuvette. As a reference, a 1 cm quartz cuvette filled with DI water was used.

The hydrodynamic diameter of both systems was determined by dynamic light scattering using Zetasizer Nano ZS (Malvern Instruments Ltd., Malvern, UK) equipped with a He-Ne laser (λ = 633 nm) at 22 ± 1 °C. For fluorescence, absorbance, and hydrodynamic diameter measurements, the ratio of the sample dilution with DI water was the same.

2.4.2. HR-TEM, STEM, and EDS

The AuBSA-Fe samples were measured by HR-TEM Titan G2 60–300 (FEI, Hillsboro, OR, USA) with an image corrector at an accelerating voltage of 300 kV. Images were taken with a BM UltraScan CCD camera (Gatan, Pleasanton, CA, USA). Energy Dispersive Spectrometry (EDS) was performed in STEM mode by a Super-X system with four silicon drift detectors (Bruker, Billerica, MA, USA). STEM images were taken with an HAADF detector 3000 (Fishione, Export, PA, USA).

2.4.3. Mössbauer Spectroscopy

A home-made Mössbauer spectrometer was used to determine the oxidation and spin state of iron atoms within AuBSA-Fe samples. A representative as-prepared and centrifuged AuBSA-Fe sample was measured with an OLTWINS Mössbauer spectrometer in the transmission mode [39], using a constant acceleration rate and ^{57}Co (Rh) source. The isomer shift values were related to the 28 μm α-Fe foil (Ritverc) measured at room temperature. By using measurements in magnetic field at low temperature, average sizes of SPIONs within AuBSA-Fe samples could be roughly estimated. The acquired Mössbauer spectra were processed using MossWinn 4.0 software [40].

2.4.4. XPS

The X-ray photoelectron spectroscopy (XPS) measurements were carried out with the PHI 5000 VersaProbe II XPS system (Physical Electronics) with a monochromatic Al-Kα source (15 kV, 50 W) and a photon energy of 1486.7 eV. All the spectra were measured in a vacuum of 1.1×10^{-7} Pa and at a room temperature of 20 °C. Dual beam charge compensation was used for all measurements. The spectra were evaluated with MultiPak software, version 9 (Ulvac—PHI, Inc., Chanhassen, MN, USA).

2.4.5. ICP-MS

To accurately determine the total Au and Fe concentrations, the validated ICP-MS method was employed. Prior to ICP-MS analysis, each sample was sonicated and consequently digested using MLS 1200 mega closed vessel microwave digestion unit (Milestone, Italy). The organic matrix was decomposed by a mixture of 4 mL of nitric acid (69%, Analpure) and hydrochloric acid (36%, Analpure) in 1:1 ratio. The digests were allowed to cool down to laboratory temperature, diluted with the ultrapure water to 25 mL in volumetric flasks, and stored at 4 °C until ICP-MS analysis. The detailed ICP-MS method description and the corresponding validation in terms of the limit of detection (LOD), the limit of quantification (LOQ), trueness, and precision are presented in the Supplementary Materials. All ICP-MS measurements were performed in six replicates, and the results are expressed as an average ± standard deviation (SD).

2.4.6. MR Relaxometry and Imaging

The MR relaxometry was used to determine the relaxivities $r_{1,2}$ of AuBSA-Fe nanocomposites (M1–M4). The relaxation times T_1 and T_2 were measured on relaxometer Bruker Minispec mq 60 (Bruker Biospin, Ettlingen, Germany) at 1.5 T, at a stabilized temperature of 37 °C throughout the whole experiment. MR sequence for T_1 measurement: Inversion recovery (IR), 20 points for fitting, 1 excitation, time of repetition (TR) = 0.01–10,000 ms, recycle delay 2 s. T_2 relaxation times were measured with Carr-Purcell-Meiboom-Gill (CPMG), TR = 5000 ms, 20,000 echoes, 1 excitation, echo time (TE) = 0.05 ms, recycle delay 2 s. The relaxivities $r_{1,2}$ were calculated via the least-squares curve fitting of R_1 and R_2 relaxation rates [s^{-1}] versus iron concentration (mM). The experimentally determined solvent relaxation rate R was subtracted as a starting value from the nanoparticle relaxation rates prior to the linear regression analysis.

The MR imaging experiments were performed on a Bruker Biospec 47/20 (Bruker, Ettlingen, Germany) at 4.7 T. T_1- and T_2-weighted MR images of M1–M4 and water (served as a control) samples in tubes were acquired. Rapid acquisition with relaxation enhancement (RARE) multi-spin echo MR sequence were used with the following parameters: T_1-weighted sequence: effective echo time (TE) = 11.6 ms, time of repetition (TR) = 587.0 ms, turbo factor (TF) = 1, scan time = 10.5 min, plane resolution (PR) = 234 × 195 µm^2, slice thickness = 0.6 mm. T_2-weighted sequence: RARE, TE = 36 ms, TR = 3300 ms, TF = 8, scan time = 11.0 min, PR = 234 × 195 µm^2, slice thickness = 0.6 mm. MR image processing and quantification were performed using ImageJ software. The signal-to-noise ratio (SNR) was calculated from images as $0.655 \times S_{sample}/\sigma_{noise}$ and contrast-to-noise ratio (CNR) was calculated from images as $0.655 \times |S_{sample} - S_{water}|/\sigma_{noise}$, where S is signal intensity in the region of interest, σ is the standard deviation of background noise, and the constant 0.655 reflects the Rician distribution of background noise in a magnitude MR image.

2.4.7. Alamar Blue Assay (Resazurin Assay)

In a typical experiment, 80 µL of cultivation medium (second column) or cell (RPE-1) suspension was added to a 96-well plate, which was afterward plaved inside the incubator (37 °C, 5% CO$_2$). After 24 h, 20 µL of DI water (second and third column), two different concentrations of gold and iron precursors, or AuBSA-Fe nanocomposites were added in the form of tri/hexaplicates. Another 24 h later, 20 µL of resazurin was introduced to each well. After 3 h of incubation, fluorescence intensity was measured on a microplate reader Synergy Mx (BioTek™, Winooski, VT, USA). The excitation and emission wavelengths were set to 540 nm and 590 nm, respectively. Cell viability (CV) was calculated according to Equation (2):

$$CV = 100 \times \frac{F_{sample} - F_{medium}}{F_{cells} - F_{medium}}, \quad (2)$$

where F is the averaged fluorescence intensity and the subscripts sample, cells, and medium indicate the measurement of fluorescence in the suspensions of sample-treated cells, non-treated cells, and the solution of cultivation medium alone, respectively.

3. Results and Discussion

The samples of AuBSA-Fe were prepared by an easy one-pot synthetic procedure performed in a sequential manner, which was newly developed by us, as described in detail in the Materials and Methods section. Essentially, ferrous and ferric ions were mixed together in the ratio of 1:2, added to Au (III) aqueous solution and then allowed to interact with BSA for a certain period. The reaction mixture was alkalized in the next step to set up conditions for simultaneous and spontaneous Au (III) reduction and SPIONs formation (i.e., precipitation of Fe ions under alkaline medium in the presence of BSA); the subsequent heating accelerated both bio-mineralization reactions. As a reference, the AuBSA sample was prepared by using the same amount of Au (III) and BSA as in AuBSA-Fe system. Thus, AuBSA and AuBSA-Fe systems differ only in the absence/presence of iron ions in their synthetic procedures, respectively. The procedures of both nanocomposite syntheses are schematically depicted in Figure 1.

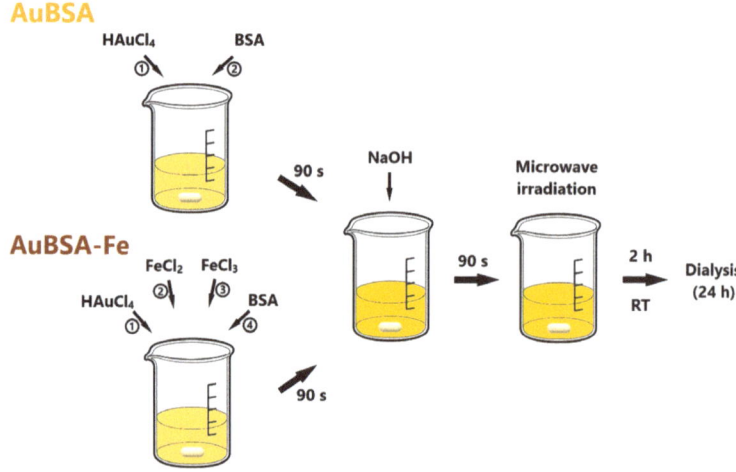

Figure 1. Schematic depiction of AuBSA and AuBSA-Fe nanocomposites.

3.1. Luminescent Properties of AuBSA-Fe in Comparison to AuBSA

There might be concerns about luminescence quenching induced by iron cations, since luminescent AuNCs have been used as sensors of Fe (III) in solution [41–43]. However, in the cited studies, BSA is not used as the template for luminescent AuNCs formation. Moreover, there is a big difference between (i) Fe cations being present in the course of luminescent AuNCs formation within BSA (this study) and (ii) Fe cations being added to well-formed luminescent AuNCs [41–43].

Prompted by this issue, we first focused our attention on the validation of luminescent properties of AuNCs in the AuBSA-Fe system inherited from AuBSA—see Figure 2 for emission spectra in the region of 500–850 nm and Figure S1 for the whole-range 3D excitation–emission maps. Obviously, the average position of the emission maximum of AuNCs remained almost unchanged when iron ions were present: 657 ± 2 nm for AuBSA and 656 ± 1 nm for AuBSA-Fe (Tables S1 and S2, respectively). The intensity of luminescence decreased slightly in AuBSA-Fe in comparison to AuBSA (Figure 2). The fluorescent quantum yield reflects this fact and is of virtually the same average value for AuBSA-Fe, 6.2 ± 0.2 (Table S2), as for AuBSA, 6.4 ± 0.1 (Table S1). This is a good sign that qualitative and quantitative luminescent features of AuNCs are not affected by the presence of iron atoms in AuBSA-Fe samples. Furthermore, one can assume that sizes and numbers of AuNCs within AuBSA-Fe and AuBSA nanocomposites are approximately the same.

3.2. Investigation of Morphology and Particle Size Distribution in Luminescent AuBSA-Fe

According to STEM image in Figure 3A, one can see relatively large aggregates exceeding several hundreds of nanometres in size; however, they consist of individual particles with sizes in units of nanometres and are frequently encountered in AuBSA-Fe systems. EDS data shown in Figure 3B,C further demonstrate that oxygen dominates in the close vicinity of iron in nanoparticulate form (e.g., Fe_xO_y), while sulphur can be co-located together with gold atoms, respectively. This supports previous results of many researchers (including us, [22]) concerning Au–S interactions within AuBSA. It also correlates well with the observation that the luminescent features of AuNCs are not severely hampered by the presence of Fe_xO_y in AuBSA-Fe. Thus, we anticipate that the same type of amino-acid residues creates the closest nano-environment of luminescent AuNCs in AuBSA-Fe as that in AuBSA systems. Since the samples for STEM/EDS are prepared by drying on a support (lacey carbon-coated Cu grid), the real particle size distribution (PSD) in the solution may differ from that observed by STEM. Therefore, it is reasonable to determine PSD directly by measuring the aqueous solutions of the samples by DLS. The average values of the hydrodynamic diameters of particles in AuBSA and AuBSA-Fe nanocomposite solutions along with polydispersity values (PDI) determined by DLS are compared in Table 1. Both samples (AuBSA as well as AuBSA-Fe) represent proper solutions without any obvious aggregate formation visible by the naked eye.

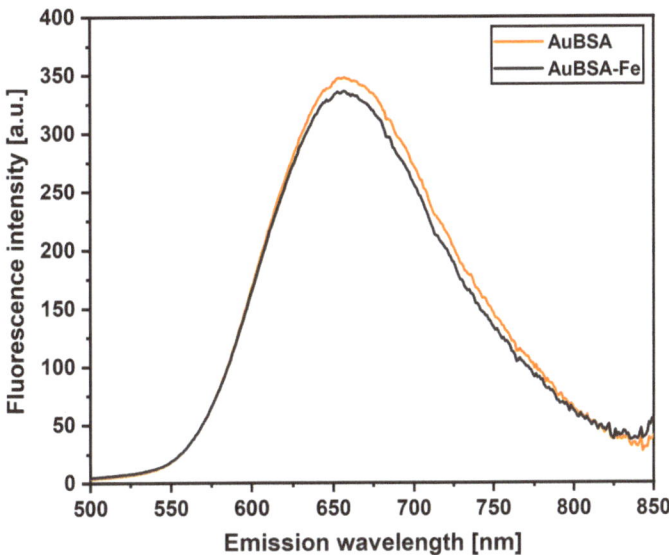

Figure 2. Comparison of fluorescence emission spectra of AuBSA (orange curve) and AuBSA-Fe (black curve) samples when excited at 480 nm. Average fluorescence spectra are shown as a result of seven independent sample preparations and their measurements.

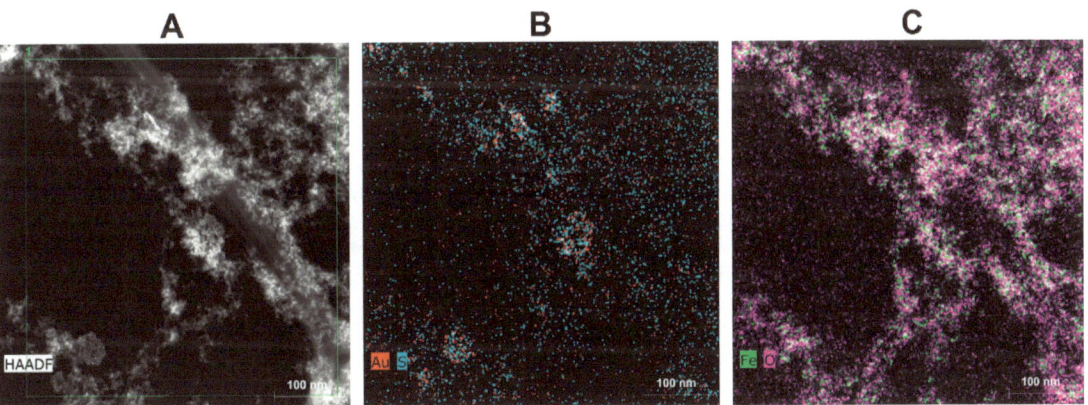

Figure 3. Scanning transmission electron microscopy (STEM) and energy dispersive spectroscopic (EDS) analysis of a representative AuBSA-Fe sample: (**A**) STEM image, scale bar of 100 nm; (**B**) Au and S spatial distribution map; and (**C**) Fe and O spatial distribution map.

Table 1. Hydrodynamic diameter (represented by Z-average) and polydispersity (PDI) of nanocomposites determined by DLS measurements.

Sample	Z-Average [nm]	PDI
AuBSA	23.9 ± 10.8	0.4 ± 0.1
AuBSA-Fe	71.2 ± 8.0	1.0 ± 0.0

Obviously, both the hydrodynamic diameter and PDI increased in AuBSA-Fe in comparison to AuBSA (Table 1). These increases in the average values (from approx. 24 nm in diameter and 0.4 polydispersity in AuBSA to 71 nm and 1.0 in AuBSA-Fe) can be ascribed to the presence of iron oxide particles and their aggregates in AuBSA-Fe because these are the only differences between the two compared systems. Further details of DLS data are shown and discussed in the Supplementary Materials (Figures S2–S4); whereas appropriate values for AuBSA and AuBSA-Fe are listed in Tables S3 and S4, respectively. Although influenced by sample drying to some extent, the STEM images of AuBSA-Fe in dried state (Figure 3A) correlate with the PSD determined for the same system by DLS measured directly in aqueous solution (liquid state).

3.3. Evidence of SPIONs in Luminescent AuBSA-Fe via Mössbauer Spectroscopy

Mössbauer spectroscopy as an iron-sensitive method has been selected to give direct evidence regarding the type of iron oxide present in AuBSA-Fe. Since relatively high concentrations of iron are required in this spectroscopy and, simultaneously, by knowing (from STEM-EDS) that iron is most dominantly distributed in nanoparticulate form at the surface of BSA, we centrifuged the AuBSA-Fe samples, a rusty pellet was carefully dried under nitrogen atmosphere and then measured. The Mössbauer spectrum of AuBSA-Fe recorded at room temperature, shown in Figure 4A, manifested itself as a doublet with an isomer shift value of 0.33 ± 0.01 mm·s^{-1} and the quadrupole splitting of 0.68 ± 0.01 mm·s^{-1}. By measuring the Mössbauer spectrum at 5 K and 5 T, as seen Figure 4B, a sextet with an isomer shift value of 0.43 ± 0.01 mm·s^{-1}, a quadrupole splitting of -0.08 ± 0.01 mm·s^{-1}, and an effective hyperfine magnetic field of 46.4 ± 0.3 T was revealed. Based on these parameters and our previous knowledge [44], the nanoparticulate form of iron in AuBSA-Fe samples can be assigned to superparamagnetic Fe (III) oxide. Furthermore, the measurements at low temperatures and under external magnetic fields showed a symmetrical environment with no preferential orientation; therefore, very small superparamagnetic iron oxide particles (SPIONs) are present in AuBSA-Fe, generally in units of nanometres. This coincides well with STEM imaging and DLS analysis.

3.4. Application of Luminescent AuBSA-Fe as MRI Contrast Agents

SPIONs are well-known as negative or T_2-weighted MRI contrast agents [23]. Therefore, we assessed MRI performance of our AuBSA-Fe samples. In Figure 5, we show the T_2-weighted MR images of four independently prepared AuBSA-Fe samples (denoted as M1–M4), containing different (increasing) concentrations of gold and iron, as determined by ICP-MS (Table S6), but keeping the same molar ratio of these metals (10:0.75). Intentionally, four independently prepared samples were concentrated to verify the reproducibility and to increase the T_2-weighted signal. Obviously, the T_2-weighted MR images of water phantoms were affected by the presence of AuBSA-Fe samples and the clear decrease in the MR signal was observed; on the other hand, and as expected, the only negligible effect was observed in T_1-weighted MR images, where the MR signal increase was low (Figure 5). The values of signal-to-noise ratio (SNR) as well as contrast-to-noise ratio (CNR) for the quantitative comparison of M1–M4 samples are listed in Figure 5. Both SNR and CNR reached values above 37 in the T_2-weighted MR images of all four variants of AuBSA-Fe samples; simultaneously, low SNR and CNR values in T_1-weighted MR images were achieved. This means that AuBSA-Fe samples represent "negative" contrast agents due to the presence of SPIONs. This is in full accordance with the literature [29,30].

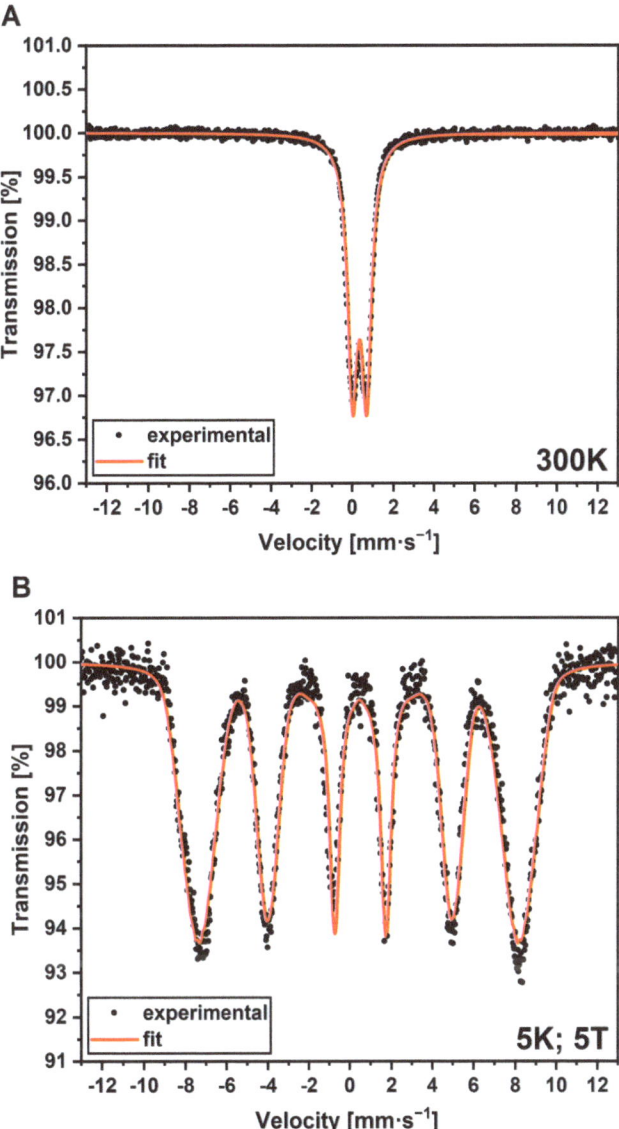

Figure 4. Mössbauer spectra of AuBSA-Fe recorded (**A**) at room temperature and (**B**) at the 5 K and 5 T external magnetic field.

Aside from the MRI imaging of water phantoms containing AuBSA-Fe samples (M1–M4), MR relaxometry was performed. The relaxation rates R_1 and R_2 were calculated as $1/T_1$ and $1/T_2$, respectively, for concentrated and diluted M1–M4 samples. Note that the real concentrations of Fe in concentrated and diluted M1–M4 samples together with the corresponding values of R_1, R_2 relaxation rates are listed in Table S7 in the Supporting Materials. Plotting the relaxation rates as a function of real iron concentration in AuBSA-Fe samples (determined by ICP-MS) resulted in the determination of relaxivities r_1 and r_2 from graphs shown in Figure 6. Evidently, the experimental R_1 values could be best fitted with a linear function (although it can be separated in two parts, according to R_2 dependence).

On the other hand, two linear functions with two different slopes are best able to fit the experimental R_2 values: 3.44 ± 0.36 L·mmol^{-1}·s^{-1} for iron concentrations equal and above 0.52 mM; 2.68 ± 0.11 L·mmol^{-1}·s^{-1} for iron concentrations below this value (Table 2). These slopes represent the characteristic r_2 relaxivity of AuBSA-Fe samples and, as such, can be compared with the relaxivity values of the commercial MRI contrast agents (e.g., in [45]). From this direct comparison, it is obvious that the r_2 relaxivity values of AuBSA-Fe samples closely approach those of several commercially available contrast agents. Importantly, the commercial MRI contrast agents do not possess luminescent properties, while AuBSA-Fe samples do. Therefore, AuBSA-Fe samples could serve as bimodal (dual) probes for MRI and fluorescence measurements.

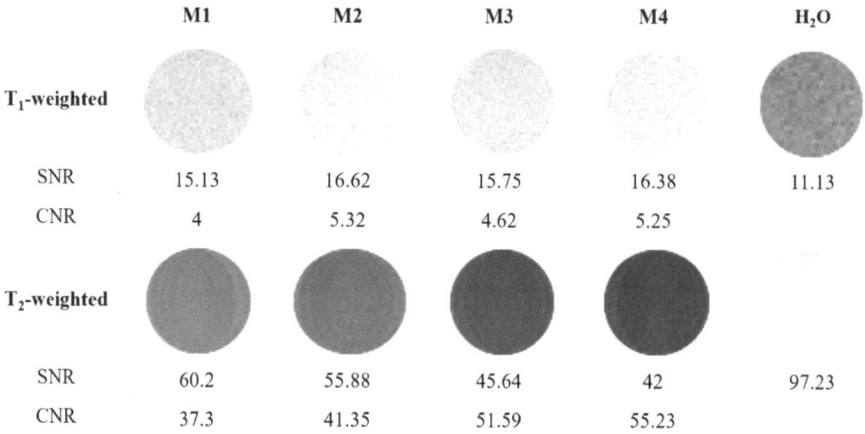

Figure 5. Magnetic resonance (MR) images of AuBSA-Fe phantoms (denoted as M1–M4) containing different Fe concentrations (807 µM Fe in M1, 1020 µM Fe in M2, 1193 µM Fe in M3, and 1249 µM Fe in M4) and water phantom (H$_2$O), measured at 4.7 T external magnetic field. T_1- and T_2-weighted MR images are shown. Note: the signal-to-noise ratio (SNR) was calculated using SNR = $0.655 \times S/\sigma$, where S is signal intensity in the region of interest (ROI), σ is the standard deviation of background noise, and the constant 0.655 reflects the Rician distribution of background noise in a magnitude MR image. Eight averages were used.

Interestingly, R_2 values may be even fitted with a quadratic function as shown for concentrated samples in Figure S5. The quadratic dependence of relaxation rates on concentration of contrast agents was observed in previous studies by different authors [46–51]. In our opinion, two plausible explanations may be adopted in the case of AuBSA-Fe samples: either the aggregation of SPIONs and the consequent inhomogeneity of magnetic fields as in [52] or the small sizes of SPIONs (evidenced for our AuBSA-Fe samples through direct visualization using STEM and/or spectroscopically through the Mössbauer effect), thus falling in a range of quadratic relaxation [53].

3.5. Stability and Biocompatibility of AuBSA-Fe Nanocomposites

An important issue in any sample applicability is their stability in time if stored under relevant conditions. Since AuBSA-Fe samples contain inorganic parts, being responsible for luminescent and MR features as well as protein (although denatured during the synthesis), generally, we stored our samples in a fridge. However, for the sake of curiosity, a sample of AuBSA-Fe was stored at room temperature over 1 year, and its X-ray photoelectron spectroscopic (XPS) spectrum measured and directly compared with that of freshly prepared AuBSA-Fe. The XPS results, shown in Figure S6 and discussed in the Supplementary Materials, confirmed the degradation of organic part, while preserving Au (0) content even in the AuBSA-Fe sample stored at room temperature. Thus, the stability of the newly developed AuBSA-Fe dual probes was verified. It can be summed up that

AuBSA-Fe, representing a stable system when stored in a fridge, could potentially be applied as fluorescent and MRI contrast agents.

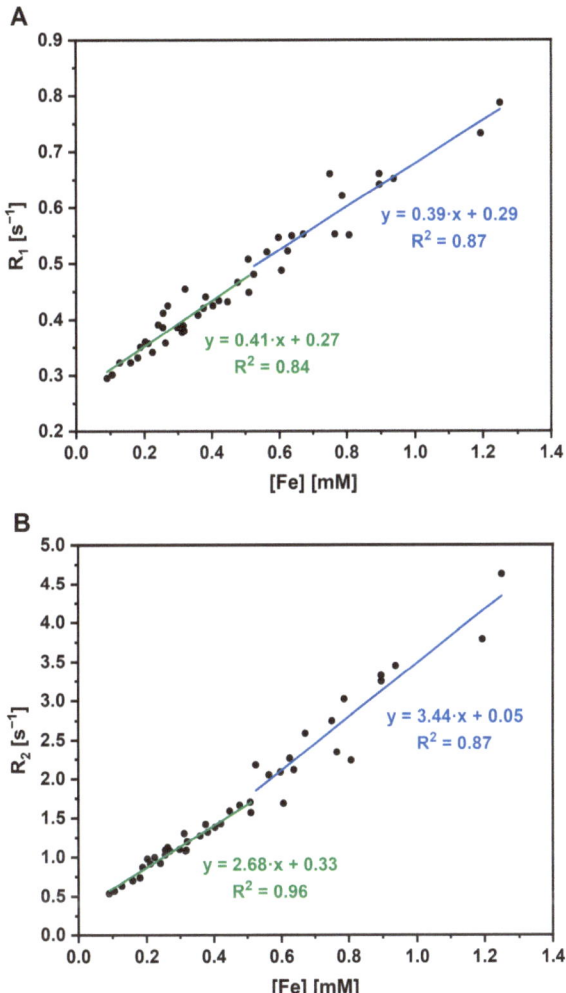

Figure 6. (**A**) Relaxation rate R_1 and (**B**) relaxation rate R_2 as functions of real iron concentrations in AuBSA-Fe samples, as determined by ICP-MS (values are listed in Table S7).

Table 2. The values of r_1 and r_2 relaxivities assessed for AuBSA-Fe samples, depending on real iron concentrations, as determined by ICP-MS. Two linear regimes are recognized by a jump around the value of 0.52 mM in Fe concentrations.

Fe Concentration [mM]	Relaxivity r_1 [L·mmol^{-1}·s^{-1}]	Relaxivity r_2 [L·mmol^{-1}·s^{-1}]
<0.52	0.41 ± 0.04	2.68 ± 0.11
≥0.52	0.39 ± 0.04	3.44 ± 0.36

Another very important issue of AuBSA-Fe nanocomposite application as a potential contrast agent is its biocompatibility. Since AuBSA-Fe nanocomposites are prepared by a synthetic approach obeying the principles of green chemistry (i.e., non-toxic reactants and aqueous environments, no abundant chemicals used), their biocompatibility can be presumed. Moreover, AuBSA nanocomposites have been tested by many authors, including us [19], for potential cytotoxicity, which was revealed to be negligible. Similarly, SPIONs were tested by several authors and manifested almost zero cytotoxicity (e.g., [25–28]). It would be thus very unusual if AuBSA-Fe nanocomposites were cytotoxic. However, the assumption of the low cytotoxicity of AuBSA-Fe was validated by using Alamar blue assay (exploiting resazurin and fluorescence measurements) in the present study. The average cell viabilities for AuBSA-Fe nanocomposites with different iron concentrations (below and/or above 0.52 mM Fe content, in correlation with MRI data) are shown in Table 3, and an example of the resazurin assay is given in Table S8.

Table 3. Results of cell viability tests.

AuBSA-Fe	Average Viability [%]
Iron concentration < 0.52 mM	78 ± 3
Iron concentration ≥ 0.52 mM	80 ± 2

Surprisingly, the average cell viability was determined to be around 80% (only) in all AuBSA-Fe nanocomposites. This value still falls in the range of non-toxic species according to ISO 10993. However, it should be pointed out that the cytotoxicity results may be false negatives because resazurin is able to interact with serum albumin, especially at elevated protein concentrations, as revealed in [54]. In which case, the final values of cell viability (here evaluated around 80%) could be underestimated with respect to reality, i.e., the biocompatibility of AuBSA-Fe nanocomposites could be much better than determined by the Alamar blue assay. It should be also noted that the MTT assay and CCK-8 kit were not employed because both are able to provide false-positive results, as discussed in [55,56]. Further experiments assessing the real cytotoxicity of AuBSA-Fe nanocomposites are in progress.

4. Conclusions

We developed an easy, reproducible, one-pot, green synthesis of a new type of potential bimodal probe, labelled as AuBSA-Fe. These AuBSA-Fe probes are based on non-toxic luminescent AuNCs (embedded in BSA), which are generated together with SPIONs simply through the alkalization of the reaction mixture. Luminescent features of AuNCs are preserved in AuBSA-Fe samples, i.e., emission maxima and quantum yields are comparable within experimental errors with those of AuBSA (serving here as a reference). Furthermore, MRI experiments confirmed the effect of AuBSA-Fe on T_2 contrast in MR images. The relaxivity values of AuBSA-Fe approach those of commercial contrast agents. The great benefit of AuBSA-Fe probes, serving as MR alternatives, lies in their simultaneous luminescent feature. Therefore, AuBSA-Fe nanocomposites (stable when stored in a fridge) represent promising bimodal probes and could be potentially applied as fluorescent and MRI contrast agents. Further experiments with AuBSA-Fe nanocomposites are envisaged, leading to the increased possibility of their use as MRI alternatives and testing their biocompatibility and stability, performed not only *in vitro* but also *in vivo*.

Supplementary Materials: The following supporting information can be downloaded at: https://www.mdpi.com/article/10.3390/nano13061027/s1, Figure S1: 3D excitation-emission maps of AuBSA (A) and AuBSA-Fe (B); Table S1: Quantum yield and position of emission maxima of AuBSA (seven independent sample preparations); Table S2: Quantum yield and position of emission maxima of AuBSA-Fe (seven independent sample preparations); Figure S2: Particle size distribution (PSD) histograms of AuBSA (orange curve) and AuBSA-Fe (black curve) based on the changes in intensity of scattered light (633 nm laser line) measured by dynamic light scattering. Trimodal PSD is observed in both samples, however, with different average values and percentage (in brackets): 266.1 ± 38.0 nm (12.9 ± 2.1%), 26.8 ± 2.4 nm (50.8 ± 1.2%), 3.0 ± 0.1 nm (27.7 ± 0.8%) for AuBSA; 351.2 ± 21.0 nm (68.7 ± 1.4%), 30.0 ± 2.9 nm (16.7 ± 0.9%), 4.4 ± 0.3 nm (10.6 ± 0.8%) for AuBSA-Fe; Table S3:

PSD of several independently measured AuBSA samples determined by DLS based on intensity and number. Average and standard deviation (SD) values are then calculated; Table S4: PSD of several independently measured AuBSA-Fe determined by DLS based on intensity and number. Average and standard deviation (SD) values are then calculated; Figure S3: Histograms of PSD of several independently measured AuBSA; Figure S4: Histograms of PSD of several independently measured AuBSA-Fe; Table S5: Validation results for ICP-MS; Table S6: Contents of Au and Fe in many independently prepared AuBSA-Fe samples as determined by ICP-MS and calculation of Au:Fe ratios in real samples; Table S7: Values of relaxation times T_1, T_2 and relaxation rates R_1, R_2 together with real iron concentrations (as determined by ICP-MS for concentrated samples, while derived from these values for diluted samples); Figure S5: Relaxation rates as a function of iron concentration in AuBSA-Fe samples (100% concentration, any dilution is omitted). Comparison of linear and nonlinear (quadratic) fits; Figure S6: (A) XPS signal of fresh AuBSA-Fe sample, Au4f region; (B) XPS signal of one-year aged AuBSA-Fe sample, Au4f region; (C) XPS signal of fresh AuBSA-Fe sample, N1s region; (D) XPS signal of one-year aged AuBSA-Fe sample, N1s region; (E) XPS signal of fresh AuBSA-Fe sample, S2p region; (F) XPS signal of one-year aged AuBSA-Fe sample, S2p region; (G) XPS signal of fresh AuBSA-Fe sample, C1s region; (H) XPS signal of one-year aged AuBSA-Fe sample, C1s region; (I) XPS signal of fresh AuBSA-Fe sample, O1s region; (J) XPS signal of one-year aged AuBSA-Fe sample, O1s region; Table S8: Table showing values of fluorescence in each well of the titration plate when cell viability tests of AuBSA-Fe nanocomposites and their precursors ($HAuCl_4$, mixture of $FeCl_2$ and $FeCl_3$) were performed in two representative iron concentrations (below and above 0.52 mM).

Author Contributions: R.O.: investigation, methodology, formal analysis, original draft—review and editing. T.P.: investigation, original draft—review and editing. O.T.: investigation. D.P.: investigation. P.N.: investigation. D.J.: funding acquisition, original draft—review and editing. K.Š.: conceptualization, resources, methodology, funding acquisition, supervision, original draft—writing and editing, original draft—review and editing. All authors have read and agreed to the published version of the manuscript.

Funding: Financial support from the Czech Science Foundation (project no. 19-03207S); from the Ministry of Health CR-DRO (Institute for Clinical and Experimental Medicine IKEM, IN00023001); from the OP RDE project "Improving schematics of Doctoral student grant competition and their pilot implementation", Reg. No. CZ.02.2.69/0.0/0.0/19_073/0016713 (Doctoral Student Grant Competition, grant number DSGC-2021-0113); and from the Internal Grant Agency of Palacký University (projects no. IGA_PrF_2022_003, IGA_PrF_2023_003) is gratefully acknowledged.

Data Availability Statement: The raw/processed data required to reproduce these findings can be requested from the authors directly.

Acknowledgments: Martin Petr is thanked for XPS measurements. Marcela Václavíková is thanked for her help with the bibliographical search and retrieval of several articles. Helena Sedláčková is thanked for her English correction of the revised version of the manuscript. All five reviewers are thanked for their valuable comments, questions, and suggestions that improved the manuscript.

Conflicts of Interest: The authors declare no conflict of interest.

References

1. Han, X.; Xu, K.; Taratula, O.; Farsad, K. Applications of Nanoparticles in Biomedical Imaging. *Nanoscale* **2019**, *11*, 799–819. [CrossRef]
2. Nienhaus, K.; Wang, H.; Nienhaus, G.U. Nanoparticles for Biomedical Applications: Exploring and Exploiting Molecular Interactions at the Nano-Bio Interface. *Mater. Today Adv.* **2020**, *5*, 100036. [CrossRef]
3. Xu, C.; Wang, Y.; Zhang, C.; Jia, Y.; Luo, Y.; Gao, X. AuGd Integrated Nanoprobes for Optical/MRI/CT Triple-Modal in Vivo Tumor Imaging. *Nanoscale* **2017**, *9*, 4620–4628. [CrossRef]
4. Pan, U.N.; Khandelia, R.; Sanpui, P.; Das, S.; Paul, A.; Chattopadhyay, A. Protein-Based Multifunctional Nanocarriers for Imaging, Photothermal Therapy, and Anticancer Drug Delivery. *ACS Appl. Mater. Interfaces* **2017**, *9*, 19495–19501. [CrossRef] [PubMed]
5. Zhao, C.; Du, T.; ur Rehman, F.; Lai, L.; Liu, X.; Jiang, X.; Li, X.; Chen, Y.; Zhang, H.; Sun, Y.; et al. Biosynthesized Gold Nanoclusters and Iron Complexes as Scaffolds for Multimodal Cancer Bioimaging. *Small* **2016**, *12*, 6255–6265. [CrossRef]
6. Pahari, S.K.; Olszakier, S.; Kahn, I.; Amirav, L. Magneto-Fluorescent Yolk–Shell Nanoparticles. *Chem. Mater.* **2018**, *30*, 775–780. [CrossRef]
7. Su, X.; Xu, Y.; Che, Y.; Liao, X.; Jiang, Y. A Type of Novel Fluorescent Magnetic Carbon Quantum Dots for Cells Imaging and Detection. *J. Biomed. Mater. Res. A* **2015**, *103*, 3956–3964. [CrossRef] [PubMed]

8. Wang, C.; Yao, Y.; Song, Q. Gold Nanoclusters Decorated with Magnetic Iron Oxide Nanoparticles for Potential Multimodal Optical/Magnetic Resonance Imaging. *J. Mater. Chem. C Mater.* **2015**, *3*, 5910–5917. [CrossRef]
9. Huang, C.-L.; Hsieh, W.-J.; Lin, C.-W.; Yang, H.-W.; Wang, C.-K. Multifunctional Liposomal Drug Delivery with Dual Probes of Magnetic Resonance and Fluorescence Imaging. *Ceram. Int.* **2018**, *44*, 12442–12450. [CrossRef]
10. Binaymotlagh, R.; Hajareh Haghighi, F.; Aboutalebi, F.; Mirahmadi-Zare, S.Z.; Hadadzadeh, H.; Nasr-Esfahani, M.-H. Selective Chemotherapy and Imaging of Colorectal and Breast Cancer Cells by a Modified MUC-1 Aptamer Conjugated to a Poly(Ethylene Glycol)-Dimethacrylate Coated Fe_3O_4–AuNCs Nanocomposite. *New J. Chem.* **2019**, *43*, 238–248. [CrossRef]
11. Sheng, J.; Jiang, X.; Wang, L.; Yang, M.; Liu, Y.-N. Biomimetic Mineralization Guided One-Pot Preparation of Gold Clusters Anchored Two-Dimensional MnO2 Nanosheets for Fluorometric/Magnetic Bimodal Sensing. *Anal. Chem.* **2018**, *90*, 2926–2932. [CrossRef]
12. Xu, Y.; Palchoudhury, S.; Qin, Y.; Macher, T.; Bao, Y. Make Conjugation Simple: A Facile Approach to Integrated Nanostructures. *Langmuir* **2012**, *28*, 8767–8772. [CrossRef]
13. Meng, L.; Ma, X.; Jiang, S.; Ji, G.; Han, W.; Xu, B.; Tian, J.; Tian, W. High-Efficiency Fluorescent and Magnetic Multimodal Probe for Long-Term Monitoring and Deep Penetration Imaging of Tumors. *J. Mater. Chem. B* **2019**, *7*, 5345–5351. [CrossRef] [PubMed]
14. Li, D.-L.; Tan, J.-E.; Tian, Y.; Huang, S.; Sun, P.-H.; Wang, M.; Han, Y.-J.; Li, H.-S.; Wu, H.-B.; Zhang, X.-M.; et al. Multifunctional Superparamagnetic Nanoparticles Conjugated with Fluorescein-Labeled Designed Ankyrin Repeat Protein as an Efficient HER2-Targeted Probe in Breast Cancer. *Biomaterials* **2017**, *147*, 86–98. [CrossRef]
15. Le, W.; Cui, S.; Chen, X.; Zhu, H.; Chen, B.; Cui, Z. Facile Synthesis of Gd-Functionalized Gold Nanoclusters as Potential MRI/CT Contrast Agents. *Nanomaterials* **2016**, *6*, 65. [CrossRef]
16. Liang, G.; Xiao, L. Gd 3+-Functionalized Gold Nanoclusters for Fluorescence–Magnetic Resonance Bimodal Imaging. *Biomater. Sci.* **2017**, *5*, 2122–2130. [CrossRef]
17. Dong, D.; Jing, X.; Zhang, X.; Hu, X.; Wu, Y.; Duan, C. Gadolinium(III)–Fluorescein Complex as a Dual Modal Probe for MRI and Fluorescence Zinc Sensing. *Tetrahedron* **2012**, *68*, 306–310. [CrossRef]
18. Guan, S.; Liang, R.; Li, C.; Wei, M. A Supramolecular Material for Dual-Modal Imaging and Targeted Cancer Therapy. *Talanta* **2017**, *165*, 297–303. [CrossRef]
19. Andrýsková, P.; Šišková, K.M.; Michetschlägerová, Š.; Jiráková, K.; Kubala, M.; Jirák, D. The Effect of Fatty Acids and BSA Purity on Synthesis and Properties of Fluorescent Gold Nanoclusters. *Nanomaterials* **2020**, *10*, 343. [CrossRef] [PubMed]
20. Hsu, N.-Y.; Lin, Y.-W. Microwave-Assisted Synthesis of Bovine Serum Albumin–Gold Nanoclusters and Their Fluorescence-Quenched Sensing of Hg^{2+} Ions. *New J. Chem.* **2016**, *40*, 1155–1161. [CrossRef]
21. Yan, L.; Cai, Y.; Zheng, B.; Yuan, H.; Guo, Y.; Xiao, D.; Choi, M.M.F. Microwave-Assisted Synthesis of BSA-Stabilized and HSA-Protected Gold Nanoclusters with Red Emission. *J. Mater. Chem.* **2012**, *22*, 1000–1005. [CrossRef]
22. Ostruszka, R.; Zoppellaro, G.; Tomanec, O.; Pinkas, D.; Filimonenko, V.; Šišková, K. Evidence of Au(II) and Au(0) States in Bovine Serum Albumin-Au Nanoclusters Revealed by CW-EPR/LEPR and Peculiarities in HR-TEM/STEM Imaging. *Nanomaterials* **2022**, *12*, 1425. [CrossRef] [PubMed]
23. Zhou, Z.; Yang, L.; Gao, J.; Chen, X. Structure-Relaxivity Relationships of Magnetic Nanoparticles for Magnetic Resonance Imaging. *Adv. Mater.* **2019**, *31*, 1804567. [CrossRef] [PubMed]
24. Babes, L.; Denizot, B.; Tanguy, G.; le Jeune, J.J.; Jallet, P. Synthesis of Iron Oxide Nanoparticles Used as MRI Contrast Agents: A Parametric Study. *J. Colloid Interface Sci.* **1999**, *212*, 474–482. [CrossRef]
25. Bajaj, A.; Samanta, B.; Yan, H.; Jerry, D.J.; Rotello, V.M. Stability, Toxicity and Differential Cellular Uptake of Protein Passivated-Fe_3O_4 Nanoparticles. *J. Mater. Chem.* **2009**, *19*, 6328. [CrossRef]
26. Li, D.; Hua, M.; Fang, K.; Liang, R. BSA Directed-Synthesis of Biocompatible Fe_3O_4 Nanoparticles for Dual-Modal T1 and T2 MR Imaging in Vivo. *Anal. Methods* **2017**, *9*, 3099–3104. [CrossRef]
27. Nosrati, H.; Sefidi, N.; Sharafi, A.; Danafar, H.; Kheiri Manjili, H. Bovine Serum Albumin (BSA) Coated Iron Oxide Magnetic Nanoparticles as Biocompatible Carriers for Curcumin-Anticancer Drug. *Bioorg. Chem.* **2018**, *76*, 501–509. [CrossRef]
28. Xu, S.; Wang, J.; Wei, Y.; Zhao, H.; Tao, T.; Wang, H.; Wang, Z.; Du, J.; Wang, P.; Qian, J.; et al. In Situ One-Pot Synthesis of Fe_2O_3@BSA Core-Shell Nanoparticles as Enhanced T1-Weighted Magnetic Resonance Imagine Contrast Agents. *ACS Appl. Mater. Interfaces* **2020**, *12*, 56701–56711. [CrossRef]
29. Wang, Y.; Xu, C.; Chang, Y.; Zhao, L.; Zhang, K.; Zhao, Y.; Gao, F.; Gao, X. Ultrasmall Superparamagnetic Iron Oxide Nanoparticle for T2-Weighted Magnetic Resonance Imaging. *ACS Appl. Mater. Interfaces* **2017**, *9*, 28959–28966. [CrossRef]
30. Li, H.; Yan, K.; Shang, Y.; Shrestha, L.; Liao, R.; Liu, F.; Li, P.; Xu, H.; Xu, Z.; Chu, P.K. Folate-Bovine Serum Albumin Functionalized Polymeric Micelles Loaded with Superparamagnetic Iron Oxide Nanoparticles for Tumor Targeting and Magnetic Resonance Imaging. *Acta Biomater.* **2015**, *15*, 117–126. [CrossRef]
31. Vismara, E.; Bongio, C.; Coletti, A.; Edelman, R.; Serafini, A.; Mauri, M.; Simonutti, R.; Bertini, S.; Urso, E.; Assaraf, Y.; et al. Albumin and Hyaluronic Acid-Coated Superparamagnetic Iron Oxide Nanoparticles Loaded with Paclitaxel for Biomedical Applications. *Molecules* **2017**, *22*, 1030. [CrossRef]
32. An, L.; Yan, C.; Mu, X.; Tao, C.; Tian, Q.; Lin, J.; Yang, S. Paclitaxel-Induced Ultrasmall Gallic Acid-Fe@BSA Self-Assembly with Enhanced MRI Performance and Tumor Accumulation for Cancer Theranostics. *ACS Appl. Mater. Interfaces* **2018**, *10*, 28483–28493. [CrossRef]

33. Tian, Q.; An, L.; Tian, Q.; Lin, J.; Yang, S. Ellagic Acid-Fe@BSA Nanoparticles for Endogenous H2S Accelerated Fe(III)/Fe(II) Conversion and Photothermal Synergistically Enhanced Chemodynamic Therapy. *Theranostics* **2020**, *10*, 4101–4115. [CrossRef]
34. Harini, G.; Balasurya, S.; Khan, S.S. Recent Advances on Gadolinium-Based Nano-Photocatalysts for Environmental Remediation and Clean Energy Production: Properties, Fabrication, Defect Engineering and Toxicity. *J. Clean Prod.* **2022**, *345*, 131139. [CrossRef]
35. Gao, F.; Qu, H.; Duan, Y.; Wang, J.; Song, X.; Ji, T.; Cao, L.; Nie, G.; Sun, S. Dopamine Coating as a General and Facile Route to Biofunctionalization of Superparamagnetic Fe_3O_4 Nanoparticles for Magnetic Separation of Proteins. *RSC Adv.* **2014**, *4*, 6657. [CrossRef]
36. Nosrati, H.; Davaran, S.; Kheiri Manjili, H.; Rezaeejam, H.; Danafar, H. Bovine Serum Albumin Stabilized Iron Oxide and Gold Bimetallic Heterodimers: Synthesis, Characterization and Stereological Study. *Appl. Organomet. Chem.* **2019**, *33*, e5155. [CrossRef]
37. Nosrati, H.; Baghdadchi, Y.; Abbasi, R.; Barsbay, M.; Ghaffarlou, M.; Abhari, F.; Mohammadi, A.; Kavetskyy, T.; Bochani, S.; Rezaeejam, H.; et al. Iron Oxide and Gold Bimetallic Radiosensitizers for Synchronous Tumor Chemoradiation Therapy in 4T1 Breast Cancer Murine Model. *J. Mater. Chem. B* **2021**, *9*, 4510–4522. [CrossRef] [PubMed]
38. Rurack, K.; Spieles, M. Fluorescence Quantum Yields of a Series of Red and Near-Infrared Dyes Emitting at 600−1000 nm. *Anal. Chem.* **2011**, *83*, 1232–1242. [CrossRef]
39. Procházka, V.; Novák, P.; Stejskal, A. Department of Experimental Physics. Mössbauer Spectrometers OLTWINS. Available online: http://oltwins.upol.cz/ (accessed on 6 February 2023).
40. Klencsár, Z.; Kuzmann, E.; Vértes, A. User-Friendly Software for Mössbauer Spectrum Analysis. *J. Radioanal. Nucl. Chem. Artic.* **1996**, *210*, 105–118. [CrossRef]
41. Zhang, J.; Cai, Y.; Razzaque, S.; Hussain, I.; Lu, Q.-W.; Tan, B. Synthesis of Water-Soluble and Highly Fluorescent Gold Nanoclusters for Fe^{3+} Sensing in Living Cells Using Fluorescence Imaging. *J. Mater. Chem. B* **2017**, *5*, 5608–5615. [CrossRef]
42. Zhang, Y.; Chen, Y.; Jiang, H.; Wang, X. Selective and Sensitive Detection of Fe^{3+} Ion in Drinking Water Using L-Glutathione Stabilized Red Fluorescent Gold Nanoclusters. *J. Nanosci. Nanotechnol.* **2016**, *16*, 12179–12186. [CrossRef]
43. Ungor, D.; Csapó, E.; Kismárton, B.; Juhász, Á.; Dékány, I. Nucleotide-Directed Syntheses of Gold Nanohybrid Systems with Structure-Dependent Optical Features: Selective Fluorescence Sensing of Fe^{3+} Ions. *Colloids Surf B Biointerfaces* **2017**, *155*, 135–141. [CrossRef] [PubMed]
44. Šišková, K.; Machala, L.; Tuček, J.; Kašlík, J.; Mojzeš, P.; Zbořil, R. Mixtures of L-Amino Acids as Reaction Medium for Formation of Iron Nanoparticles: The Order of Addition into a Ferrous Salt Solution Matters. *Int. J. Mol. Sci.* **2013**, *14*, 19452–19473. [CrossRef]
45. Rohrer, M.; Bauer, H.; Mintorovitch, J.; Requardt, M.; Weinmann, H.-J. Comparison of Magnetic Properties of MRI Contrast Media Solutions at Different Magnetic Field Strengths. *Investig. Radiol.* **2005**, *40*, 715–724. [CrossRef] [PubMed]
46. Stanisz, G.J.; Henkelman, R.M. Gd-DTPA Relaxivity Depends on Macromolecular Content. *Magn. Reson. Med.* **2000**, *44*, 665–667. [CrossRef]
47. Bjørnerud, A.; Johansson, L.O.; Briley-Saebø, K.; Ahlström, H.K. Assessment of T1 and T2* Effects in Vivo and Ex Vivo Using Iron Oxide Nanoparticles in Steady State-Dependence on Blood Volume and Water Exchange. *Magn. Reson. Med.* **2002**, *47*, 461–471. [CrossRef]
48. Van Osch, M.J.P.; Vonken, E.P.A.; Viergever, M.A.; van der Grond, J.; Bakker, C.J.G. Measuring the Arterial Input Function with Gradient Echo Sequences. *Magn. Reson. Med.* **2003**, *49*, 1067–1076. [CrossRef]
49. Zhao, J.M.; Clingman, C.S.; Närväinen, M.J.; Kauppinen, R.A.; van Zijl, P.C.M. Oxygenation and Hematocrit Dependence of Transverse Relaxation Rates of Blood at 3T. *Magn. Reson. Med.* **2007**, *58*, 592–597. [CrossRef]
50. Calamante, F.; Connelly, A.; van Osch, M.J.P. Nonlinear ΔR2* Effects in Perfusion Quantification Using Bolus-Tracking MRI. *Magn. Reson. Med.* **2009**, *61*, 486–492. [CrossRef]
51. Patil, V.; Jensen, J.H.; Johnson, G. Intravascular Contrast Agent T2* Relaxivity in Brain Tissue. *NMR Biomed.* **2013**, *26*, 392–399. [CrossRef]
52. Ta, H.T.; Li, Z.; Wu, Y.; Cowin, G.; Zhang, S.; Yago, A.; Whittaker, A.K.; Xu, Z.P. Effects of Magnetic Field Strength and Particle Aggregation on Relaxivity of Ultra-Small Dual Contrast Iron Oxide Nanoparticles. *Mater. Res. Express* **2017**, *4*, 116105. [CrossRef]
53. Weisskoff, R.; Zuo, C.S.; Boxerman, J.L.; Rosen, B.R. Microscopic Susceptibility Variation and Transverse Relaxation: Theory and Experiment. *Magn. Reson. Med.* **1994**, *31*, 601–610. [CrossRef] [PubMed]
54. Goegan, P.; Johnson, G.; Vincent, R. Effects of Serum Protein and Colloid on the AlamarBlue Assay in Cell Cultures. *Toxicol. In Vitr.* **1995**, *9*, 257–266. [CrossRef] [PubMed]
55. Funk, D.; Schrenk, H.-H.; Frei, E. Serum Albumin Leads to False-Positive Results in the XTT and the MTT Assay. *Biotechniques* **2007**, *43*, 178–186. [CrossRef]
56. Neufeld, B.H.; Tapia, J.B.; Lutzke, A.; Reynolds, M.M. Small Molecule Interferences in Resazurin and MTT-Based Metabolic Assays in the Absence of Cells. *Anal. Chem.* **2018**, *90*, 6867–6876. [CrossRef] [PubMed]

Disclaimer/Publisher's Note: The statements, opinions and data contained in all publications are solely those of the individual author(s) and contributor(s) and not of MDPI and/or the editor(s). MDPI and/or the editor(s) disclaim responsibility for any injury to people or property resulting from any ideas, methods, instructions or products referred to in the content.

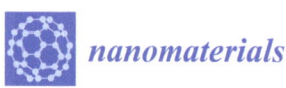

Review

Metal-Polymer Nanoconjugates Application in Cancer Imaging and Therapy

André Q. Figueiredo [1], Carolina F. Rodrigues [1], Natanael Fernandes [1], Duarte de Melo-Diogo [1], Ilídio J. Correia [1,*] and André F. Moreira [1,2,*]

[1] CICS-UBI—Health Sciences Research Centre, Universidade da Beira Interior, Av. Infante D. Henrique, 6200-506 Covilhã, Portugal
[2] CPIRN-UDI/IPG—Centro de Potencial e Inovação em Recursos Naturais, Unidade de Investigação para o Desenvolvimento do Interior do Instituto Politécnico da Guarda, Avenida Dr. Francisco de Sá Carneiro, No. 50, 6300-559 Guarda, Portugal
* Correspondence: icorreia@ubi.pt (I.J.C.); afmoreira@fcsaude.ubi.pt (A.F.M.); Tel.: +351-275-329-002 (I.J.C.)

Abstract: Metallic-based nanoparticles present a unique set of physicochemical properties that support their application in different fields, such as electronics, medical diagnostics, and therapeutics. Particularly, in cancer therapy, the plasmonic resonance, magnetic behavior, X-ray attenuation, and radical oxygen species generation capacity displayed by metallic nanoparticles make them highly promising theragnostic solutions. Nevertheless, metallic-based nanoparticles are often associated with some toxicological issues, lack of colloidal stability, and establishment of off-target interactions. Therefore, researchers have been exploiting the combination of metallic nanoparticles with other materials, inorganic (e.g., silica) and/or organic (e.g., polymers). In terms of biological performance, metal-polymer conjugation can be advantageous for improving biocompatibility, colloidal stability, and tumor specificity. In this review, the application of metallic-polymer nanoconjugates/nanohybrids as a multifunctional all-in-one solution for cancer therapy will be summarized, focusing on the physicochemical properties that make metallic nanomaterials capable of acting as imaging and/or therapeutic agents. Then, an overview of the main advantages of metal-polymer conjugation as well as the most common structural arrangements will be provided. Moreover, the application of metallic-polymer nanoconjugates/nanohybrids made of gold, iron, copper, and other metals in cancer therapy will be discussed, in addition to an outlook of the current solution in clinical trials.

Keywords: metallic nanoparticles; metal-polymer nanoconjugates; cancer; photothermal effect

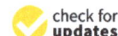

Citation: Figueiredo, A.Q.; Rodrigues, C.F.; Fernandes, N.; de Melo-Diogo, D.; Correia, I.J.; Moreira, A.F. Metal-Polymer Nanoconjugates Application in Cancer Imaging and Therapy. *Nanomaterials* **2022**, *12*, 3166. https://doi.org/10.3390/nano12183166

Academic Editor: Horacio Cabral

Received: 26 August 2022
Accepted: 9 September 2022
Published: 13 September 2022

Publisher's Note: MDPI stays neutral with regard to jurisdictional claims in published maps and institutional affiliations.

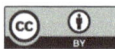

Copyright: © 2022 by the authors. Licensee MDPI, Basel, Switzerland. This article is an open access article distributed under the terms and conditions of the Creative Commons Attribution (CC BY) license (https://creativecommons.org/licenses/by/4.0/).

1. Introduction

The manipulation of matter at the nanoscale led to the development of various nanomaterials, based on polymers, lipids, ceramics, or metals, that exhibit exciting properties for improving the performance of electronics, medical diagnostics, and therapeutics [1,2]. Particularly, the application of nanoparticles for cancer therapy led to the development of new alternatives from therapeutics (i.e., drug delivery, photothermal and photodynamic effects) to diagnostic and imaging, leveraging the innate ability of these materials to accumulate in the tumor tissue [3–5].

In this field, the application of metallic-based nanomaterials (e.g., gold, iron, silver, and copper) has been capturing more attention in recent years due to their characteristic physical (e.g., magnetic behavior, plasmonic resonance, and imaging capacity) and chemical (e.g., radical oxygen species (ROS) generation, and catalytic activity enhancement) properties, which render them as platforms suitable for creating multifunctional cancer therapeutics [2,6–9]. Moreover, there are several methodologies described for the synthesis of metallic nanoparticles, such as physical or chemical vapor deposition, sol-gel methods, chemical reduction, hydrothermal methods, solvothermal method, laser ablation, and green synthesis processes, allowing the selection of the process most compatible with the available laboratory/industrial conditions and desired physicochemical properties [10–13]. Additionally, metallic nanomaterials surface functionalization, a strategy often used to refine the therapeutics pharmacokinetics, can be performed by well-known and defined methodologies [14]. Thus, the metallic nanomaterials' theranostic potential provides an all-in-one solution for cancer diagnosis, therapy, and real-time monitoring, which ultimately can improve the therapeutic outcome of anticancer therapy [15,16]. This is the rationale behind various metallic-based nanomaterials under clinical trials, such as Aurolase®, Nanotherm®, and Magnablate®.

Nevertheless, despite the wide number of publications showing the appealing features of metallic-based nanomaterials, their translation into the clinic is still very limited [17]. Such is widely associated with some toxicological issues, lack of colloidal stability, and the establishment of off-target interactions [18]. Additionally, when subjected to high-energy radiations, the metallic nanoparticles often undergo reshaping processes or are even degraded leading to the loss of their therapeutic potential [19]. Therefore, researchers have been exploring the combination of metallic nanoparticles with other materials, inorganic (e.g., silica) and/or organic (e.g., polymers). Particularly, the combination of the metallic nanoparticles' physicochemical properties with the superior biological performance of synthetic or natural polymers emerges as a valuable and straightforward approach to develop more effective anti-cancer therapeutics [16,20]. In this review, the application of metallic-polymer nanoconjugates/nanohybrids as a multifunctional all-in-one solution for cancer therapy will be summarized. Initially, the physicochemical properties rendering the metallic nanomaterials' potential to act as imaging and/or therapeutic agents will be summarized. Then, an overview of the main advantages of metal-polymer conjugation as well as the most common structural arrangements will be provided. Moreover, the application of metallic-polymer nanoconjugates/nanohybrids made of gold, iron, copper, and others in cancer therapy will be discussed, in addition to an outlook of the current solution in clinical trials.

2. Metallic Nanoparticles Applications and Therapies

Nanosized metals present optical and electrical properties that differentiate them from other nanomaterials, supporting their application in biomedicine, such as the development of biosensors (e.g., diagnosis of viruses using colloidal gold nanoparticles), bioimaging agents (e.g., iron oxide-based contrast agents), catalysts, mechanical reinforcement, and drug delivery system or other therapeutics. Moreover, these unique characteristics can be explored to create more effective antitumoral nanomedicines. The high density and X-ray attenuation capacity of metallic nanoparticles allow them the intrinsic capacity to be applied as contrast agents for bioimaging applications [21]. Up to now, several studies available in the literature have already shown that metallic nanoparticles provide a higher contrast enhancement in X-ray computed tomography (CT) imaging than the iodine-based contrast agents conventionally used in the clinic [22–26]. On the other hand, nanosized metals, such as gold, silver, and copper, show a pronounced plasmonic resonance phenomenon, i.e., the collective oscillation of the conduction band electrons in metal-based nanomaterials in response to the incident photons [27]. This interaction can lead to light absorption or scattering and is dependent on the size, morphology, distance, and dielectric constant of the metallic nanoparticles and surrounding medium [28–30]. In turn, the excited surface electrons can decay to the ground state via different processes (e.g., electron-to-photon, electron-to-electron, and electron-to-phonon energy conversion), the two most common events being the release of the absorbed energy in the form of light or heat [31]. The former is often explored to enhance the quantum efficiency and photostability of fluorophores, allowing the detection of lower quantities of biomarkers used in biosensing or bioimaging [32]. The latter is the foundation stone for the application of metallic nanoparticles in cancer hyperthermia/photothermal therapy [33]. However, it is essential to tailor the nanomaterials to interact specifically with near-infrared (NIR) radiation, a region of the spectra where the major biological components (e.g., collagen, hemoglobin, and water) have the lowest or insignificant absorption [34]. This will reduce the off-target interactions and guarantee a site-specific activation of the metallic nanomaterials. Then, the heat generated by the light-nanoparticles interaction can mediate the destruction of the cancer cells [35,36]. The elevation of the tumor temperature to values superior to 45 °C provokes irreversible damage to cancer cells (e.g., DNA degradation, cell membrane disruption, protein denaturation), leading to cell death (i.e., tumor ablation). Otherwise, if mild temperature increases are achieved (i.e., between 40 and 45 °C), the cell damage is less pronounced and often reversed by the cell repair mechanisms [5,37,38]. Nevertheless, this creates a time window during which the cancer cells are more sensitive to the action of other therapeutic modalities such as chemotherapy [39]. Furthermore, metallic nanomaterials, such as those composed of iron, nickel, and cobalt, can also present magnetic properties, also allowing their application as contrast agents (magnetic resonance imaging (MRI)) and in tumor magnetic hyperthermia [40]. This capacity to be magnetically manipulated by external magnetic fields is also explored to guide these metallic nanomaterials in the human body and promote a tumor-specific accumulation [41,42]. At the tumor site, the utilization of alternating magnetic fields will promote the nanoparticles' vibration and consequently a localized temperature increase will be obtained [43].

Metallic nanomaterials have also shown the capacity to mediate the formation of ROS [18]. This oxidative stress can influence several cellular processes/structures, e.g., intracellular calcium concentrations, activate transcription factors, induce DNA damage, and lipid peroxidation (cell membrane disruption), and increased amounts of ROS are highly cytotoxic [18]. The mechanism of ROS generation by metallic nanomaterials is influenced by their physicochemical properties (e.g., size, chemical structure, surface area, and charge) [44]. Generally, metallic nanomaterials act as the reactant or catalyst for the reduction of molecular oxygen to water, which yields the production of ROS, such as superoxide radicals and hydroxyl radicals [45]. The ROS generation of metallic nanomaterials can be further boosted by light absorption [46]. During this process, the electrons transit to higher energy bands, facilitating the reaction with water or molecular oxygen and consequently the ROS generation, a process denominated by photodynamic effect [47,48].

Despite the imaging and therapeutic potential of metallic nanoparticles, the in vivo application and translation to the clinic are severely hindered by their low colloidal stability, high reactivity, the formation of the protein corona, and high cytotoxicity [49–51]. Therefore, to overcome these limitations, researchers have been combining the superior physicochemical features of metallic nanoparticles with the increased biological properties (e.g., biocompatibility, enhanced blood circulation time, targeting capacity) of synthetic and natural polymers, often referred to as metal-polymer nanocomplexes or nanohybrids.

3. Metal-Polymer Based Nanomaterials

The metal-polymer nanocomplexes or nanohybrids are a class of nanomaterials that aim to address the biological bottlenecks of the metallic nanoparticles' administration in humans. For that purpose, several strategies have been explored to create these new nanomaterials (Figure 1), namely the (i) surface coating of metallic cores (e.g., physical linkage and layer-by-layer), (ii) entrapment of metallic cores within polymeric matrices (e.g., nanoparticle in situ growth or post-synthesis entrapment), and (iii) the utilization of polymeric capsules [52–54]. One of the main rationales behind the introduction of polymers is to increase the colloidal stability of metallic nanoparticles and avoid protein adsorption during the nanoparticles' circulation in the blood [55,56].

Highly hydrophilic polymers are often associated with improvements in the nanoparticles' blood circulation time, namely by minimizing the nanoparticle-protein interaction, avoiding nanoparticles' aggregation as well as the size and charge changes, and reducing the recognition by the immune cells [57,58]. For this purpose, polymers, such as poly(ethylene glycol) (PEG), poly(oxazolines) (POX), and poly(zwitterion)s, have been excelling in enhancing the nanoparticles' blood circulation [59]. The PEG and POX antifouling properties, which are attributed to two main events, (i) the steric repulsion and (ii) the water barrier, impede the nanoparticles–proteins interaction, avoiding the formation of a protein corona that negatively impacts the nanomaterials' biological performance [60,61]. In turn, the zwitterionic polymers present overall electrostatic neutrality and high chain hydration that confer to them a stealthing capacity [62,63]. The higher blood circulation times associated with the utilization of these polymers will increase the nanomaterials' probability to accumulate and interact with the tumor cells, which can be essential for achieving superior antitumoral effects [64]. On the other hand, the natural and synthetic polymers can also imprint a stimuli-responsive (e.g., pH, temperature, and enzymatic) behaviour on the metallic-based nanomaterials, which can be particularly advantageous for controlling drug delivery [33,65–68]. In this regard, the heat generated by the nanomaterials (e.g., PTT and magnetic hyperthermia) can be also explored to induce phase changes in the polymers (e.g., Poly(N-isopropylacrylamide) (PNIPAM)) or increase their solubility, which will trigger the drug release [68,69]. Additionally, at the tumor site, the metal-polymer nanocomplexes/nanohybrids will also have an impact on the physiological conditions that can be explored to trigger the drug release, such as an acidic pH, overexpression of certain enzymes (e.g., matrix metalloproteinases), and an increased RedOx environment [65,67,70]. Apart from the passive accumulation of the nanomaterials at the tumor site, usually dependent on the enhanced permeability and retention (EPR) effect, the polymers or other targeting moieties can confer a specific recognition of molecules overexpressed in the tumor tissue [5,71]. This higher specificity towards cancer cells will favor the accumulation of nanomaterials in these areas as well as the nanomaterials–cancer cell interaction [72]. Therefore, the metal–polymer nanocomplexes or nanohybrids show the potential to create novel and more effective anticancer therapeutics. In the following section, the application of metallic–polymer nanoconjugates/nanohybrids made of gold, iron, copper, and others in cancer therapy will be overviewed, showing the therapeutic modalities that each metal nanoparticle allows to explore.

3.1. Gold-Polymer Conjugates

Gold nanoparticles are one of the most explored metallic nanomaterials for biomedical applications, from bioimaging to drug delivery [73–75]. The applicability of gold nanomaterials in bioimaging is demonstrated in different works in the literature, principally as a contrast agent for CT imaging [76]. For example, Xi and co-workers observed that, when an X-ray beam of 100 KeV is used, gold nanoparticles present an absorption coefficient two-times superior to that obtained with iodine (a conventional contrast agent used in the clinic) [77]. In turn, the pronounced surface plasmon resonance of gold nanoparticles has been supporting the development of novel photothermal therapies for cancer therapy (Table 1). This phenomenon can be fine-tuned to enhance the gold nanoparticles' absorption in the NIR region (700–1100 nm) by optimizing the nanoparticles' size and/or shape (e.g., spheres, cages, stars, and rods) [37,78]. Per se, the application of gold nanospheres in cancer photothermal therapy (PTT) is limited since its absorption peak is in the 500–550 nm region [79]. However, the organization of gold nanospheres in nanoclusters or shells renders a shift in the absorption spectra to the NIR region [2,5]. This change in the gold nanoparticles' optical properties is attributed to the coupling of the plasmon resonance of adjacent gold nanospheres [80]. Therefore, the fine-tuning of the gold nanoclusters or shells' absorption spectra can be achieved by optimizing the nanospheres' size and interparticle distance [2]. In turn, the surface plasmon resonance in non-spherical gold nanoparticles varies with the nanoparticle surface [81,82]. For example, the two different surfaces in gold nanorods, longitudinal and transversal surfaces, originate two absorption bands. The transversal surface leads to an absorption band in the 500–550 nm region of the spectra, whereas the longitudinal surface originates an absorption peak that can be fine-tuned from the visible to the NIR region of the spectra [83,84]. This peak generated by the longitudinal surface resonance is determined by the aspect ratio of gold nanorods (i.e., quotient between length and width) [85]. Otherwise, the surface plasmon resonance of gold nanostars is defined by the particle's core size, the number of tips, as well as the tips' length and width [2]. Therefore, the gold nanoparticles' plasticity and fine-tunning ability to present a high absorption efficiency in the NIR region of the spectra propelled their application in the cancer PTT. Nevertheless, despite the theragnostic potential of gold nanoparticles, their direct application in the human body is hindered by their high affinity to establish interactions with thiol groups, which favors the interaction with different biomolecules and lead to the nanoparticles' aggregation [80]. Moreover, the gold nanoparticles can also be degraded when exposed to high-energy radiations, such as those used in CT imaging and PTT, causing the loss of their bioactivity [86]. Furthermore, several reports in the literature also describe that gold nanoparticles are strongly accumulated in the kidneys, causing nephrotoxicity, and may also trigger the lysis of red blood cells [78]. To address these issues, researchers have been exploring the development of gold-polymer nanocomplexes or nanohybrids to increase colloidal stability, biocompatibility, and even tumor specificity.

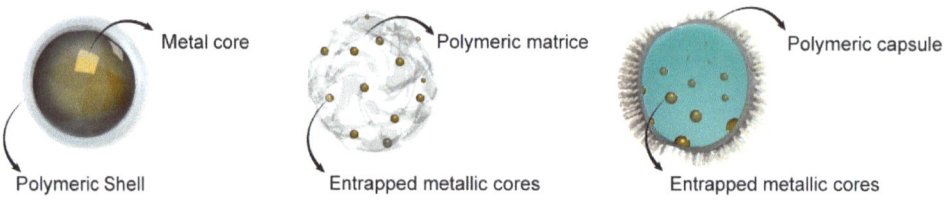

Figure 1. Overview of the properties of metallic nanoparticles, advantages of the polymers' inclusion, and representation of the most common structural organizations of the metal-polymer nanohybrids/complexes.

Table 1. Gold-based metallic-polymer nanoconjugates/nanohybrids, their physicochemical properties, and therapeutic applications (N.D.—non disclosed, N.A.—not applicable).

Metal	Morphology	Modification	Size (nm)	Surface Charge (mV)	Loading	In Vitro	In Vivo	Application	Ref.
Gold	Rods	UCST polymer (P(AAm-co-AN)-DDAT), metalloproteinase 2 (MMP-2)-sensitive peptides	Length ≈ 48.04; Width ≈ 12.08	N.D.	Doxorubicin (DOX)	HepG2 cells	HepG2 tumor-bearing mice	PTT (λex = 808 nm) and chemotherapy	[33]
		Mesoporous silica; D-α-Tocopherol polyethylene glycol 1000 succinate (TPGS), and Hyaluronic acid (HA)	Length ≈ 85; Width ≈ 64	−3 ± 5 and −10 ± 4 for TPGS/HA ratios of 1:1 and 4:1, respectively	N.A.	HeLa cells	N.A.	PTT (λex = 780 nm)	[86]
		Mesoporous silica, HA, and polyethyleneimine (PEI)	Length: 88 ± 5; Width: 63 ± 5;	−10 ± 2	Acridine Orange (AO)	HeLa cells	N.A.	PTT (λex = 750 nm) and chemotherapy	[87]
	Spheres	Poly(ethylene glycol) (PEG) and Lactoferrin (LF)	5	N.D.	N.A.	Caco-2, U87MG cells	GBM tumor-bearing mice	PTT (λex = 532 nm)	[54]
	Stars	Polydopamine (PDA) and Folic acid (FA)	149 ± 3	−19 ± 2.7	DOX	MCF-7, MCF-7/ADR, NIH/3T3, and HaCaT cells	MCF-7/ADR bearing mice	PTT (λex ≈ 800 nm) and chemotherapy	[56]
		Dendritic polyglycerol (dPG) and HA	68.1	13.9	Retinoic acid (RA)	MDA-MB-231 cells	4T1 tumor-bearing mice	PTT (λex ≈ 800 nm) and chemotherapy	[88]
		PEG and CD133 antibody	≈120	−22.47	IR780/DTX	PC3 cells	PC3 tumor-bearing mice	PTT (λex = 810 nm), PDT, and chemotherapy	[89]
	Cages	Poly(acrylic acid) (p_A) or Poly(NIPAM-co-AM) (p_N)	for p_A(Au) ≈130; N.D. for p_N(Au)	≈−4 for p_A(Au) formulation at pH 7.4; N.D. for p_N(Au) formulation	p_A(Au)-loaded with Erl and p_N(Au) loaded with DOX	A431 or MCF-7 cells	A431 or MCF-7 tumor-bearing mice	PTT (λex ≈ 800 nm for both formulations) and chemotherapy	[68]
		PVP, PEG, and anti-heat shock protein (HSP) monoclonal antibody	61.2 ± 4.85	−8.2 ± 1.25	N.A.	4T1	4T1 tumor-bearing mice	PTT (λex ≈ 808 nm)	[90]

Abbreviations—PDT: Photodynamic Therapy; PTT: Photothermal Therapy.

Peng and colleagues demonstrated the applicability of gold-based nanomaterials in bioimaging by following the biodistribution and tumor accumulation of PEGylated dendrimer-entrapped gold nanospheres [91]. In fact, the authors reported that these nanomaterials have an attenuation intensity higher than Omnipaque (an iodine-based contrast agent), which allowed them to follow the PEGylated dendrimer-entrapped gold nanoparticles in the blood circulation, after intravenous injection, as well as to perform the CT imaging of SPC-A1 xenograft tumors. Moreover, the authors reported that the PEGylated dendrimer-entrapped gold nanoparticles had a half-decay time in the blood circulation of 31.76 h, which was 2.5 times higher than that of bare gold nanorods previously reported. Furthermore, Gu et al. produced RGD-modified mPEG-PLGA nanocapsules containing gold nanoclusters and indocyanine green for the imaging and PTT of breast cancer [92]. The loaded mPEG-PLGA nanocapsules were formed via a water-in-oil-in-water emulsion using sonication, where (i) the first emulsion consisted of the water phase with gold nanoclusters and the oil phase with indocyanine green and the mPEG-PLGA. In the second emulsion, the mPEG-PLGA nanocapsules were further modified with poly(vinyl alcohol) and poly(acrylic acid), allowing the subsequent functionalization with RGD peptide via carbodiimide chemistry. The authors demonstrated that both one-photon and two-photon imaging techniques could be used to follow the nanocapsules in 4T1 tumor-bearing BALB/c mice. Moreover, the RGD-modified nanocapsules showed a preferential accumulation in

U87-MG cancer cells (overexpressing αvβ3 integrins), when compared to MCF-7 cancer cells (low expression of αvβ3 integrins), leading to the almost complete ablation of the cancer cells after irradiation with a NIR laser (808 nm, 2 W cm^{-2}, for 5 min). Feng and co-workers developed two different tumor-targeted gold nanocages for the combinatorial chemo-PTT of breast cancer [68]. For that purpose, pH-responsive gold nanocages were formulated via electrostatic interaction between the poly(acrylic acid) and the surface of the particles, entrapping the gold particles in the polymeric chains (p_AAu nanoparticles) and loaded with Erlotinib (Erl), an epidermal growth factor receptor (EGFR) inhibitor. In turn, temperature-responsive gold nanocages were produced by reacting them with the thiol-terminated N-isopropylacrylamide (NIPAM) and acrylamide (AM) (p(NIPAM-co-AM) co-polymer (p_NAu nanoparticles) and subsequently loaded with doxorubicin (Dox). The p_AAu nanoparticles showed a pH-triggered Erl release due to the protonation of poly(acrylic acid) in acidic pH (i.e., loosening of the polymeric barrier), 4.5%, 24.8%, 44.1%, or 66.3% Erl released after 6 h at pH 7.4, 6.5, 6, or 5. Otherwise, the Dox-loaded p_NAu nanoparticles were responsive to the irradiation with a NIR laser (808 nm, 0.5 W cm^{-2}, for 10 min) and consequent increase in temperature (i.e., superior to 45 °C, a value higher than the lower critical solution temperature). The authors reported 46.2% of Dox released in 10 h, after a 10 min NIR laser irradiation, contrasting with the 5% detected in the absence of NIR irradiation. The in vivo studies performed in MCF-7 and A431 tumor-bearing mice demonstrated a passive and preferential accumulation in the tumor tissue (Figure 2). Moreover, the combinatorial therapy led to the reduction of A431 tumors' size by 98%, after 14 days, whereas in MCF-7 tumors (low expression of EGFR), these nanomaterials only slowed the tumor growth.

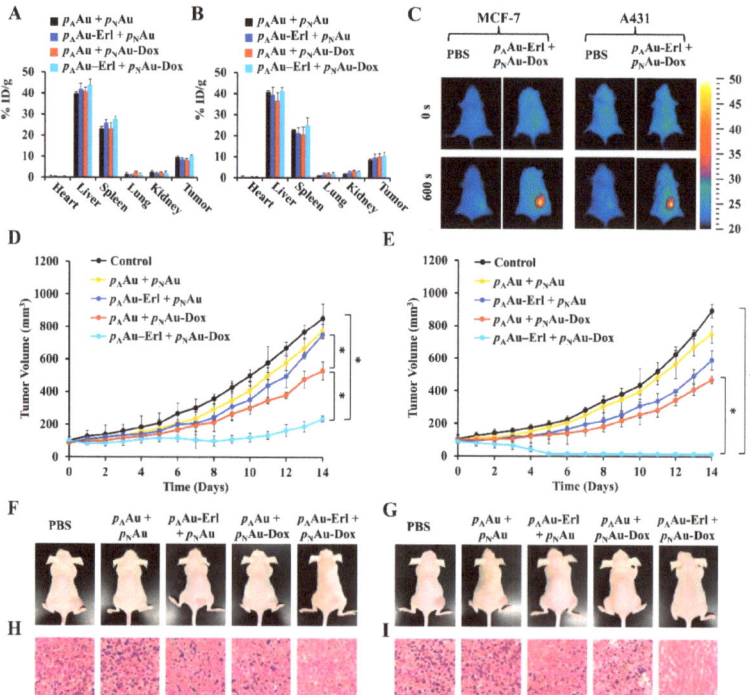

Figure 2. In vivo evaluation of the p_AAu-Erl plus p_NAu-Dox antitumoral efficacy. Biodistribution analysis of p_AAu + p_NAu, p_AAu-Erl + p_NAu, p_AAu + p_NAu-Dox, and p_AAu–Erl + p_NAu-Dox (12.4 Au mg kg^{-1} of mouse, Erl:Dox = 1:1) in MCF-7 (**A**) and A431 (**B**) tumor-bearing mice. Infrared thermal images of MCF-7 and A431 tumor-bearing mice before and after NIR laser irradiation

(808 nm, 0.5 W cm^{-2}, for 10 min) (**C**). Analysis of the tumor growth curve in MCF-7 (**D**) and A431 (**E**) tumor-bearing mice. * $p < 0.05$ analysed by ANOVA. Photos and histological analysis of MCF-7 (**F,H**) and A431 (**G,I**) tumor-bearing mice. Reprinted with permission from [68]. Copyright (2019) Elsevier.

3.2. Iron-Polymer Conjugates

The utilization of iron oxide nanoparticles can be explored in different biomedical applications, such as drug delivery, hyperthermia, and magnetic resonance imaging. Similar to gold nanoparticles, iron oxide can be produced in different shapes, such as spherical, rod-like, and cubical [93,94]. These nanoparticles (Fe_2O_3 and Fe_3O_4), when their size is inferior to 20 nm, present a superparamagnetic behavior at room temperature, i.e., the magnetization of the nanoparticles is close to 0 in the absence of an external magnetic field [95,96]. The iron oxide nanoparticles magnetism allows for widespread application in cancer therapy (Table 2), namely as contrast agents for magnetic resonance imaging: Feridex®, Resovist®, and Endorem®. The data available in the literature indicate that iron oxide nanoparticles are less toxic than the conventionally used gadolinium-based contrast agents, without presenting significant losses in imaging capacity [95]. Moreover, the magnetic properties of iron oxide nanoparticles have also been explored to direct the accumulation of the nanoparticles, specifically towards the tumor tissue, and in certain cases mediate a hyperthermic effect [97,98]. The former explores the application of an external magnetic field to guide the nanoparticles and promote their accumulation in the target tissue [99]. The latter employs an alternating magnetic field to induce the oscillation of iron oxide nanoparticles, which in turn generate heat [97]. This hyperthermic effect is dependent on the magnetic properties of the nanoparticles as well as on the frequency and intensity of the alternating magnetic field [100,101]. However, the biological application of iron oxide nanoparticles is hindered by their limited colloidal stability, tending to agglomerate when in contact with biological fluids [102]. With this in mind, Xu et al. prepared GSH-responsive hyaluronic acid-coated small iron oxide nanoparticles (HIONPs) for the diagnosis of liver metastases [103]. The nanoparticles were formed via a one-pot method, promoting the oxidation of ferrous ions to create iron oxide nanoparticles that were coated with hyaluronic acid modified with dopamine through the establishment phenol−metal coordination interactions. The in vitro measurements in a 0.52 T NMR instrument showed that the HIONPs have a longitudinal proton relaxivity (r_1) of 41.3 Fe mM^{-1} s^{-1}, indicating the applicability of HIONPs as T_1 MRI contrast agents. This was confirmed using a 3 T MR scanner where the HIONPs led to higher T_1-weighted magnetic resonance signals and lower T_2-weighted magnetic resonance signals when the Fe concentration increased from 0 to 0.2 mM. Moreover, the application of HIONPs (Fe—0.03 mmol kg^{-1}) in mice with B16F10, 4T1, and CT26 liver metastases allowed the metastases detection via MRI, showing the highest contrast-to-noise ratio 1 h after injection. This capacity is attributed to the higher GSH concentration in the mice liver tissue (i.e., 11 to 76-times higher) when compared to the tumor/metastases. The higher GSH concentration promotes the removal of the hyaluronic acid coating and consequent nanoparticle aggregation, which led to a significant decrease in the r_1 value. In this way, the hepatic tissues became dark whereas the tumor/metastases are bright in the MRI. Moreover, the authors also described that the HIONPs presented a higher imaging capacity than Primovist® (Gd-based imaging agent), where the metastases and surrounding liver tissue presented a similar contrast-to-noise ratio. In another work, Xiao and co-workers developed ultrathin vesicles with multimodal imaging capacity for the combinatorial chemo-PTT of cancer [104]. For that purpose, ultrasmall superparamagnetic iron oxide nanoparticles, cisplatin, and liquid perfluorohexane were encapsulated in PLGA nanovesicles, followed by the formation of an ultrathin silica layer to prevent leakage. Then, the surface of the particles was modified with polyaniline (a photothermal agent) and functionalized with R8-RGD. In these nanoparticles, the iron oxide acted as a

T_2-weighted magnetic resonance contrast agent, with a transverse relaxivity (r_2) value of 258.5 Fe mM^{-1} s^{-1}, three times superior to the iron oxide nanoparticles alone. Moreover, the in vivo studies in A549 tumor-bearing mice showed that the administration of the PLGA vesicles containing the iron oxide nanoparticles allows the monitoring of the changes in the tumor cellularity via MRI. Additionally, the chemo-photothermal combinatorial treatment led to a significant regression, close to 97%, of the tumor volume in 21 days. Chen and colleagues produced a dual-targeted magnetic iron oxide nanoparticle for the imaging and hyperthermia of breast tumors (Figure 3) [105]. The iron oxide nanoparticles were coated with a DSPE-PEG2000 shell and then modified with RGDyK (neovascular endothelium targeting) and D-glucosamine (glucose transporter affinity) via carbodiimide chemistry. The authors observed that the combination of magnetic and active targeting approaches resulted in the best contrast effect on T_2-weighted MRI from 3 to 48 h, showing the tumor region completely dark due to the accumulation of the nanoparticles. The tumor/normal tissue signal ratio at 48 h for active targeting strategies was 0.6 whereas for the magnetic plus active targeting combination this value was inferior to 0.3, showing a higher difference in the signal obtained in the tumor and normal tissues. Moreover, the utilization of alternating current magnetic fields (1.485 × 10^9 Am^{-1} s^{-1}), focused on the tumor region, induced a temperature increase to 44 °C, which successfully slowed the growth of 4T1 tumors when compared to the control group (i.e., the relative tumor volume of 500% and 200% for control and iron oxide groups, respectively).

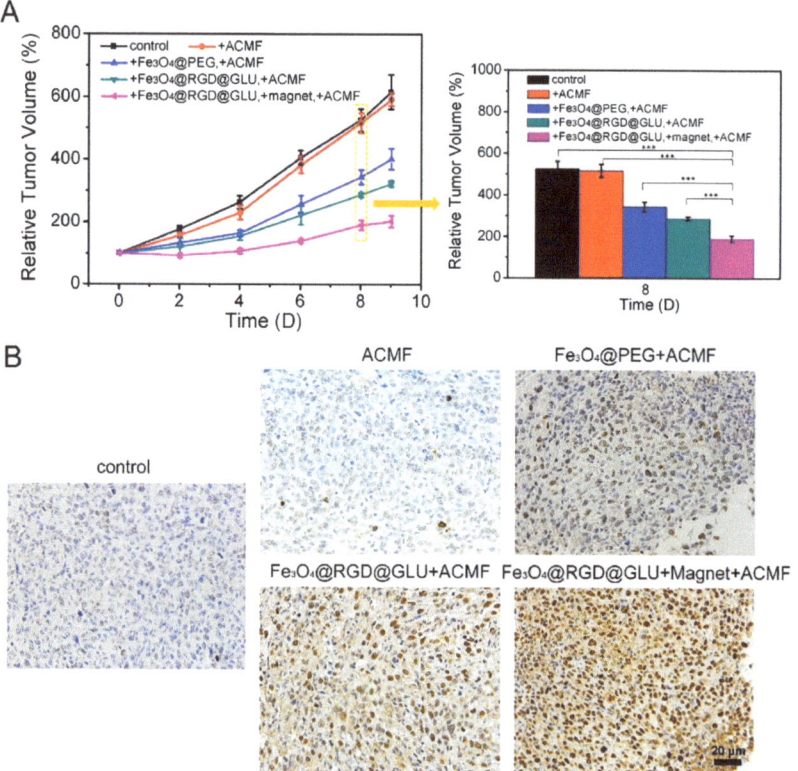

Figure 3. Analysis of the tumor growth curves for 10 days after treatment with iron oxide nanomaterials, mean ± SE and $n = 5$ (**A**). TUNEL histological analysis of mice tumors at day 9. Statistical significance is represented by the asterisk (*** $p < 0.001$). TUNEL assay for mice tumors on day 9 following various treatments (**B**). Reprinted with permission from [105]. Copyright (2019) Elsevier.

Table 2. Iron-based metallic-polymer nanoconjugates/nanohybrids, their physicochemical properties, and therapeutic applications (N.D.—non disclosed, N.A.—not applicable).

Metal	Morphology	Modification	Size (nm)	Surface Charge (mV)	Loading	Longitudinal/Transverse Proton Relaxivity	In Vitro	In Vivo	Applications	Ref.
Iron	Ring	GO (graphene oxide) and CREKA (Cys-Arg-Glu-Lys-Ala)	223.3	22 ± 0.4	N.A.	N.D.	4T1 cells	4T1 tumor-bearing mice	MTD and MTT	[6]
		HA conjugated with dopamine (HA-DA)	60.7	−16	N.A.	r1: 41.3 mM^{-1}	A549, HepG2, CT26, B16F10, and 4T1 cells	A549, B16F10, and CT26 tumor-bearing mice	MRI	[103]
		PLGA, silica, Polyaniline (PANI), and R8-RGD	206	22.8	Cisplatin	r2: 258.5 mM^{-1} s^{-1}	A549 cells	A549 tumor-bearing mice	PTT (Strong Absorption in NIR region), MRI, and chemotherapy	[104]
		PEG, RGD, D-Glucosamine	32.31 ± 0.71	−30.2 ± 0.76	N.A.	r2: 554 mM^{-1} s^{-1}	4T1 cells	4T1 tumor-bearing mice	MRI and hyperthermia	[105]
	Spheres	PEI, PLGA, and HA	159.5 ± 2.3	−9.1	Olaparib (Olb)	Saturation magnetizations: 21.08 emu/g	MDA-MB-231 cells	MDA-MB-231 tumor-bearing mice	RMF and chemotherapy	[106]
		PLGA, gold shell, and Herceptin	285.7 ± 81.4	N.D.	DOX	r2: 345.31 ± 23.06 mM^{-1} s^{-1}	BT474, MCF, and BT474/Adr cells	BT474 tumor-bearing mice	MRI, PTT (λex ≈ 750–800 nm), and chemotherapy	[107]
		AS1411 and PLGA	201.87 ± 1.60	−10.67 ± 0.25	N.A.	N.D.	MCF-7 cells	MCF-7 tumor-bearing mice	PA/US imaging and PTT (λex = 635 nm),	[108]
		HA-SS-PLA	≈11	N.D.	PTX	N.D.	HeLa cells	HeLa tumor-bearing mice	Chemotherapy	[109]
	Sheets	PDA (polydopamine), and rGO (reduced graphene oxide)	251	−27.5	N.A.	N.D.	MCF-7 cells	N.A.	MRI, PTT (Strong Absorption in NIR region), and PDT	[110]

Abbreviations—MRI: Magnetic Resonance Imaging; MTD: Magnetothermodynamic therapy; MTT: Magnetothermal Therapy; PA: Photoacoustic Imaging; PDT: Photodynamic Therapy; PTT: Photothermal Therapy; RMF: Rotating Magnetic Field Therapy; US: Ultrasound Imaging.

3.3. Copper-Polymer Conjugates

Copper nanomaterials have emerged in recent years as promising inorganic nanoparticles for biomedical applications (Table 3). Copper is a transition metal and can be engineered to form various nanomaterials, such as copper oxides, copper selenides, and copper sulfides [111–113]. Among them, copper sulfides have been the most explored due to the simple synthesis process and high NIR absorbing capacity, allowing their application in cancer PTT [37]. On the other hand, the copper nanomaterials can also be used as Fenton-like reagents mediating the formation of ROS (chemodynamic therapy) [114]. Moreover, the generation of ROS can also be stimulated under light irradiation (photodynamic therapy (PDT)) [115]. However, copper is often defined as more toxic than iron and gold, which makes the release of copper ions in the human body undesirable [116,117]. With that in mind, Li et al. showed that the surface functionalization with an amphiphilic polymer, poly(isobutylene-alt-maleic anhydride) (PMA), enhances the colloidal stability of copper telluride nanoparticles without visible agglomeration for periods longer than one month [118]. Furthermore, in vitro studies performed in 3T3 fibroblasts showed significant cytotoxicity after irradiation with a NIR laser (830 nm, 0.5 mW cm^{-2}, for 2 s). In another work, Li and colleagues developed a PEGylated copper sulfide nanoparticle for the simultaneous PDT and PTT of lung cancer (Figure 4) [119]. For that purpose, thiolated-PEG was reacted with the copper sulfide nanoparticles rendering the PEGylated nanoparticles. The authors observed that the nanoparticles' irradiation (30 µg mL^{-1}) with a NIR laser (808 nm, 1 W cm^{-2}, for 10 min) reaches temperatures superior to 42 °C. Moreover, the authors also observed the continuous quenching of the p-nitrosodimethylaniline (RNO) absorption under NIR irradiation, indicating the generation of ROS during this period. Moreover, the in vivo studies in SPC-A-1 tumor-bearing mice showed that the combination of PDT and PTT decreases tumor growth, observing a 5% increase in the tumor volume at day 14 after administering PEGylated copper sulfide nanoparticles (30 µg mL^{-1}) plus NIR. Similarly, Shi et al. produced a PEGylated copper sulfide nanoparticle modified with RGD to target metastatic gastric cancer [120]. The nanoparticles were formed by the reaction of thiolated-PEG-COOH and copper sulfide, followed by the RGD modification using carbodiimide chemistry. The obtained nanoparticles showed computed-tomography contrast capacity similar to the Iodixanol (a clinically used contrast agent). Furthermore, the irradiation of the nanoparticles (60 µg mL^{-1}) with a NIR laser (808 nm, 1 W cm^{-2}, for 5 min) led to a temperature increase to 60 °C. In the in vivo studies, the authors observed that the RGD-modified PEGylated copper sulfide nanoparticles allowed the identification of MKN45 tumors and metastasis in sentinel lymph nodes through T_2-weighted magnetic resonance images. Moreover, the NIR laser irradiation (808 nm, 1 W cm^{-2}, for 10 min) promoted the increase in tumor/metastases temperature to 57 °C, leading to the complete ablation of the metastatic MKN45 tumors (sentinel lymph nodes weight similar to the healthy ones, 2.5 mg).

Table 3. Copper-based metallic-polymer nanoconjugates/nanohybrids, their physicochemical properties, and therapeutic applications (N.D.—non disclosed, N.A.—not applicable).

Metal	Morphology	Modification	Size (nm)	Surface Charge (mV)	Loading	In Vitro	In Vivo	Applications	Ref.
Copper	Spheres	Lanthanide-doped nanoparticles and PEG	45	N.D.	N.A.	HeLa cells	Cervical cancer tumor xenograft	NIR-II luminescence imaging/CT/MRI, CDT, and PDT	[121]
		p-(OEOMA-co-MEMA)	285	−17.2	TAPP	CT26 cells	CT26 tumor-bearing mice	PA/PI, PTT (Band from visible to NIR), PDT, and SDT	[122]
		DSPE-PEG modified with Lanreotide	186.1 ± 5.2	−16.4 ± 0.1	Docetaxel	PC-3 cells	PC-3 tumor-bearing mice	PA, PI, PTT (Band between 700 and 1000 nm), PDT, and chemotherapy	[123]

Table 3. Cont.

Metal	Morphology	Modification	Size (nm)	Surface Charge (mV)	Loading	In Vitro	In Vivo	Applications	Ref.
		PLGA, PDA, and PEG	288 (Higher MW-PLGA); 257 (Lower MW-PLGA)	−18.7 (Higher MW-PLGA); −22.2 (Lower MW-PLGA)	N.A.	Cal-33 cells	N.A.	MRI, PTT (N.D.), and chemotherapy	[124]
		HA/PEI	330.7	16.9	Disulfiram	Eca109	Eca109 tumor-bearing mice	Chemotherapy and FL	[125]
		PEG-NH$_2$ and PCL-SS-P(DPA/GMA/MP)	151.5 ± 2.2	−17.1 ± 1.7	Dox	L929 and 4T1	4T1 tumor-bearing mice	PTT (Strong absorption in the NIR region), and chemotherapy	[126]
		HA and PDA	106	−19.43	Dox	HeLa and 4T1	4T1 tumor-bearing mice	PA, PTT (N.D), CDT, and chemotherapy	[127]
	Framework	Pluronic F127	186.4 ± 16.7	−1.2 ± 0.1	O$_2$	4T1 and HeLa cells	4T1 tumor-bearing mice	PDT (Band from visible to NIR)	[128]
	Cubes	BSA and PEG-FA	60	N.A.	N.A.	HepG2 cells	N.A.	PTT (Band from visible to NIR) and chemotherapy	[129]

Abbreviations—CT: Computed Tomography; PA: Photoacoustic Imaging; PDT; Photodynamic Therapy; PTT: Photothermal Therapy; SDT: Sonodynamic Therapy.

3.4. Other Metal-Polymer Nanoconjugates

Apart from the previously presented gold-, iron-, and copper-based nanomaterials, other metals have also been explored to create novel and more effective anticancer therapeutics (Table 4). Zinc-based nanoparticles, particularly zinc oxide (ZnO), are considered relatively biocompatible and generally regarded as safe. These nanoparticles present photoluminescence properties and a band gap that facilitates the interaction with oxygen and hydroxyl ions prompting the generation of superoxide and hydroxyl radicals (Table 4) [130,131]. Moreover, this ROS generation shows a certain selectivity towards cancer cells, decreasing the potential for inducing side effects [132]. Song and co-workers functionalized ZnO nanoparticles with polyvinylpyrrolidone for application in the imaging and therapy of colon cancer [133]. These authors reported that the surface functionalization maintained the stability of nanoparticles for 14 days, whereas non-coated ZnO nanoparticles aggregated after three days, without impacting the ROS generation capacity. Moreover, the authors also observed that the administration of the polyvinylpyrrolidone coated ZnO nanoparticles, at a concentration of 50 µg mL^{-1}, reduced the viability of SW480 cancer cells to 54% due to ROS generation. In turn, the ROS generation was boosted by the irradiation with UV light, with cell viability of 15% at a concentration of 50 µg mL^{-1} (IC$_{50}$ of 21.688 µg mL^{-1}). This PDT capacity was also observed in the SW480 tumor-bearing mice, where the nanoparticles plus light treatment slowed the tumor growth for 28 days, a tumor inhibition rate of 61.1%.

Platinum (Pt) is a catalytic noble metal that has been explored in cancer therapy, namely in the form of chemotherapeutic drugs containing platinum atoms, such as cisplatin and derivatives [134]. The utilization of platinum nanoparticles is focused on the release of platinum ions that will induce DNA damage and provoke cell death [135]. Additionally, the platinum nanoparticles can also mediate the generation of ROS or act as photothermal agents [136,137]. Chen and colleagues developed PEGylated porous platinum nanoparticles loaded with Dox for application in breast cancer therapy [138]. In the synthesis process, Pluronic F127 was used as a surfactant for the platinum nanoparticles and then reacted with thiolated-mPEG. This surface modification enhanced the solubility and stability of the platinum nanoparticles. Moreover, the authors also reported that the presence of a 10 mHz square wave AC field (10 mA) further enhanced the ROS generation capacity. In turn, the combination of Dox delivery and ROS generation induced the regression of 4T1 tumors, showing a tumor growth inhibition of 95.5% after 14 days. Zhu and co-workers prepared sodium hyaluronate stabilized platinum nanoparticles (HA/Pt) for mediating a photothermal effect [139]. Apart from the nanoparticle stabilization, the HA functionalization increased the nanoparticles' specificity towards the MDA-MB231 cancer cells (overexpression of CD44), when compared to the uptake by NIH3T3 cells (low expression of CD44). Furthermore, the in vivo studies in MDA-MB231 tumor-bearing mice revealed that upon irradiation with a NIR laser (808 nm, 1 W cm^{-1}, for 10 min), the HA/Pt nanoparticles induced an increase in the temperature of the tumor to 44 °C, which translated to a reduction in the tumor growth for 14 days.

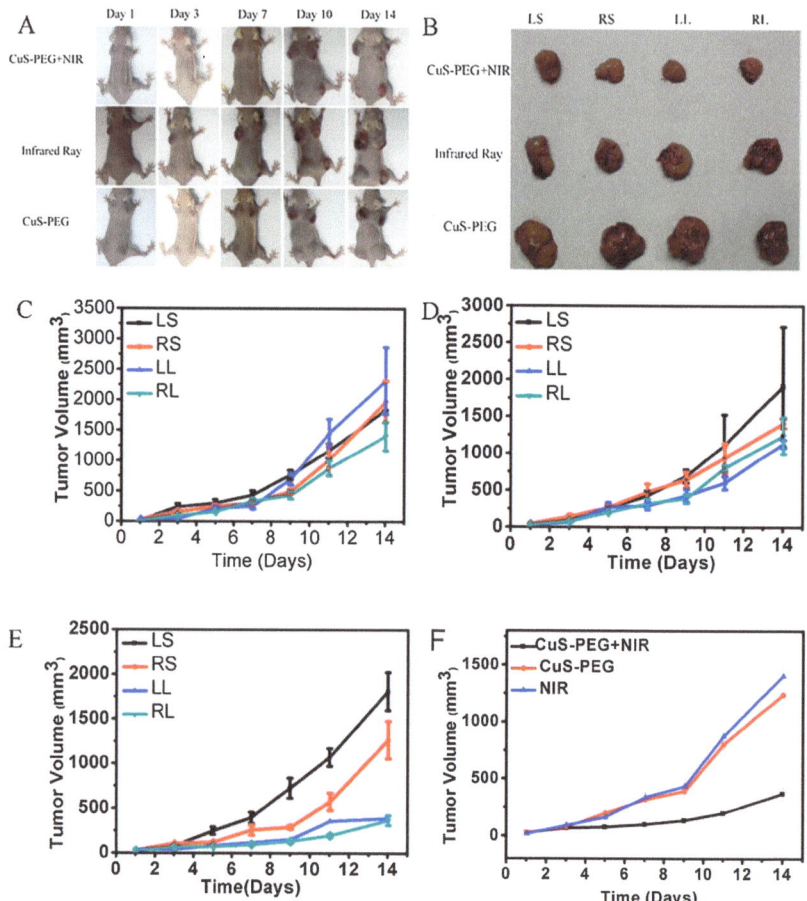

Figure 4. Photos of the tumor-bearing mice at 1, 3, 7, 10 and 14 days (**A**) and SPC-A-1 tumors at day 14 (**B**) after the treatment of the nanomaterials. Tumor growth curves in the control group; 0 µL CuS-PEG in LS, 30 µL CuS-PEG in the RS, 50 µL of CuS-PEG in the LL, and 100 µL CuS-PEG in the RL (**C**). Tumor growth curves in the NIR—irradiated group; 0 µL NS in the LS, 30 µL NS in the RS, 50 µL NS in the LL, and 100 µL NS CuS-PEG in the RL (**D**). Tumor growth curves in the CuS-PEG + NIR group, 100 µL NS in the LS, 30 µL CuS-PEG in the RS, 50 µL CuS-PEG in the LL, and 100 µL CuS-PEG in the RL (**E**). Tumor growth volume curve comparison for 100 µL (30 µg/mL) CuS-PEG +NIR in the RL; 100 µL (30 µg/mL) CuS-PEG in the RL, and 100 µL NS in the RL (**F**). LS—left shoulder administration; RS—right shoulder administration; LL—left leg administration; RL—right leg administration; NS—normal saline solution. Reprinted with permission from [111]. Copyright (2017) Elsevier.

Silver (Ag) is a noble metal with vast applications, being widely applied in the biomedical field as an antimicrobial agent [140]. The silver nanoparticles can mediate ROS formation and consequently induce lipid peroxidation, protein oxidation, and DNA damage [141,142]. Park and co-workers developed indocyanine green-loaded silver nanoparticles functionalized with PEG and BSA for application in cancer PTT [143]. The BSA was used to stabilize the produced silver nanoparticles, followed by the reaction with NHS-PEG for obtaining the functionalized silver nanoparticles. The authors reported that the PEG-BSA silver nanoparticles were stable in solution for at least five days after the synthesis. Moreover, the combination of indocyanine green-silver nanoparticles resulted in a more stable photothermal effect, reaching temperatures of $\approx$45 °C even after three irradiations with a NIR laser (885 nm, 1.3 W, for 10 min). The in vivo studies performed in B16F10 tumor-bearing mice showed a preferential accumulation in the liver, kidney, and tumors and upon irradiation (885 nm, 0.95 W for 20 min), the tumors' temperature reached 49 °C. This photothermal effect led to the tumors' ablation after four days.

Table 4. Summary of the Platinum/Silver/Zinc-based metallic-polymer nanoconjugates/nanohybrids, their physicochemical properties, and therapeutic applications (N.D.—non disclosed, N.A.—not applicable).

Metal	Morphology	Modification	Size (nm)	Surface Charge (mV)	Loading	In Vitro	In Vivo	Applications	Ref.
Platinum	Spheres	PDA and Folate	$\approx$100	N.A.	Indocyanine Green (ICG)	MCF-7	Breast cancer tumor xenograft	PA, FL, PTT (λex $\approx$ 700–800 nm), and PDT	[136]
		PEG	120	-14.6	DOX	4T1	4T1 tumor-bearing mice	EDT and chemotherapy	[138]
		HA	38 ± 6	-31 ± 1	N.A.	MDA-MB-231 (CD44+) and PC9 (CD44-)	MDA-MB-231 tumor-bearing mice	PI and PTT (N.D.)	[139]
		PEG	119.7	-1.6 ± 0.4	Cisplatin and IR780	4T1	4T1 tumor-bearing mice/Hepatocellular Carcinoma Patient Derived Xenograft	PI, FL, PTT (λex = 780 nm), and chemotherapy	[144]
Silver	Globular irregular shape	BSA and PEG	131.5 ± 2.7	-34.68 ± 0.6	ICG	B16F10 cells	B16F10 tumor-bearing mice	PTT (λex $\approx$ 790 nm)	[143]
	Spheres	Polythiourea and PEG	25–30	N.D.	N.A.	A549	A549 tumor-bearing mice	FL	[145]
		HA	104 ± 6.2	-30	N.A.	4T1	4T1 tumor-bearing mice	FL and RT	[146]
	Dots	FA modified DSPE-PEG$_{2000}$	200	-30.84	N.A.	HeLa and A549 cells	HeLa tumor-bearing mice	FL/PA imaging and PTT (Strong absorption in the visible and NIR region)	[147]
Zinc	Spheres	PVP40	$\approx$5	-3.6	N.A.	SW480 and HEK293T cells	SW480 tumor-bearing mice	PDT (N.D.)	[133]
		PDA	$\approx$175	-21.7	DOX and DNAzyme	A549 cells	A549 tumor-bearing mice	FL, PI, GT, PTT (N.D.), and chemotherapy	[148]
		PEG and RGD	112.0 ± 3.2	-14.6 ± 5.2	PTX	4T1 cells	4T1 tumor-bearing mice	MRI, NIRFI, and chemotherapy	[149]
		PEG and PLGA	PLGA-ZnNPc-NP = 141; PLGA-ZnPc-NPs = 152	PLGA-ZnNPc-NPs = 4.8; PLGA-ZnPc-NPs = 5.1	N.A.	MCF-7 cells	DMBA-induced breast cancer-bearing mice	FL and PDT (N.D.)	[150]

Abbreviations—CDT: Chemodynamic Therapy; EDT: Electrodynamic Therapy; FL: Fluorescence Imaging; GT: Gene Therapy; MRI: Magnetic Resonance Imaging; NIRFI: Near Infrared Fluorescence Imaging; PA: Photoacoustic Imaging; PDT: Photodynamic Therapy; PI: Photothermal Imaging; PTT: Photothermal Therapy; RT: Radiotherapy.

3.5. Clinical Trials

Since the 1990s, more than 50 nanomedicines have been approved by the Food and Drug Administration (FDA) and are currently on the market [151]. However, in the last decade, only a small number of formulations successfully reached the clinic for cancer treatment, a fact that is in part related to the poor pharmacokinetics of the nanomaterials [152]. The latest data indicate that less than 1% of the administered nanoparticles reach the tumor site [153]. Nevertheless, most of the approved nanomedicines are based on liposomes, protein nanoparticles, nano-emulsions, and metal oxide nanoparticles.

Particularly, iron oxide nanoparticles' clinical utility is demonstrated by the FDA approval for application in cancer diagnosis, hyperthermia, and iron deficiency anemia. Among them, it is worth highlighting the various contrast agents based on iron oxide nanoparticles commercially available for MRI, such as Feridex®, Resovist®, and Endorem®. Moreover, there are more systems under clinical trial, such as Magnablate® and Nanotherm® (Table 5). The former is an iron oxide nanoparticle developed for magneto-hyperthermia applications that underwent a Phase 0 clinical trial (ClinicalTrials.gov Identifier: NCT02033447), with 12 participants, for the thermoablation of prostate cancer (no results are yet available) [154]. In turn, Nanotherm® is also based on an aqueous suspension of iron oxide nanoparticles and was already approved by the European Medicines Agency (EMA) for brain tumor treatment [37]. Moreover, recently, a new clinical trial (ClinicalTrials.gov Identifier: NCT05010759; still recruiting) was announced to study the application of Nanotherm® in the ablation of prostate carcinoma.

Regarding gold-based nanoparticles, to this date, two promising nanomedicines are currently in clinical trials [151]. AuroLase® uses the particles denominated as AuroShell®, a PEGylated silica-gold nanoshell with ≈150 nm in size, for the laser-activated thermal ablation of solid tumors, metastatic lung tumors, and cancer prostatic tissue [151,155]. In the clinical trial (ClinicalTrials.gov Identifier: NCT01679470), a single dose of AuroShell® was administered to promote the ablation of primary and/or metastatic lung tumors, still, to this date, no results were posted [156]. There is a second clinical trial (ClinicalTrials.gov Identifier: NCT00848042) involving the utilization of this nanomedicine for the treatment of patients with refractory and/or recurrent head and neck tumors. The patients were subjected to one or more doses of laser irradiation (808 nm) [30,33]. The participants were divided into three groups: (i) five participants, Auroshell® dose 4.5 mL kg^{-1}, laser potency 3.5 W; (ii) five participants, Auroshell® dose 7.5 mL kg^{-1}, laser potency 4.5 W; (iii) one participant, Auroshell® dose 7.5 mL kg^{-1}, laser potency 5 W. However, no data were published to assess the effect on the targeted tumors. In a more recent clinical trial (ClinicalTrials.gov Identifier: NCT02680535), the Auroshell® nanoparticles were tested in combination with the MRI/Ultrasound fusion technology to promote the focal ablation of neoplastic prostate tissue. The extension of this clinical trial is still active (ClinicalTrials.gov Identifier: NCT04240639), however no data have been found describing the evolution of the targeted tumors. The NU-0129® is another gold-based nanomedicine under clinical trial (ClinicalTrials.gov Identifier: NCT03020017). This nanoparticle is formed by a spherical gold nanoparticle conjugated with siRNA oligonucleotides for targeting BCL2L12 oncogene in glioblastoma multiforme or gliosarcoma treatment applications [151,157]. The early results showed that the NU-0129® nanoparticles can cross the blood–brain barrier without unexpected adverse effects, still pending the data regarding antitumoral efficacy [158].

Table 5. Summary of clinical trials comprising metallic-polymer nanoconjugates/nanohybrids (N.A.—not applicable).

Name	Description	Application	Administration Route	Type of Cancer	Clinical Trials Identifier (Phase)	Results	Ref.
Magnablate®	Iron oxide nanoparticles	Magnetic Hyperthermia	Intratumoral	Prostate Cancer	NCT02033447 (Early Phase I): Completed	No results yet available	[154]
Nanotherm®	Iron oxide nanoparticles	Magnetic Hyperthermia	Intratumoral	Brain tumor	Approved by the EMA in 2010		[37]
			Intratumoral	Prostate Carcinoma	NCT05010759: Still recruiting (Phase not applicable)	No results yet available	N.A.

Table 5. Cont.

Name	Description	Application	Administration Route	Type of Cancer	Clinical Trials Identifier (Phase)	Results	Ref.
AuroLase®	PEGylated silica-gold nanoshell (AuroShell®)	Laser-activated termal ablation	Intravenous	Metastic lung tumors	NCT01679470: Phase not applicable	No results yet available	[156]
				Refractory and/or recurrent head and neck tumors	NCT00848042: Phase not applicable	No results yet available	N.A.
		Laser-activated termal ablation combined with MRI/US fusion technology for focal ablation		Neoplastic Prostate tissue	NCT02680535 and NCT04240639 (extension of the previous): Phase not applicable	No results yet available	N.A.
NU-0129®	Spherical gold nanoparticle conjugated with siRNA oligonucleotides	Targeting BCL2L12 oncogene	Intravenous	Glioblastoma multiforme or Gliosarcoma Treatment	NCT03020017: Completed	No results provide about the antitumor efficacy	[158]

Abbreviations—EMA: European Medicines Agency; MRI: Magnetic Resonance Imaging; US: Ultrasound Imaging.

4. Conclusions

Metallic-based nanomaterials have been showing promising results in a variety of cancer-related applications, from imaging to the ablation of tumors. Nevertheless, several of these nanomedicines remain in a preclinical stage, an exception being the application of iron oxide-derived nanomaterials in the imaging of tumors.

In this review, the unique set of physicochemical properties that make the metallic nanoparticles highly promising for biomedical applications is described. The high density and X-ray attenuation capacity make these nanomaterials natural contrast agents for conventional imaging techniques such as CT. Moreover, the surface plasmon resonance and/or the magnetism allow the utilization of hyperthermia treatments (e.g., PTT and magneto-hyperthermia). Therefore, the conjugation with natural and/or synthetic polymers can further increase the biological performance of the metallic nanoparticles by enhancing the colloidal stability and blood circulation time as well as conferring additional specificity to the cancer cells. Nevertheless, there remain significant challenges to overcome and effectively translate the metallic-polymer nanoconjugates/nanohybrids to the clinic. Additional studies on the biosafety and long-term fate of these nanomaterials are still missing. Moreover, the optimization and scale-up of the production methods are mandatory to decrease batch-to-batch variability. Furthermore, regulatory agencies should create a comprehensive set of guidelines for the translation of metallic nanoparticles to the clinic.

In summary, the metallic-polymer nanoconjugates/nanohybrids have the potential to support the development of more effective and multifunctional all-in-one nanomedicines, with the capacity to diagnose and treat the tumor as well as monitor in real-time its response to the treatment. Such raw potential of metallic-polymer nanoconjugates/nanohybrids presents an area of opportunity for both researchers and industrial partners (e.g., pharmaceutics) to develop a new generation of nanomedicines for cancer therapy. Moreover, it is worthwhile to notice that the physicochemical properties of metallic-polymer nanoconjugates/nanohybrids can also be explored to create innovative solutions in the biomedical field, such as biosensors, antimicrobial agents, and tissue regeneration.

Author Contributions: Conceptualization, A.F.M.; methodology, A.Q.F., N.F., C.F.R. and A.F.M.; software, A.Q.F., C.F.R. and A.F.M.; validation, A.F.M. and I.J.C.; formal analysis, A.F.M. and D.d.M.-D.; investigation, A.Q.F., N.F. and C.F.R.; resources, A.F.M., I.J.C. and D.d.M.-D.; data curation, A.Q.F., N.F. and C.F.R.; writing—original draft preparation, A.Q.F., N.F., C.F.R. and A.F.M.; writing—review and editing, A.F.M., I.J.C. and D.d.M.-D.; visualization, I.J.C. and D.d.M.-D.; supervision, A.F.M. and I.J.C.; project administration, I.J.C.; funding acquisition, I.J.C. All authors have read and agreed to the published version of the manuscript.

Funding: This research was funded by the Foundation for Science and Technology (FCT), through funds from the State Budget, and by the European Regional Development Fund (ERDF), under the Portugal 2020 Program, through the Regional Operational Program of the Center (Centro2020), through the Project with the reference UIDB/00709/2020, CENTRO-01-0145-FEDER-028989 and POCI-01-0145-FEDER-031462. The funder had no role in the decision to publish or in the preparation of the manuscript.

Data Availability Statement: The data presented in this article are available at request from the corresponding author.

Acknowledgments: Carolina F. Rodrigues acknowledges her Ph.D. fellowship from FCT (SFRH/BD/144680/2019). Duarte de Melo-Diogo acknowledges FCT for the financial support given through a Junior Researcher contract (2021.00590.CEECIND). Natanael Fernandes acknowledges the individual fellowship from UBI-Banco Santander/Totta. The funders had no role in the decision to publish or in the preparation of the manuscript.

Conflicts of Interest: The authors declare no financial or commercial conflict of interest.

References

1. Aghebati-Maleki, A.; Dolati, S.; Ahmadi, M.; Baghbanzhadeh, A.; Asadi, M.; Fotouhi, A.; Yousefi, M.; Aghebati-Maleki, L. Nanoparticles and cancer therapy: Perspectives for application of nanoparticles in the treatment of cancers. *J. Cell. Physiol.* **2020**, *235*, 1962–1972. [CrossRef] [PubMed]
2. Goncalves, A.S.C.; Rodrigues, C.F.; Moreira, A.F.; Correia, I.J. Strategies to improve the photothermal capacity of gold-based nanomedicines. *Acta Biomater.* **2020**, *116*, 105–137. [CrossRef] [PubMed]
3. Guimaraes, R.S.; Rodrigues, C.F.; Moreira, A.F.; Correia, I.J. Overview of stimuli-responsive mesoporous organosilica nanocarriers for drug delivery. *Pharmacol. Res.* **2020**, *155*, 104742. [CrossRef] [PubMed]
4. Huang, N.; Liu, Y.; Fang, Y.; Zheng, S.; Wu, J.; Wang, M.; Zhong, W.; Shi, M.; Xing, M.; Liao, W. Gold Nanoparticles Induce Tumor Vessel Normalization and Impair Metastasis by Inhibiting Endothelial Smad2/3 Signaling. *ACS Nano* **2020**, *14*, 7940–7958. [CrossRef]
5. Rodrigues, C.F.; Alves, C.G.; Lima-Sousa, R.; Moreira, A.F.; de Melo-Diogo, D.; Correia, I.J. Inorganic-based drug delivery systems for cancer therapy. In *Advances and Avenues in the Development of Novel Carriers for Bioactives and Biological Agents*; Academic Press: Cambridge, MA, USA, 2020; pp. 283–316.
6. Liu, X.; Yan, B.; Li, Y.; Ma, X.; Jiao, W.; Shi, K.; Zhang, T.; Chen, S.; He, Y.; Liang, X.; et al. Graphene Oxide-Grafted Magnetic Nanorings Mediated Magnetothermodynamic Therapy Favoring Reactive Oxygen Species-Related Immune Response for Enhanced Antitumor Efficacy. *ACS Nano* **2020**, *14*, 1936–1950. [CrossRef]
7. Li, G.; Zhong, X.; Wang, X.; Gong, F.; Lei, H.; Zhou, Y.; Li, C.; Xiao, Z.; Ren, G.; Zhang, L. Titanium carbide nanosheets with defect structure for photothermal-enhanced sonodynamic therapy. *Bioact. Mater.* **2022**, *8*, 409–419. [CrossRef]
8. Loh, X.J.; Lee, T.C.; Dou, Q.; Deen, G.R. Utilising inorganic nanocarriers for gene delivery. *Biomater. Sci.* **2016**, *4*, 70–86. [CrossRef]
9. Liou, G.Y.; Storz, P. Reactive oxygen species in cancer. *Free Radic. Res.* **2010**, *44*, 479–496. [CrossRef]
10. Tricoli, A.; Righettoni, M.; Teleki, A. Semiconductor gas sensors: Dry synthesis and application. *Angew. Chem. Int. Ed.* **2010**, *49*, 7632–7659. [CrossRef]
11. Huynh, K.H.; Pham, X.H.; Kim, J.; Lee, S.H.; Chang, H.; Rho, W.Y.; Jun, B.H. Synthesis, Properties, and Biological Applications of Metallic Alloy Nanoparticles. *Int. J. Mol. Sci.* **2020**, *21*, 5174. [CrossRef]
12. Amendola, V.; Meneghetti, M. Laser ablation synthesis in solution and size manipulation of noble metal nanoparticles. *Phys. Chem. Chem. Phys.* **2009**, *11*, 3805–3821. [CrossRef]
13. Annamalai, J.; Murugan, P.; Ganapathy, D.; Nallaswamy, D.; Atchudan, R.; Arya, S.; Khosla, A.; Barathi, S.; Sundramoorthy, A.K. Synthesis of various dimensional metal organic frameworks (MOFs) and their hybrid composites for emerging applications—A review. *Chemosphere* **2022**, *298*, 134184. [CrossRef]
14. Hu, P.; Chen, L.; Kang, X.; Chen, S. Surface Functionalization of Metal Nanoparticles by Conjugated Metal-Ligand Interfacial Bonds: Impacts on Intraparticle Charge Transfer. *Acc. Chem. Res.* **2016**, *49*, 2251–2260. [CrossRef]
15. Neha, D.; Momin, M.; Khan, T.; Gharat, S.; Ningthoujam, R.S.; Omri, A. Metallic nanoparticles as drug delivery system for the treatment of cancer. *Expert Opin. Drug Deliv.* **2021**, *18*, 1261–1290. [CrossRef]

16. Xu, J.J.; Zhang, W.C.; Guo, Y.W.; Chen, X.Y.; Zhang, Y.N. Metal nanoparticles as a promising technology in targeted cancer treatment. *Drug Deliv.* **2022**, *29*, 664–678. [CrossRef]
17. Anselmo, A.C.; Mitragotri, S. A Review of Clinical Translation of Inorganic Nanoparticles. *AAPS J.* **2015**, *17*, 1041–1054. [CrossRef]
18. Canaparo, R.; Foglietta, F.; Limongi, T.; Serpe, L. Biomedical Applications of Reactive Oxygen Species Generation by Metal Nanoparticles. *Materials* **2020**, *14*, 53. [CrossRef]
19. Gonzalez-Rubio, G.; Guerrero-Martinez, A.; Liz-Marzan, L.M. Reshaping, Fragmentation, and Assembly of Gold Nanoparticles Assisted by Pulse Lasers. *Acc. Chem. Res.* **2016**, *49*, 678–686. [CrossRef]
20. Bhatia, S. Natural Polymers vs Synthetic Polymer. In *Natural Polymer Drug Delivery Systems*; Springer: Cham, Switzerland, 2016; pp. 95–118.
21. Aslan, N.; Ceylan, B.; Koç, M.M.; Findik, F. Metallic nanoparticles as X-ray computed tomography (CT) contrast agents: A review. *J. Mol. Struct.* **2020**, *1219*, 128599. [CrossRef]
22. Liu, Y.; Ai, K.; Lu, L. Nanoparticulate X-ray computed tomography contrast agents: From design validation to in vivo applications. *Acc. Chem. Res.* **2012**, *45*, 1817–1827. [CrossRef]
23. Cheheltani, R.; Ezzibdeh, R.M.; Chhour, P.; Pulaparthi, K.; Kim, J.; Jurcova, M.; Hsu, J.; Blundell, C.; Litt, H.; Ferrari, V.A.; et al. Tunable, biodegradable gold nanoparticles as contrast agents for computed tomography and photoacoustic imaging. *Biomaterials* **2016**, *102*, 87–97. [CrossRef] [PubMed]
24. De La Vega, J.C.; Esquinas, P.L.; Gill, J.K.; Jessa, S.; Gill, B.; Thakur, Y.; Saatchi, K.; Hafeli, U.O. Comparison of Rhenium and Iodine as Contrast Agents in X-ray Imaging. *Contrast Media Mol. Imaging* **2021**, *2021*, 1250360. [CrossRef] [PubMed]
25. Berger, M.; Bauser, M.; Frenzel, T.; Hilger, C.S.; Jost, G.; Lauria, S.; Morgenstern, B.; Neis, C.; Pietsch, H.; Sülzle, D.; et al. Hafnium-Based Contrast Agents for X-ray Computed Tomography. *Inorg. Chem.* **2017**, *56*, 5757–5761. [CrossRef] [PubMed]
26. Bae, K.T.; McDermott, R.; Gierada, D.S.; Heiken, J.P.; Nolte, M.A.; Takahashi, N.; Hong, C. Gadolinium-enhanced computed tomography angiography in multi-detector row computed tomography. *Acad. Radiol.* **2004**, *11*, 61–68. [CrossRef]
27. Werts, M.H.V.; Allix, F.; Francais, O.; Frochot, C.; Griscom, L.; Le Pioufle, B.; Loumaigne, M.; Midelet, J. Manipulation and Optical Detection of Colloidal Functional Plasmonic Nanostructures in Microfluidic Systems. *IEEE J. Sel. Top. Quantum Electron.* **2014**, *20*, 102–114.
28. Wang, L.; Hasanzadeh Kafshgari, M.; Meunier, M. Optical Properties and Applications of Plasmonic-Metal Nanoparticles. *Adv. Funct. Mater.* **2020**, *30*, 2005400. [CrossRef]
29. Noguez, C. Surface Plasmons on Metal Nanoparticles: The Influence of Shape and Physical Environment. *J. Phys. Chem. C* **2007**, *111*, 3806–3819. [CrossRef]
30. Liz-Marzán, L.M. Tailoring Surface Plasmons through the Morphology and Assembly of Metal Nanoparticles. *Langmuir* **2006**, *22*, 32–41. [CrossRef]
31. Liang, J.; Liu, H.; Yu, J.; Zhou, L.; Zhu, J. Plasmon-enhanced solar vapor generation. *Nanophotonics* **2019**, *8*, 771–786. [CrossRef]
32. Jeong, Y.; Kook, Y.M.; Lee, K.; Koh, W.G. Metal enhanced fluorescence (MEF) for biosensors: General approaches and a review of recent developments. *Biosens. Bioelectron.* **2018**, *111*, 102–116. [CrossRef]
33. Lin, Q.; Jia, M.; Fu, Y.; Li, B.; Dong, Z.; Niu, X.; You, Z. Upper-Critical-Solution-Temperature Polymer Modified Gold Nanorods for Laser Controlled Drug Release and Enhanced Anti-Tumour Therapy. *Front. Pharm.* **2021**, *12*, 738630. [CrossRef]
34. de Melo-Diogo, D.; Pais-Silva, C.; Dias, D.R.; Moreira, A.F.; Correia, I.J. Strategies to Improve Cancer Photothermal Therapy Mediated by Nanomaterials. *Adv. Healthc. Mater.* **2017**, *6*, 1700073. [CrossRef]
35. Bettaieb, A.; Wrzal, K.P.; Averill-Bates, D.A. Hyperthermia: Cancer Treatment and Beyond. *Cancer Treat. Conv. Innov. Approaches* **2013**, 257–283. [CrossRef]
36. Zhang, Y.; Zhan, X.; Xiong, J.; Peng, S.; Huang, W.; Joshi, R.; Cai, Y.; Liu, Y.; Li, R.; Yuan, K.; et al. Temperature-dependent cell death patterns induced by functionalized gold nanoparticle photothermal therapy in melanoma cells. *Sci. Rep.* **2018**, *8*, 8720. [CrossRef]
37. Fernandes, N.; Rodrigues, C.F.; Moreira, A.F.; Correia, I.J. Overview of the application of inorganic nanomaterials in cancer photothermal therapy. *Biomater. Sci.* **2020**, *8*, 2990–3020. [CrossRef]
38. Xing, Y.; Cai, Z.; Xu, M.; Ju, W.; Luo, X.; Hu, Y.; Liu, X.; Kang, T.; Wu, P.; Cai, C.; et al. Raman observation of a molecular signaling pathway of apoptotic cells induced by photothermal therapy. *Chem. Sci.* **2019**, *10*, 10900–10910. [CrossRef]
39. Jiang, Z.; Li, T.; Cheng, H.; Zhang, F.; Yang, X.; Wang, S.; Zhou, J.; Ding, Y. Nanomedicine potentiates mild photothermal therapy for tumor ablation. *Asian J. Pharm. Sci.* **2021**, *16*, 738–761. [CrossRef]
40. Rudakov, G.A.; Tsiberkin, K.B.; Ponomarev, R.S.; Henner, V.K.; Ziolkowska, D.A.; Jasinski, J.B.; Sumanasekera, G. Magnetic properties of transition metal nanoparticles enclosed in carbon nanocages. *J. Magn. Magn. Mater.* **2019**, *472*, 34–39. [CrossRef]
41. Soheilian, R.; Choi, Y.S.; David, A.E.; Abdi, H.; Maloney, C.E.; Erb, R.M. Toward Accumulation of Magnetic Nanoparticles into Tissues of Small Porosity. *Langmuir* **2015**, *31*, 8267–8274. [CrossRef]
42. Guo, X.; Li, W.; Luo, L.; Wang, Z.; Li, Q.; Kong, F.; Zhang, H.; Yang, J.; Zhu, C.; Du, Y.; et al. External Magnetic Field-Enhanced Chemo-Photothermal Combination Tumor Therapy via Iron Oxide Nanoparticles. *ACS Appl. Mater. Interfaces* **2017**, *9*, 16581–16593. [CrossRef]
43. Farzin, A.; Etesami, S.A.; Quint, J.; Memic, A.; Tamayol, A. Magnetic Nanoparticles in Cancer Therapy and Diagnosis. *Adv. Healthc. Mater.* **2020**, *9*, e1901058. [CrossRef] [PubMed]

44. Sengul, A.B.; Asmatulu, E. Toxicity of metal and metal oxide nanoparticles: A review. *Environ. Chem. Lett.* **2020**, *18*, 1659–1683. [CrossRef]
45. Wu, H.; Yin, J.J.; Wamer, W.G.; Zeng, M.; Lo, Y.M. Reactive oxygen species-related activities of nano-iron metal and nano-iron oxides. *J. Food Drug Anal.* **2014**, *22*, 86–94. [CrossRef] [PubMed]
46. Yuan, P.; Ding, X.; Yang, Y.Y.; Xu, Q.-H. Metal Nanoparticles for Diagnosis and Therapy of Bacterial Infection. *Adv. Healthc. Mater.* **2018**, *7*, 1701392. [CrossRef]
47. Juarranz, Á.; Jaén, P.; Sanz-Rodríguez, F.; Cuevas, J.; González, S. Photodynamic therapy of cancer. Basic principles and applications. *Clin. Transl. Oncol.* **2008**, *10*, 148–154. [CrossRef]
48. Wilson, B.C. Photodynamic Therapy for Cancer: Principles. *Can. J. Gastroenterol.* **2002**, *16*, 743109. [CrossRef]
49. Vinković Vrček, I.; Pavičić, I.; Crnković, T.; Jurašin, D.; Babič, M.; Horák, D.; Lovric, M.; Ferhatovic, L.; Curlin, M.; Gajovic, S. Does surface coating of metallic nanoparticles modulate their interference with in vitro assays? *RSC Adv.* **2015**, *5*, 70787–70807. [CrossRef]
50. Rajendran, K.; Pujari, L.; Krishnamoorthy, M.; Sen, S.; Dharmaraj, D.; Karuppiah, K.; Ethiraj, K. Toxicological evaluation of biosynthesised hematite nanoparticles in vivo. *Colloids Surf. B Biointerfaces* **2021**, *198*, 111475. [CrossRef]
51. García-Álvarez, R.; Hadjidemetriou, M.; Sánchez-Iglesias, A.; Liz-Marzán, L.M.; Kostarelos, K. In vivo formation of protein corona on gold nanoparticles. The effect of their size and shape. *Nanoscale* **2018**, *10*, 1256–1264. [CrossRef]
52. Thambiraj, S.; Vijayalakshmi, R.; Ravi Shankaran, D. An effective strategy for development of docetaxel encapsulated gold nanoformulations for treatment of prostate cancer. *Sci. Rep.* **2021**, *11*, 2808. [CrossRef]
53. Hada, A.M.; Craciun, A.M.; Focsan, M.; Borlan, R.; Soritau, O.; Todea, M.; Astilean, S. Folic acid functionalized gold nanoclusters for enabling targeted fluorescence imaging of human ovarian cancer cells. *Talanta* **2021**, *225*, 121960. [CrossRef]
54. Kim, H.S.; Lee, S.J.; Lee, D.Y. Milk protein-shelled gold nanoparticles with gastrointestinally active absorption for aurotherapy to brain tumor. *Bioact. Mater.* **2022**, *8*, 35–48. [CrossRef]
55. Mapanao, A.K.; Santi, M.; Voliani, V. Combined chemo-photothermal treatment of three-dimensional head and neck squamous cell carcinomas by gold nano-architectures. *J. Colloid Interface Sci.* **2021**, *582*, 1003–1011. [CrossRef]
56. You, Y.H.; Lin, Y.F.; Nirosha, B.; Chang, H.T.; Huang, Y.F. Polydopamine-coated gold nanostar for combined antitumor and antiangiogenic therapy in multidrug-resistant breast cancer. *Nanotheranostics* **2019**, *3*, 266–283. [CrossRef]
57. Sheng, Y.; Liu, C.; Yuan, Y.; Tao, X.; Yang, F.; Shan, X.; Zhou, H.; Xu, F. Long-circulating polymeric nanoparticles bearing a combinatorial coating of PEG and water-soluble chitosan. *Biomaterials* **2009**, *30*, 2340–2348. [CrossRef]
58. Li, B.; Xie, J.; Yuan, Z.; Jain, P.; Lin, X.; Wu, K.; Jiang, S. Mitigation of Inflammatory Immune Responses with Hydrophilic Nanoparticles. *Angew. Chem. Int. Ed.* **2018**, *57*, 4527–4531. [CrossRef]
59. Lowe, S.; O'Brien-Simpson, N.M.; Connal, L.A. Antibiofouling polymer interfaces: Poly(ethylene glycol) and other promising candidates. *Polym. Chem.* **2015**, *6*, 198–212. [CrossRef]
60. Yu, Y.; Luan, Y.; Dai, W. Dynamic process, mechanisms, influencing factors and study methods of protein corona formation. *Int. J. Biol. Macromol.* **2022**, *205*, 731–739. [CrossRef]
61. Feng, W.; Zhu, S.; Ishihara, K.; Brash, J.L. Protein resistant surfaces: Comparison of acrylate graft polymers bearing oligo-ethylene oxide and phosphorylcholine side chains. *Biointerphases* **2006**, *1*, 50. [CrossRef]
62. He, M.; Gao, K.; Zhou, L.; Jiao, Z.; Wu, M.; Cao, J.; You, X.; Cai, Z.; Su, Y.; Jiang, Z. Zwitterionic materials for antifouling membrane surface construction. *Acta Biomater.* **2016**, *40*, 142–152. [CrossRef]
63. Zhang, Y.; Liu, Y.; Ren, B.; Zhang, D.; Xie, S.; Chang, Y.; Yang, J.; Wu, J.; Xu, L.; Zheng, J. Fundamentals and applications of zwitterionic antifouling polymers. *J. Phys. D Appl. Phys.* **2019**, *52*, 403001. [CrossRef]
64. Liu, X.; Li, H.; Chen, Y.; Jin, Q.; Ren, K.; Ji, J. Mixed-Charge Nanoparticles for Long Circulation, Low Reticuloendothelial System Clearance, and High Tumor Accumulation. *Adv. Healthc. Mater.* **2014**, *3*, 1439–1447. [CrossRef]
65. Wu, L.; Lin, B.; Yang, H.; Chen, J.; Mao, Z.; Wang, W.; Gao, C. Enzyme-responsive multifunctional peptide coating of gold nanorods improves tumor targeting and photothermal therapy efficacy. *Acta Biomater.* **2019**, *86*, 363–372. [CrossRef] [PubMed]
66. Li, W.; Cao, Z.; Yu, L.; Huang, Q.; Zhu, D.; Lu, C.; Lu, A.; Liu, Y. Hierarchical drug release designed Au @PDA-PEG-MTX NPs for targeted delivery to breast cancer with combined photothermal-chemotherapy. *J. Nanobiotechnol.* **2021**, *19*, 143. [CrossRef] [PubMed]
67. Sathiyaseelan, A.; Saravanakumar, K.; Mariadoss, A.V.A.; Wang, M.H. pH-controlled nucleolin targeted release of dual drug from chitosan-gold based aptamer functionalized nano drug delivery system for improved glioblastoma treatment. *Carbohydr. Polym.* **2021**, *262*, 117907. [CrossRef] [PubMed]
68. Feng, Y.; Cheng, Y.; Chang, Y.; Jian, H.; Zheng, R.; Wu, X.; Xu, K.; Wang, L.; Ma, X.; Li, X.; et al. Time-staggered delivery of erlotinib and doxorubicin by gold nanocages with two smart polymers for reprogrammable release and synergistic with photothermal therapy. *Biomaterials* **2019**, *217*, 119327. [CrossRef]
69. Wang, N.; Shi, J.; Wu, C.; Chu, W.; Tao, W.; Li, W.; Yuan, X. Design of DOX-GNRs-PNIPAM@PEG-PLA Micelle With Temperature and Light Dual-Function for Potent Melanoma Therapy. *Front. Chem.* **2020**, *8*, 599740. [CrossRef]
70. Li, D.; Zhang, R.; Liu, G.; Kang, Y.; Wu, J. Redox-Responsive Self-Assembled Nanoparticles for Cancer Therapy. *Adv. Healthc. Mater.* **2020**, *9*, 2000605. [CrossRef]
71. Shi, Y.; van der Meel, R.; Chen, X.; Lammers, T. The EPR effect and beyond: Strategies to improve tumor targeting and cancer nanomedicine treatment efficacy. *Theranostics* **2020**, *10*, 7921–7924. [CrossRef]

72. Acharya, S.; Sahoo, S.K. PLGA nanoparticles containing various anticancer agents and tumour delivery by EPR effect. *Adv. Drug Deliv. Rev.* **2011**, *63*, 170–183. [CrossRef]
73. Yucel, O.; Sengelen, A.; Emik, S.; Onay-Ucar, E.; Arda, N.; Gurdag, G. Folic acid-modified methotrexate-conjugated gold nanoparticles as nano-sized trojans for drug delivery to folate receptor-positive cancer cells. *Nanotechnology* **2020**, *31*, 355101. [CrossRef]
74. Mulens-Arias, V.; Nicolas-Boluda, A.; Pinto, A.; Balfourier, A.; Carn, F.; Silva, A.K.A.; Pocard, M.; Gazeau, F. Tumor-Selective Immune-Active Mild Hyperthermia Associated with Chemotherapy in Colon Peritoneal Metastasis by Photoactivation of Fluorouracil-Gold Nanoparticle Complexes. *ACS Nano* **2021**, *15*, 3330–3348. [CrossRef]
75. Guo, J.; Rahme, K.; He, Y.; Li, L.L.; Holmes, J.D.; O'Driscoll, C.M. Gold nanoparticles enlighten the future of cancer theranostics. *Int. J. Nanomed.* **2017**, *12*, 6131–6152. [CrossRef]
76. Cole, L.E.; Ross, R.D.; Tilley, J.M.R.; Vargo-Gogola, T.; Roeder, R.K. Gold nanoparticles as contrast agents in x-ray imaging and computed tomography. *Nanomedicine* **2015**, *10*, 321–341. [CrossRef]
77. Xi, D.; Dong, S.; Meng, X.; Lu, Q.; Meng, L.; Ye, J. Gold nanoparticles as computerized tomography (CT) contrast agents. *RSC Adv.* **2012**, *2*, 12515. [CrossRef]
78. Capek, I. Polymer decorated gold nanoparticles in nanomedicine conjugates. *Adv. Colloid Interface Sci.* **2017**, *249*, 386–399. [CrossRef]
79. Guo, C.; Hall, G.N.; Addison, J.B.; Yarger, J.L. Gold nanoparticle-doped silk film as biocompatible SERS substrate. *RSC Adv.* **2015**, *5*, 1937–1942. [CrossRef]
80. Fernandes, N.; Rodrigues, C.F.; de Melo-Diogo, D.; Correia, I.J.; Moreira, A.F. Optimization of the GSH-Mediated Formation of Mesoporous Silica-Coated Gold Nanoclusters for NIR Light-Triggered Photothermal Applications. *Nanomaterials* **2021**, *11*, 1946. [CrossRef]
81. Fernandes, J.; Kang, S. Numerical Study on the Surface Plasmon Resonance Tunability of Spherical and Non-Spherical Core-Shell Dimer Nanostructures. *Nanomaterials* **2021**, *11*, 1728. [CrossRef]
82. Xu, H.; Käll, M. Modeling the optical response of nanoparticle-based surface plasmon resonance sensors. *Sens. Actuators B Chem.* **2002**, *87*, 244–249. [CrossRef]
83. Bouhelier, A.; Bachelot, R.; Lerondel, G.; Kostcheev, S.; Royer, P.; Wiederrecht, G.P. Surface plasmon characteristics of tunable photoluminescence in single gold nanorods. *Phys. Rev. Lett* **2005**, *95*, 267405. [CrossRef] [PubMed]
84. Chandrasekaran, R.; Lee, A.S.W.; Yap, L.W.; Jans, D.A.; Wagstaff, K.M.; Cheng, W. Tumor cell-specific photothermal killing by SELEX-derived DNA aptamer-targeted gold nanorods. *Nanoscale* **2016**, *8*, 187–196. [CrossRef] [PubMed]
85. Shi, W.; Casas, J.; Venkataramasubramani, M.; Tang, L. Synthesis and Characterization of Gold Nanoparticles with Plasmon Absorbance Wavelength Tunable from Visible to Near Infrared Region. *ISRN Nanomater.* **2012**, *2012*, 659043. [CrossRef]
86. Jacinto, T.A.; Rodrigues, C.F.; Moreira, A.F.; Miguel, S.P.; Costa, E.C.; Ferreira, P.; Correia, I.J. Hyaluronic acid and vitamin E polyethylene glycol succinate functionalized gold-core silica shell nanorods for cancer targeted photothermal therapy. *Colloids Surf. B Biointerfaces* **2020**, *188*, 110778. [CrossRef]
87. F Rodrigues, C.; Fernandes, N.; de Melo-Diogo, D.; Ferreira, P.; J Correia, I.; F Moreira, A. HA/PEI-coated acridine orange-loaded gold-core silica shell nanorods for cancer-targeted photothermal and chemotherapy. *Nanomedicine* **2021**, *16*, 2569–2586. [CrossRef]
88. Pan, Y.; Ma, X.; Liu, C.; Xing, J.; Zhou, S.; Parshad, B.; Schwerdtle, T.; Li, W.; Wu, A.; Haag, R. Retinoic Acid-Loaded Dendritic Polyglycerol-Conjugated Gold Nanostars for Targeted Photothermal Therapy in Breast Cancer Stem Cells. *ACS Nano* **2021**, *15*, 15069–15084. [CrossRef]
89. Tan, H.; Hou, N.; Liu, Y.; Liu, B.; Cao, W.; Zheng, D.; Li, W.; Liu, Y.; Xu, B.; Wang, Z.; et al. CD133 antibody targeted delivery of gold nanostars loading IR820 and docetaxel for multimodal imaging and near-infrared photodynamic/photothermal/chemotherapy against castration resistant prostate cancer. *Nanomedicine* **2020**, *27*, 102192. [CrossRef]
90. Cheng, Y.; Bao, D.; Chen, X.; Wu, Y.; Wei, Y.; Wu, Z.; Li, F.; Piao, J.G. Microwave-triggered/HSP-targeted gold nano-system for triple-negative breast cancer photothermal therapy. *Int. J. Pharm.* **2021**, *593*, 120162. [CrossRef]
91. Peng, C.; Zheng, L.; Chen, Q.; Shen, M.; Guo, R.; Wang, H.; Cao, X.; Zhang, G.; Shi, X. PEGylated dendrimer-entrapped gold nanoparticles for in vivo blood pool and tumor imaging by computed tomography. *Biomaterials* **2012**, *33*, 1107–1119. [CrossRef]
92. Gu, W.; Zhang, Q.; Zhang, T.; Li, Y.; Xiang, J.; Peng, R.; Liu, J. Hybrid polymeric nano-capsules loaded with gold nanoclusters and indocyanine green for dual-modal imaging and photothermal therapy. *J. Mater. Chem. B* **2016**, *4*, 910–919. [CrossRef]
93. Alkhayal, A.; Fathima, A.; Alhasan, A.H.; Alsharaeh, E.H. PEG Coated Fe_3O_4/RGO Nano-Cube-Like Structures for Cancer Therapy via Magnetic Hyperthermia. *Nanomaterials* **2021**, *11*, 2398. [CrossRef]
94. Ebrahiminezhad, A.; Zare-Hoseinabadi, A.; Sarmah, A.K.; Taghizadeh, S.; Ghasemi, Y.; Berenjian, A. Plant-Mediated Synthesis and Applications of Iron Nanoparticles. *Mol. Biotechnol.* **2018**, *60*, 154–168. [CrossRef]
95. Zhi, D.; Yang, T.; Yang, J.; Fu, S.; Zhang, S. Targeting strategies for superparamagnetic iron oxide nanoparticles in cancer therapy. *Acta Biomater.* **2020**, *102*, 13–34. [CrossRef]
96. Palanisamy, S.; Wang, Y.M. Superparamagnetic iron oxide nanoparticulate system: Synthesis, targeting, drug delivery and therapy in cancer. *Dalton Trans.* **2019**, *48*, 9490–9515. [CrossRef]
97. Habra, K.; McArdle, S.E.B.; Morris, R.H.; Cave, G.W.V. Synthesis and Functionalisation of Superparamagnetic Nano-Rods towards the Treatment of Glioblastoma Brain Tumours. *Nanomaterials* **2021**, *11*, 2157. [CrossRef]

98. Vangijzegem, T.; Stanicki, D.; Laurent, S. Magnetic iron oxide nanoparticles for drug delivery: Applications and characteristics. *Expert Opin. Drug Deliv.* **2019**, *16*, 69–78. [CrossRef]
99. Liu, J.F.; Jang, B.; Issadore, D.; Tsourkas, A. Use of magnetic fields and nanoparticles to trigger drug release and improve tumor targeting. *WIREs Nanomed. Nanobiotechnol.* **2019**, *11*, e1571. [CrossRef]
100. Shah, R.R.; Davis, T.P.; Glover, A.L.; Nikles, D.E.; Brazel, C.S. Impact of magnetic field parameters and iron oxide nanoparticle properties on heat generation for use in magnetic hyperthermia. *J. Magn. Magn. Mater.* **2015**, *387*, 96–106. [CrossRef]
101. Obaidat, I.M.; Issa, B.; Haik, Y. Magnetic Properties of Magnetic Nanoparticles for Efficient Hyperthermia. *Nanomaterials* **2015**, *5*, 63–89. [CrossRef]
102. Boyer, C.; Whittaker, M.R.; Bulmus, V.; Liu, J.; Davis, T.P. The design and utility of polymer-stabilized iron-oxide nanoparticles for nanomedicine applications. *NPG Asia Mater.* **2010**, *2*, 23–30. [CrossRef]
103. Xu, X.; Zhou, X.; Xiao, B.; Xu, H.; Hu, D.; Qian, Y.; Hu, H.; Zhou, Z.; Liu, X.; Gao, J.; et al. Glutathione-Responsive Magnetic Nanoparticles for Highly Sensitive Diagnosis of Liver Metastases. *Nano Lett.* **2021**, *21*, 2199–2206. [CrossRef]
104. Xiao, Z.; You, Y.; Liu, Y.; He, L.; Zhang, D.; Cheng, Q.; Wang, D.; Chen, T.; Shi, C.; Luo, L. NIR-Triggered Blasting Nanovesicles for Targeted Multimodal Image-Guided Synergistic Cancer Photothermal and Chemotherapy. *ACS Appl. Mater. Interfaces* **2021**, *13*, 35376–35388. [CrossRef] [PubMed]
105. Chen, L.; Wu, Y.; Wu, H.; Li, J.; Xie, J.; Zang, F.; Ma, M.; Gu, N.; Zhang, Y. Magnetic targeting combined with active targeting of dual-ligand iron oxide nanoprobes to promote the penetration depth in tumors for effective magnetic resonance imaging and hyperthermia. *Acta Biomater.* **2019**, *96*, 491–504. [CrossRef] [PubMed]
106. Zhang, Y.; Hu, H.; Tang, W.; Zhang, Q.; Li, M.; Jin, H.; Huang, Z.; Cui, Z.; Xu, J.; Wang, K.; et al. A multifunctional magnetic nanosystem based on "two strikes" effect for synergistic anticancer therapy in triple-negative breast cancer. *J. Control. Release* **2020**, *322*, 401–415. [CrossRef] [PubMed]
107. Zheng, D.; Wan, C.; Yang, H.; Xu, L.; Dong, Q.; Du, C.; Du, J.; Li, F. Her2-Targeted Multifunctional Nano-Theranostic Platform Mediates Tumor Microenvironment Remodeling and Immune Activation for Breast Cancer Treatment. *Int. J. Nanomed.* **2020**, *15*, 10007–10028. [CrossRef]
108. He, Y.; Wang, M.; Fu, M.; Yuan, X.; Luo, Y.; Qiao, B.; Cao, J.; Wang, Z.; Hao, L.; Yuan, G. Iron(II) phthalocyanine Loaded and AS1411 Aptamer Targeting Nanoparticles: A Nanocomplex for Dual Modal Imaging and Photothermal Therapy of Breast Cancer. *Int. J. Nanomed.* **2020**, *15*, 5927–5949. [CrossRef]
109. Ding, X.; Jiang, W.; Dong, L.; Hong, C.; Luo, Z.; Hu, Y.; Cai, K. Redox-responsive magnetic nanovectors self-assembled from amphiphilic polymer and iron oxide nanoparticles for a remotely targeted delivery of paclitaxel. *J. Mater. Chem. B* **2021**, *9*, 6037–6043. [CrossRef]
110. Lin, C.H.; Chen, Y.C.; Huang, P.I. Preparation of Multifunctional Dopamine-Coated Zerovalent Iron/Reduced Graphene Oxide for Targeted Phototheragnosis in Breast Cancer. *Nanomaterials* **2020**, *10*, 1957. [CrossRef]
111. Yun, B.; Zhu, H.; Yuan, J.; Sun, Q.; Li, Z. Synthesis, modification and bioapplications of nanoscale copper chalcogenides. *J. Mater. Chem. B* **2020**, *8*, 4778–4812. [CrossRef]
112. Zhou, M.; Tian, M.; Li, C. Copper-Based Nanomaterials for Cancer Imaging and Therapy. *Bioconjugate Chem.* **2016**, *27*, 1188–1199. [CrossRef]
113. Rubilar, O.; Rai, M.; Tortella, G.; Diez, M.C.; Seabra, A.B.; Duran, N. Biogenic nanoparticles: Copper, copper oxides, copper sulphides, complex copper nanostructures and their applications. *Biotechnol. Lett.* **2013**, *35*, 1365–1375. [CrossRef]
114. Tian, H.; Zhang, M.; Jin, G.; Jiang, Y.; Luan, Y. Cu-MOF chemodynamic nanoplatform via modulating glutathione and H_2O_2 in tumor microenvironment for amplified cancer therapy. *J. Colloid Interface Sci.* **2021**, *587*, 358–366. [CrossRef]
115. Wang, S.; Riedinger, A.; Li, H.; Fu, C.; Liu, H.; Li, L.; Liu, T.; Tan, L.; Barthel, M.J.; Pugliese, G.; et al. Plasmonic Copper Sulfide Nanocrystals Exhibiting Near-Infrared Photothermal and Photodynamic Therapeutic Effects. *ACS Nano* **2015**, *9*, 1788–1800. [CrossRef]
116. Egorova, K.S.; Ananikov, V.P. Which Metals are Green for Catalysis? Comparison of the Toxicities of Ni, Cu, Fe, Pd, Pt, Rh, and Au Salts. *Angew. Chem. Int. Ed.* **2016**, *55*, 12150–12162. [CrossRef]
117. Letelier, M.E.; Sánchez-Jofré, S.; Peredo-Silva, L.; Cortés-Troncoso, J.; Aracena-Parks, P. Mechanisms underlying iron and copper ions toxicity in biological systems: Pro-oxidant activity and protein-binding effects. *Chem. Biol. Interact.* **2010**, *188*, 220–227. [CrossRef]
118. Li, W.; Zamani, R.; Gil, P.R.; Pelaz, B.; Ibáñez, M.; Cadavid, D.; Shavel, A.; Alvarez-Puebla, R.A.; Parak, W.J.; Arbiol, J.; et al. CuTe Nanocrystals: Shape and Size Control, Plasmonic Properties, and Use as SERS Probes and Photothermal Agents. *J. Am. Chem. Soc.* **2013**, *135*, 7098–7101. [CrossRef]
119. Li, L.; Rashidi, L.H.; Yao, M.; Ma, L.; Chen, L.; Zhang, J.; Zhang, Y.; Chen, W. CuS nanoagents for photodynamic and photothermal therapies: Phenomena and possible mechanisms. *Photodiagn. Photodyn.* **2017**, *19*, 5–14. [CrossRef]
120. Shi, H.; Yan, R.; Wu, L.; Sun, Y.; Liu, S.; Zhou, Z.; He, J.; Ye, D. Tumor-targeting CuS nanoparticles for multimodal imaging and guided photothermal therapy of lymph node metastasis. *Acta Biomater.* **2018**, *72*, 256–265. [CrossRef]
121. Xu, J.; Shi, R.; Chen, G.; Dong, S.; Yang, P.; Zhang, Z.; Niu, N.; Gai, S.; He, F.; Fu, Y.; et al. All-in-One Theranostic Nanomedicine with Ultrabright Second Near-Infrared Emission for Tumor-Modulated Bioimaging and Chemodynamic/Photodynamic Therapy. *ACS Nano* **2020**, *14*, 9613–9625. [CrossRef]

122. Liang, S.; Deng, X.; Chang, Y.; Sun, C.; Shao, S.; Xie, Z.; Xiao, X.; Ma, P.; Zhang, H.; Cheng, Z.; et al. Intelligent Hollow Pt-CuS Janus Architecture for Synergistic Catalysis-Enhanced Sonodynamic and Photothermal Cancer Therapy. *Nano Lett.* **2019**, *19*, 4134–4145. [CrossRef]
123. Poudel, K.; Thapa, R.K.; Gautam, M.; Ou, W.; Soe, Z.C.; Gupta, B.; Ruttala, H.B.; Thuy, H.N.; Dai, P.C.; Jeong, J.-H.; et al. Multifaceted NIR-responsive polymer-peptide-enveloped drug-loaded copper sulfide nanoplatform for chemo-phototherapy against highly tumorigenic prostate cancer. *Nanomedicine* **2019**, *21*, 102042. [CrossRef] [PubMed]
124. Maor, I.; Asadi, S.; Korganbayev, S.; Dahis, D.; Shamay, Y.; Schena, E.; Azhari, H.; Saccomandi, P.; Weitz, I.S. Laser-induced thermal response and controlled release of copper oxide nanoparticles from multifunctional polymeric nanocarriers. *Sci. Technol. Adv. Mater.* **2021**, *22*, 218–233. [CrossRef] [PubMed]
125. Xu, R.; Zhang, K.; Liang, J.; Gao, F.; Li, J.; Guan, F. Hyaluronic acid/polyethyleneimine nanoparticles loaded with copper ion and disulfiram for esophageal cancer. *Carbohydr. Polym.* **2021**, *261*, 117846. [CrossRef] [PubMed]
126. Wu, Z.; Zhang, P.; Wang, P.; Wang, Z.; Luo, X. Using copper sulfide nanoparticles as cross-linkers of tumor microenvironment responsive polymer micelles for cancer synergistic photo-chemotherapy. *Nanoscale* **2021**, *13*, 3723–3736. [CrossRef]
127. Xiao, Z.; Zuo, W.; Chen, L.; Wu, L.; Liu, N.; Liu, J.; Jin, Q.; Zhao, Y.; Zhu, X. H_2O_2 Self-Supplying and GSH-Depleting Nanoplatform for Chemodynamic Therapy Synergetic Photothermal/Chemotherapy. *ACS Appl. Mater. Interfaces* **2021**, *13*, 43925–43936. [CrossRef]
128. Cai, X.; Xie, Z.; Ding, B.; Shao, S.; Liang, S.; Pang, M.; Lin, J. Monodispersed Copper(I)-Based Nano Metal-Organic Framework as a Biodegradable Drug Carrier with Enhanced Photodynamic Therapy Efficacy. *Adv. Sci.* **2019**, *6*, 1900848. [CrossRef]
129. Fang, X.L.; Akrofi, R.; Yang, H.; Chen, Q.Y. The NIR inspired nano-CuSMn(II) composites for lactate and glycolysis attenuation. *Colloids Surf. B Biointerfaces* **2019**, *181*, 728–733. [CrossRef]
130. Yu, X.; Yu, J.; Cheng, B.; Huang, B. One-Pot Template-Free Synthesis of Monodisperse Zinc Sulfide Hollow Spheres and Their Photocatalytic Properties. *Chem. A Eur. J.* **2009**, *15*, 6731–6739. [CrossRef]
131. Wang, C.-C.; Wang, S.; Xia, Q.; He, W.; Yin, J.-J.; Fu, P.P.; Li, J.-H. Phototoxicity of Zinc Oxide Nanoparticles in HaCaT Keratinocytes-Generation of Oxidative DNA Damage During UVA and Visible Light Irradiation. *J. Nanosci. Nanotechnol.* **2013**, *13*, 3880–3888. [CrossRef]
132. Akhtar, M.J.; Ahamed, M.; Kumar, S.; Khan, M.M.; Ahmad, J.; Alrokayan, S.A. Zinc oxide nanoparticles selectively induce apoptosis in human cancer cells through reactive oxygen species. *Int. J. Nanomed.* **2012**, *7*, 845–857.
133. Song, T.; Qu, Y.; Ren, Z.; Yu, S.; Sun, M.; Yu, X.; Yu, X. Synthesis and Characterization of Polyvinylpyrrolidone-Modified ZnO Quantum Dots and Their In Vitro Photodynamic Tumor Suppressive Action. *Int. J. Mol. Sci.* **2021**, *22*, 8106. [CrossRef]
134. Riddell, I.A.; Lippard, S.J. Cisplatin and Oxaliplatin: Our Current Understanding of Their Actions. *Met. Ions Life Sci.* **2018**, *18*, 1–42.
135. Asharani, P.V.; Xinyi, N.; Hande, M.P.; Valiyaveettil, S. DNA damage and p53-mediated growth arrest in human cells treated with platinum nanoparticles. *Nanomedicine* **2009**, *5*, 51–64. [CrossRef]
136. Cao, H.; Yang, Y.; Liang, M.; Ma, Y.; Sun, N.; Gao, X.; Li, J. Pt@polydopamine nanoparticles as nanozymes for enhanced photodynamic and photothermal therapy. *Chem. Commun.* **2021**, *57*, 255–258. [CrossRef]
137. Pedone, D.; Moglianetti, M.; De Luca, E.; Bardi, G.; Pompa, P.P. Platinum nanoparticles in nanobiomedicine. *Chem. Soc. Rev.* **2017**, *46*, 4951–4975. [CrossRef]
138. Chen, T.; Gu, T.; Cheng, L.; Li, X.; Han, G.; Liu, Z. Porous Pt nanoparticles loaded with doxorubicin to enable synergistic Chemo-/Electrodynamic Therapy. *Biomaterials* **2020**, *255*, 120202. [CrossRef]
139. Zhu, Y.; Li, W.; Zhao, X.; Zhou, Z.; Wang, Y.; Cheng, Y.; Huang, Q.; Zhang, Q. Hyaluronic Acid-Encapsulated Platinum Nanoparticles for Targeted Photothermal Therapy of Breast Cancer. *J. Biomed. Nanotechnol.* **2017**, *13*, 1457–1467. [CrossRef]
140. Zhang, X.F.; Liu, Z.G.; Shen, W.; Gurunathan, S. Silver Nanoparticles: Synthesis, Characterization, Properties, Applications, and Therapeutic Approaches. *Int. J. Mol. Sci.* **2016**, *17*, 1534. [CrossRef]
141. Kim, S.; Ryu, D.-Y. Silver nanoparticle-induced oxidative stress, genotoxicity and apoptosis in cultured cells and animal tissues. *J. Appl. Toxicol.* **2013**, *33*, 78–89. [CrossRef]
142. Holmila, R.J.; Vance, S.A.; King, S.B.; Tsang, A.W.; Singh, R.; Furdui, C.M. Silver Nanoparticles Induce Mitochondrial Protein Oxidation in Lung Cells Impacting Cell Cycle and Proliferation. *Antioxidants* **2019**, *8*, 552. [CrossRef]
143. Park, T.; Lee, S.; Amatya, R.; Cheong, H.; Moon, C.; Kwak, H.D.; Min, K.A.; Shin, M.C. ICG-Loaded PEGylated BSA-Silver Nanoparticles for Effective Photothermal Cancer Therapy. *Int. J. Nanomed.* **2020**, *15*, 5459–5471. [CrossRef]
144. Zhang, J.; Zhao, B.; Chen, S.; Wang, Y.; Xiao, H. Near-Infrared Light Irradiation Induced Mild Hyperthermia Enhances Glutathione Depletion and DNA Interstrand Cross-Link Formation for Efficient Chemotherapy. *ACS Nano* **2020**, *14*, 14831–14845. [CrossRef]
145. Awasthi, P.; An, X.; Xiang, J.; Kalva, N.; Shen, Y.; Li, C. Facile synthesis of noncytotoxic PEGylated dendrimer encapsulated silver sulfide quantum dots for NIR-II biological imaging. *Nanoscale* **2020**, *12*, 5678–5684. [CrossRef]
146. Chong, Y.; Huang, J.; Xu, X.; Yu, C.; Ning, X.; Fan, S.; Zhang, Z. Hyaluronic Acid-Modified Au-Ag Alloy Nanoparticles for Radiation/Nanozyme/Ag+ Multimodal Synergistically Enhanced Cancer Therapy. *Bioconjugate Chem.* **2020**, *31*, 1756–1765. [CrossRef]
147. Zhang, X.-S.; Xuan, Y.; Yang, X.-Q.; Cheng, K.; Zhang, R.-Y.; Li, C.; Tan, F.; Cao, Y.-C.; Song, X.-L. A multifunctional targeting probe with dual-mode imaging and photothermal therapy used in vivo. *J. Nanobiotechnology* **2018**, *16*, 42. [CrossRef]

148. Liu, M.; Peng, Y.; Nie, Y.; Liu, P.; Hu, S.; Ding, J.; Zhou, W. Co-delivery of doxorubicin and DNAzyme using ZnO@polydopamine core-shell nanocomposites for chemo/gene/photothermal therapy. *Acta Biomater.* **2020**, *110*, 242–253. [CrossRef]
149. Sun, Y.; Yan, C.; Xie, J.; Yan, D.; Hu, K.; Huang, S.; Liu, J.; Zhang, Y.; Gu, N.; Xiong, F. High-Performance Worm-like Mn-Zn Ferrite Theranostic Nanoagents and the Application on Tumor Theranostics. *ACS Appl. Mater. Interfaces* **2019**, *11*, 29536–29548. [CrossRef] [PubMed]
150. Thakur, N.S.; Patel, G.; Kushwah, V.; Jain, S.; Banerjee, U.C.; Thakur, N.S. Facile development of biodegradable polymer-based nanotheranostics: Hydrophobic photosensitizers delivery, fluorescence imaging and photodynamic therapy. *J. Photochem. Photobiol. B* **2019**, *193*, 39–50. [CrossRef] [PubMed]
151. Anselmo, A.C.; Mitragotri, S. Nanoparticles in the clinic: An update post COVID-19 vaccines. *Bioeng. Transl. Med.* **2021**, *6*, e10246. [CrossRef] [PubMed]
152. Rodallec, A.; Benzekry, S.; Lacarelle, B.; Ciccolini, J.; Fanciullino, R. Pharmacokinetics variability: Why nanoparticles are not just magic-bullets in oncology. *Crit. Rev. Oncol. Hematol.* **2018**, *129*, 1–12. [CrossRef] [PubMed]
153. Wilhelm, S.; Tavares, A.J.; Dai, Q.; Ohta, S.; Audet, J.; Dvorak, H.F.; Chan, W.C.W. Analysis of nanoparticle delivery to tumours. *Nat. Rev. Mater.* **2016**, *1*, 16014. [CrossRef]
154. Shi, J.; Kantoff, P.W.; Wooster, R.; Farokhzad, O.C. Cancer nanomedicine: Progress, challenges and opportunities. *Nat. Rev. Cancer* **2017**, *17*, 20–37. [CrossRef]
155. Rastinehad, A.R.; Anastos, H.; Wajswol, E.; Winoker, J.S.; Sfakianos, J.P.; Doppalapudi, S.K.; Carrick, M.R.; Knauer, C.J.; Taouli, B.; Lewis, S.C. Gold nanoshell-localized photothermal ablation of prostate tumors in a clinical pilot device study. *Proc. Natl. Acad. Sci. USA* **2019**, *116*, 18590–18596. [CrossRef]
156. Bayda, S.; Hadla, M.; Palazzolo, S.; Riello, P.; Corona, G.; Toffoli, G.; Rizzolio, F. Inorganic Nanoparticles for Cancer Therapy: A Transition from Lab to Clinic. *Curr. Med. Chem.* **2018**, *25*, 4269–4303. [CrossRef]
157. Kumthekar, P.; Ko, C.H.; Paunesku, T.; Dixit, K.; Sonabend, A.M.; Bloch, O.; Tate, M.; Schwartz, M.; Zuckerman, L.; Lezon, R. A first-in-human phase 0 clinical study of RNA interference-based spherical nucleic acids in patients with recurrent glioblastoma. *Sci. Transl. Med.* **2021**, *13*, eabb3945. [CrossRef]
158. Kumthekar, P.; Rademaker, A.; Ko, C.; Dixit, K.; Schwartz, M.A.; Sonabend, A.M.; Sharp, L.; Lukas, R.V.; Stupp, R.; Horbinski, C.; et al. A phase 0 first-in-human study using NU-0129: A gold base spherical nucleic acid (SNA) nanoconjugate targeting BCL2L12 in recurrent glioblastoma patients. *J. Clin. Oncol.* **2019**, *37* (Suppl. S15), 3012. [CrossRef]

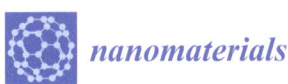

Article

Evaluation of Dosimetric Effect of Bone Scatter on Nanoparticle-Enhanced Orthovoltage Radiotherapy: A Monte Carlo Phantom Study

Afia Sadiq [1] and James C. L. Chow [2,3,*]

1 Department of Medical Physics, Toronto Metropolitan University, Toronto, ON M5B 2K3, Canada
2 Radiation Medicine Program, Princess Margaret Cancer Centre, University Health Network, Toronto, ON M5G 1X6, Canada
3 Department of Radiation Oncology, University of Toronto, Toronto, ON M5T 1P5, Canada
* Correspondence: james.chow@rmp.uhn.ca; Tel.: +1-416-946-4501

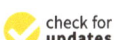

Citation: Sadiq, A.; Chow, J.C.L. Evaluation of Dosimetric Effect of Bone Scatter on Nanoparticle-Enhanced Orthovoltage Radiotherapy: A Monte Carlo Phantom Study. *Nanomaterials* 2022, 12, 2991. https://doi.org/10.3390/nano12172991

Academic Editor: Witold Łojkowski

Received: 23 June 2022
Accepted: 26 August 2022
Published: 29 August 2022

Publisher's Note: MDPI stays neutral with regard to jurisdictional claims in published maps and institutional affiliations.

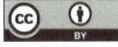

Copyright: © 2022 by the authors. Licensee MDPI, Basel, Switzerland. This article is an open access article distributed under the terms and conditions of the Creative Commons Attribution (CC BY) license (https://creativecommons.org/licenses/by/4.0/).

Abstract: In nanoparticle (NP)-enhanced orthovoltage radiotherapy, bone scatter affected dose enhancement at the skin lesion in areas such as the forehead, chest wall, and knee. Since each of these treatment sites have a bone, such as the frontal bone, rib, or patella, underneath the skin lesion and this bone is not considered in dose delivery calculations, uncertainty arises in the evaluation of dose enhancement with the addition of NPs in radiotherapy. To investigate the impact of neglecting the effect of bone scatter, Monte Carlo simulations based on heterogeneous phantoms were carried out to determine and compare the dose enhancement ratio (DER), when a bone was and was not present underneath the skin lesion. For skin lesions with added NPs, Monte Carlo simulations were used to calculate the DER values using different elemental NPs (gold, platinum, silver, iodine, as well as iron oxide), in varying NP concentrations (3–40 mg/mL), at two different photon beam energies (105 and 220 kVp). It was found that DER values at the skin lesion increased with the presence of bone when there was a higher atomic number of NPs, a higher NP concentration, and a lower photon beam energy. When comparing DER values with and without bone, using the same NP elements, NP concentration, and beam energy, differences were found in the range 0.04–3.55%, and a higher difference was found when the NP concentration increased. By considering the uncertainty in the DER calculation, the effect of bone scatter became significant to the dose enhancement (>2%) when the NP concentration was higher than 18 mg/mL. This resulted in an underestimation of dose enhancement at the skin lesion, when the bone underneath the tumour was neglected during orthovoltage radiotherapy.

Keywords: nanoparticle; nanoparticle-enhancement orthovoltage radiotherapy; skin radiotherapy; bone scatter; Monte Carlo simulation; dose enhancement; dose enhancement ratio

1. Introduction

The killing of cancer cells can effectively be improved with addition of heavy-atom nanoparticles (NPs), such as gold NPs. Studies have shown that these NPs not only increase the radiation dose delivered to the target/tumour, but also increase imaging contrast [1,2]. With enhanced image contrast the target can be better visualized by the radiation oncologist during target contouring. This results in more precise and accurate treatment planning in radiotherapy [3,4]. The reason for the dose enhancement is that the addition of the NPs makes the tumour more radiosensitive, meaning the compositional atomic number (Z) of the tumour cell is increased with the NP uptake [5]. As a result, when the tumour is irradiated, there is an enhancement of photoelectric effect. The enhanced yield of photoelectric electrons increases the energy deposition in the tumour cell, which in turn gives higher cancer control or killing effect [6].

The first study to use a high-Z radiosensitizer was carried out by Regulla et al. [7], who placed thin gold foil (150 μm) at depth in a polymethylmethacrylate slab, to increase the dose applied to mouse embryo fibroblasts. It was found that the cell kill rate increased by 45% in the presence of the gold foil. Furthermore, in a preclinical study, gold NPs of 1 nm diameter were applied to mice injected with subcutaneous EMT-6 mammary carcinomas. Radiotherapy using the 250 kVp photon beam was delivered to the tumours. The one-year survival curve before the addition of the gold NPs was 20%, but with the gold NPs it was 86% [8]. The gold was non-toxic and was cleared from the mice through the kidneys. Based on this study, researchers have developed a good understanding of the radiosensitization properties of high-Z NPs in dose enhancement [9,10]. In the above study, mammographic images were taken to observe the uptake of the NPs in the cells. From these images, it was shown that the rate of NP uptake was faster in cancerous cells than in healthy cells [11]. The cellular uptake of NP occurred mainly through energy-dependent receptor-mediated endocytosis. This resulted in the NPs accumulating in the endosome–lysosomes [12]. Following this preliminary study, Hainfeld et al. performed a preclinical experiment on the addition of gold NPs for radio-resistant brain squamous carcinoma [13]. It was found that by varying dose fractionation, radiation beam energy, and radiation dosimetry, adding gold NPs could increase the treatment outcome of aggressive squamous cell carcinoma. In a follow-up study to Hainfeld et al. [8], Monte Carlo simulations were performed to further quantify the dose enhancement properties of gold NPs. With the help of Monte Carlo codes (e.g., BEAM and DOSXYZ combined with EGS4), the dose enhancement ratio (DER) due to the addition of gold NPs was quantified based on several parameters; photon beam energies of 140 kVp, 4 MV, and 6 MV spectra with and without flattening filters, and gold NP concentrations of 7, 18, and 30 mg/mL [14]. These studies inspired many researchers to investigate the role of NPs in radiotherapy, using different types of radiation beams and delivery methods [15–18]. This has included skin therapy using orthovoltage photon beams [19].

According to the World Health Organization, the incidence of skin cancers has been increasing over the past few decades, with around 2–3 million cases occurring annually around the world [20]. With early detection and treatment, skin cancer is highly treatable, with radiotherapy being the favoured option. Radiotherapy can have a 90% success rate on skin cancers, with few to no side effects. The side effects are usually mild and last for a few weeks, until healthy cells grow back [21]. Generally, skin cancer is treated using orthovoltage photon beams. Orthovoltage radiotherapy refers to treatment using photon beam energies in the 100–300 kVp range. These kV photon beams are produced by an orthovoltage x-ray unit with a treatment cone and cutout, to conform the beams to the target of skin lesion. The radiation dose at the target skin surface is prescribed by the radiation oncologist. The required monitoring unit or treatment time is calculated by the radiotherapists and medical physicists using pre-measured dose data such as backscatter factor, relative exposure factor, and percentage depth dose [22]. Such calculations can be carried out manually using dose data tables or automatically using computer software [23].

In this study, we focused on the effect of bone scatter on dose enhancement, when NPs were added to skin lesions in NP-enhanced orthovoltage radiotherapy. Since the monitoring unit or treatment time calculation neglects the bone underneath the skin lesion in certain sites including the forehead, cheek, chest wall, and knee, the effect of bone scatter is neglected in the prescription dosimetry. When a skin lesion in the above sites is irradiated by a kV photon beam, a loss of backscatter occurs as the bone's inhomogeneity reduces the surface dose in the treatment. In current treatment modalities, dose reduction is not considered in the dose calculation. Thus, there may be an overestimation of the prescribed dose. Butson et al. [24] measured dose reduction caused by bone inhomogeneity, using a Gulmay D3300 X-ray machine (Gulmay Medical, Surrey, UK). In that study, an Attix parallel plate ionization chamber and EBT GAFCHROMIC film were used when taking measurements. Butson et al. [24] found that in some cases the presence of bone affected the backscattered dose by up to 12.5% of the surface dose (cone size diameter = 10 cm and 100 kVp beam).

Monte Carlo simulations are suitable for predicting macroscopically and nanoscopically the radiation dosimetry in NP-enhanced radiotherapy [25]. The Monte Carlo method is a mathematical algorithm based on random sampling to predict a numerical solution when the absolute solution is very difficult to determine. Different Monte Carlo codes such as the EGSnrc and Geant4 have been used and proved to be effective in NP dosimetry [26,27]. Studies have investigated dose enhancement, image contrast enhancement, and DNA damage in NP-enhanced radiotherapy using various radiation beams such as photon, proton, or electron beams [28–30]. Since the accuracy of a Monte Carlo simulation depends on the number of histories, a long computing time is therefore an issue in the simulation when aiming to obtain an accurate result. With recent advances in high-performance computing, the difficulty of long computing time was solved by using new computing technologies including cell-processor, cloud, and grid computing [31]. In this current study, Monte Carlo simulations were carried out to determine the DER at the skin lesion, when the bone underneath the skin was or was not neglected during NP-enhanced orthovoltage radiotherapy. This study focuses on predicting the physical dose enhanced at the skin lesion, using Monte Carlo simulation. The biological dose that affects cancer-cell killing and clinical outcome is not within the scope of this study [32,33].

2. Materials and Methods
2.1. Monte Carlo Simulation

For the Monte Carlo simulation using Electron Gamma Shower, the National Research Council (EGSnrc) code developed by the National Research Council of Canada was used to predict the radiation dose in this study [34]. The simulations were carried out using photon beams of 105 kVp (HVL: 3.2 mm Al) and 220 kVp (HVL: 1.7 mm Cu), produced by a Gulmay D3550 X-ray unit (Gulmay Medical, Surrey, UK) for gold, platinum, silver, iodine, and iron oxide NPs. The EGSnrc code is a software toolkit for performing Monte Carlo simulations of ionising radiation travelling through varying materials. It was developed in Canada, and is an improved version of the EGS package from the 1970s that was developed at the Stanford Linear Accelerator Centre [35]. As the name suggests, the program models certain "showers" that are generated as a result of electrons and photons transported in a medium. The EGSnrc code contains numerous applications that employ radiation physics to calculate specific quantities. These codes have been developed by numerous authors in order to support the large user community. The applications of the EGSnrc can be divided into two categories; Fortran codes and C++ codes (egs++). The Fortran codes consist of many applications, including the BEAMnrc and DOSXYZnrc that were used in this study [36].

Monte Carlo simulations are well-known as the benchmark for predicting radiation dosimetry in heterogeneous materials such as soft tissue, lung, bone, and metal [35]. The simulation has been used successfully to study metal and bone scatter in radiotherapy, and dose enhancement at the tumour in NP-enhanced radiotherapy involving kV and MV photon beams [37]. In this study, a Monte Carlo simulation using the macroscopic approach was carried out to predict dose enhancement at the skin lesion, when the bone underneath the tumour was or was not considered in the simulation model. In current skin-therapy practice regarding the dose prescribed at the patient's skin, any bone underneath the lesion is neglected. Results from the simulation were used to assess the impact of bone scatter on the dose enhancement in NP-enhanced orthovoltage radiotherapy.

2.2. Simulation Model and Geomtry

The simulation geometry using two heterogeneous phantoms is shown in Figure 1. Figure 1a shows a phantom with a layer of soft tissue (skin lesion) on top of a bone with thickness equal to 1 cm. The thickness of the skin lesion was equal to 0.2 cm. The bone was on top of a slab of soft tissue with a thickness of 8.8 cm. The dimensions of the phantom were $10 \times 10 \times 10$ cm^3 and it was designed to mimic a forehead treatment site. The phantom surface (skin) was placed in contact with a circular treatment cone of 5 cm diameter with source-to-surface distance equal to 20 cm. The cone was made of copper, steel, and poly(methyl methacrylate). The 105 and 220 kVp photon beams were generated by the Gulmay D3550 X-ray unit (Gulmay Medical, Surrey, UK) to irradiate the phantom. The kV photon beams were based on the Monte Carlo phase-space files of the treatment unit with the corresponding beam energy, quality, and geometry [38]. The phase-space files were generated using the EGSnrc-based BEAMnrc code [39]. For the heterogeneities in the phantom, the ICRUBONE521ICRU from the PEGS4 cross-section data file was selected to mimic the bone, and the ICRPTISSUE521ICRU was selected to mimic the skin lesion and soft tissue [34]. These standard materials are available in the PEGS4 data library in the simulation code. To simulate the skin lesion with the addition of NPs and model the material with NPs, cross-section datasets for various NP concentrations were created using the EGSnrc-based PEGS4 code. The datasets contained physical information of particle interactions of gold, platinum, silver, iodine, and iron oxide NPs at concentrations of 3, 7, 18, 30, and 40 mg/mL [19]. This range of concentration was selected according to small-animal experiments in nanoparticle-enhanced radiotherapy [8]. It was assumed that there was no biological washout of NPs during the simulation. Radiation dose was calculated at the skin lesion layer using the DOSXYZnrc code [40], and 150 million histories were run for each simulation. Under this number of histories, the uncertainty of calculated dose in the simulation was less than 1%. The energy cut-offs for the electron and photon transport were set to 521 and 1 keV, respectively. In the simulation, the PRESTA II was used for the electron-step algorithm, and the feature options of spin effect, bound Compton scattering, Rayleigh scattering, atomic relaxation, and electron impact ionization were all employed in the simulation using the kV photon beams [34]. For this phantom (Figure 1a), various kinds of doses were added at the skin lesion layer: with and without addition of NPs, with various metallic elements, and with various concentrations and photon beam energies. To investigate the dependence of dose enhancement on the effect of bone scatter, Figure 1b mimicked the case when the bone underneath the skin lesion was neglected in radiotherapy. In Figure 1b, the bone layer in Figure 1a was replaced by soft tissue. This is the clinical situation when the monitor unit or treatment time is calculated with the dose prescribed at the patient's skin [22]. In this event, the material underneath the skin lesion was assumed to be soft tissue or water during the treatment. The same simulations were carried out as per the phantom in Figure 1a. By comparing the dose enhancements at the skin lesions in Figure 1a,b, the difference of dose enhancement due to the presence of bone scatter was determined.

2.3. Dose Enhancement Ratio (DER)

The dose enhancement in the presence of NPs at the skin lesion is expressed as DER [41]:

$$\text{Does Enhancement Ration (DER)} = \frac{\text{Does at the skin lesion with nanoparticle addition}}{\text{Dose at the skin lesion without nanoparticle addition}} \quad (1)$$

When there was no NP added to the skin lesion in the simulation model, the material of the skin layer was set to soft tissue. This resulted in a DER value calculation of one. Because the addition of NPs can increase the dose at the skin lesion layer due to the enhancement of photoelectric effect, the dose at the skin lesion was higher than the same layer without added NPs. This caused the DER value exceed one, reflecting the dose enhancement.

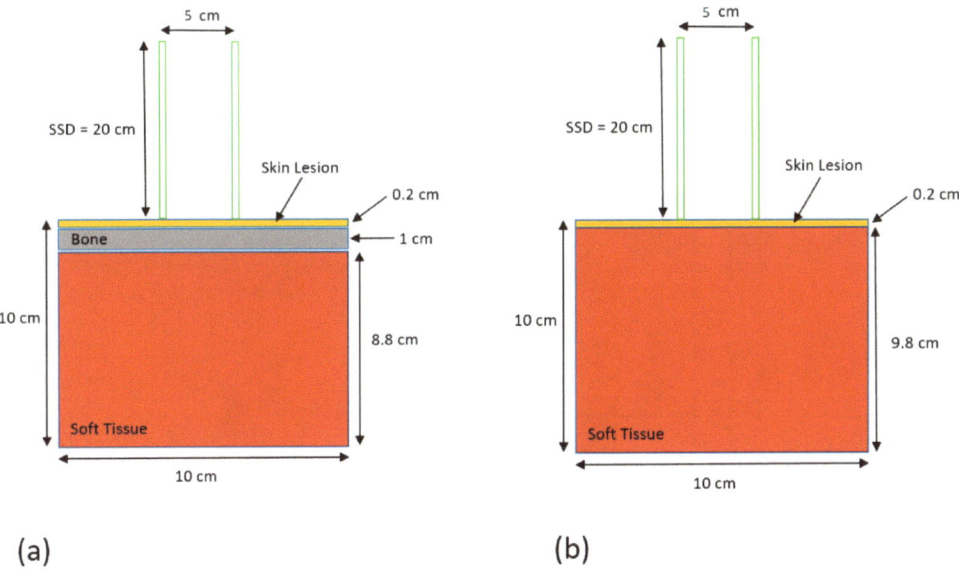

Figure 1. Schematic diagrams (not to scale) showing the heterogeneous phantoms used in Monte Carlo simulations, (**a**) with and (**b**) without a bone between the skin lesion and the soft tissue. The dimensions of the phantoms were equal to $10 \times 10 \times 10$ cm^3. The phantoms were irradiated by the 105 and 220 kVp photon beams with circular cone applicator (5 cm diameter) attached to the phantom's surface. The source-to-surface distance (SSD) was equal to 20 cm, mimicking the clinical dose delivery.

3. Results

The relationships between DER and NP concentration with variable presence of bone and photon beam energy are shown in Figure 2a–e, for the gold, platinum, silver, iodine, and iron oxide NPs. The uncertainty of the calculated DER was equal to 2% based on the radiation dose determined from Monte Carlo simulation. It can be seen in Figure 2 that all DER values were higher than one, showing that the addition of NPs to the skin lesion enhanced the dose during orthovoltage radiotherapy. The maximum DER value shown in Figure 2a was 5.91, for the phantom with bone irradiated by the 105 kVp photon beam. This DER value was larger than the maximum DER values of 5.75, 5.05, 4.81, and 2.05 shown in Figure 2b–e with the same phantom geometry and beam energy. Similarly, the minimum DER values were 3.83, 3.79, 3.43, 3.04, and 1.31 for the gold, platinum, silver, iodine, and iron oxide NPs, respectively, in the phantom without bone irradiated by the 220 kVp photon beam (Figure 2). The differences of DER with and without the presence of bone, shown in Figure 2, were calculated for different NPs, NP concentrations, and photon beam energies. These results are shown in Table 1. The differences of DER for the gold, platinum, silver, iodine, and iron oxide NPs ranged from 0.04–2.08, 0.06–2.01, 0.16–2.22, 0.37–2.79, and 0.06–0.62 using the 105 kVp photon beam, and 0.77–2.98, 0.61–3.08, 1.55–3.55, 1.17–3.23, and 0.4–2.12 using the 220 kVp beam, respectively.

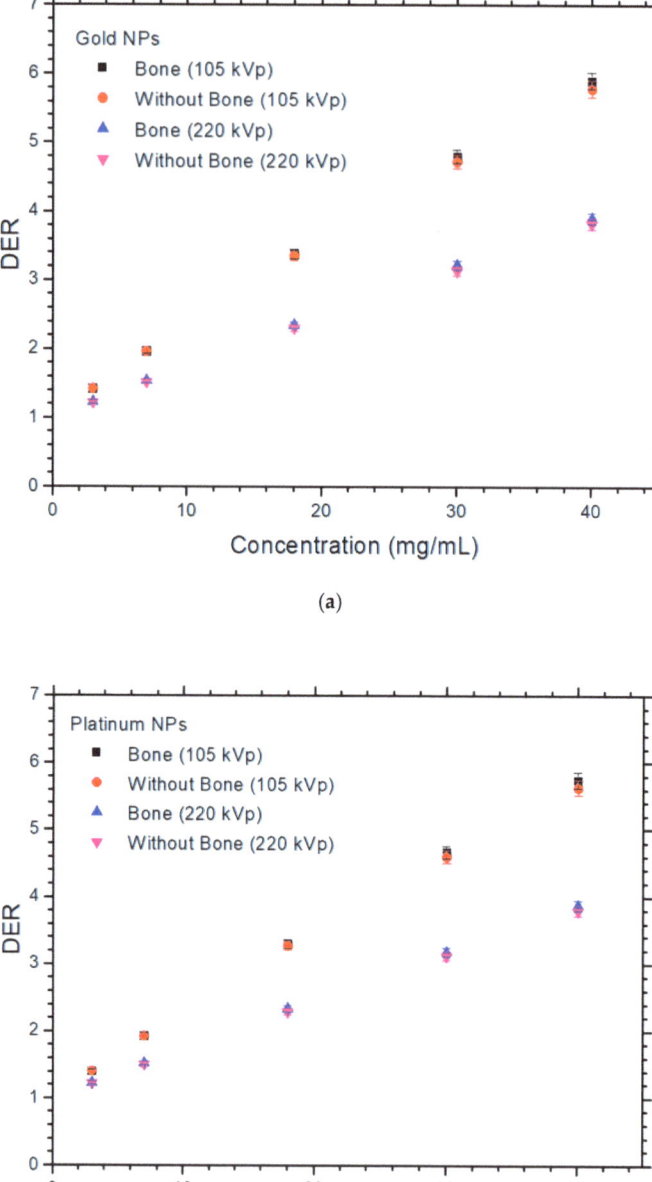

Figure 2. Cont.

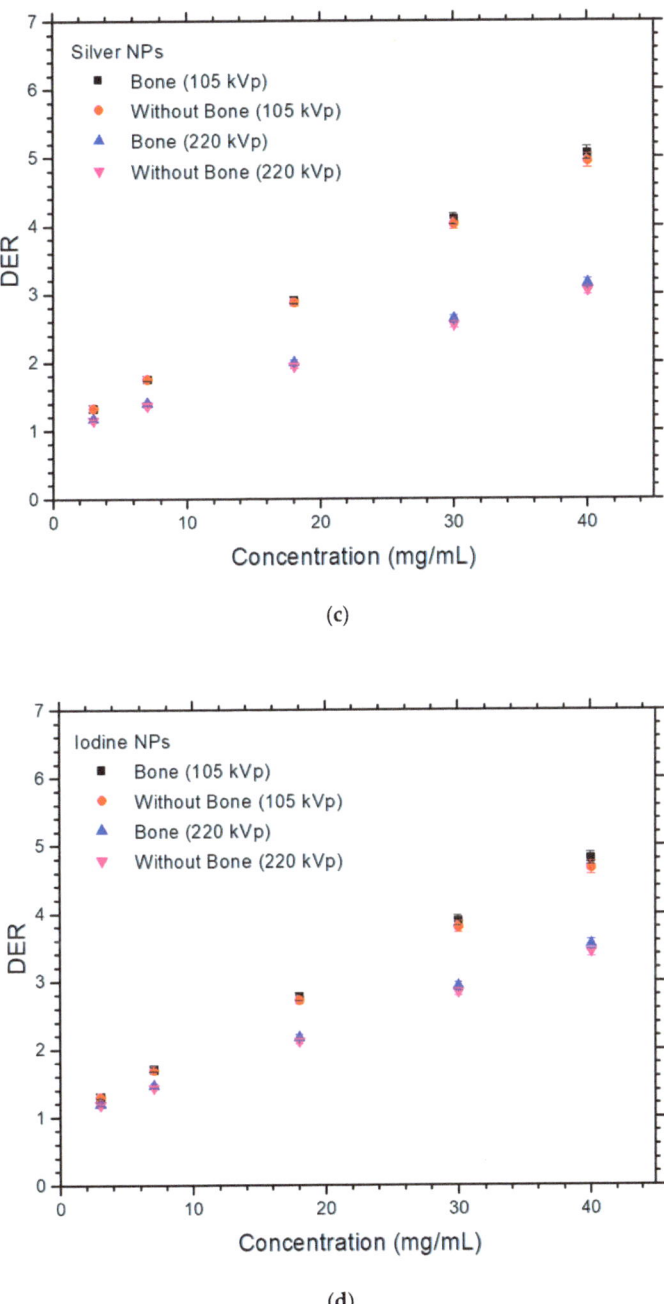

(c)

(d)

Figure 2. *Cont.*

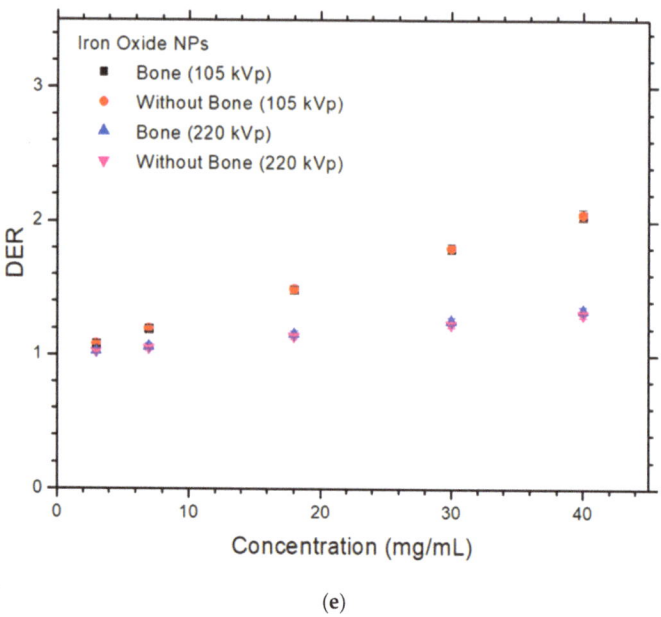

(e)

Figure 2. Relationships of dose enhancement ratio and NP concentration (mg/mL) with variations of photon beam energies (105 and 220 kVp) and presence of bone for (**a**) gold, (**b**) platinum, (**c**) silver, (**d**) iodine, and (**e**) iron oxide NPs in Monte Carlo simulations.

Table 1. Difference of DER (%) between bone under the skin and no bone under the skin in the Monte Carlo simulation, using various NPs, NP concentrations, and photon beam energies. Differences of DER values are marked in bold where statistically significant ($p < 0.05$).

Photon Beam Energy	105 kVp					220 kVp				
Concentration (mg/mL)	Gold NP	Platinum NP	Silver NP	Iodine NP	Iron Oxide NP	Gold NP	Platinum NP	Silver NP	Iodine NP	Iron Oxide NP
3	0.04	0.06	0.16	0.37	0.06	0.77	0.61	1.55	1.17	0.40
7	0.18	0.14	0.43	0.93	0.14	1.27	1.38	2.32	1.87	0.95
18	0.75	0.71	1.06	1.74	0.29	1.94	2.07	2.77	2.51	1.49
30	1.49	1.46	1.67	2.33	0.47	2.61	2.86	3.29	2.98	1.93
40	2.08	2.01	2.22	2.79	0.62	2.98	3.08	3.55	3.23	2.12

4. Discussion

4.1. Dependences of DER on the NP and NP Concentration

For the different elemental NPs used in this study, it is found that gold NPs performed best with maximum DER value of 5.9 using the maximum NP concentration (40 mg/mL) for the phantom with bone (Figure 1a) irradiated by the 105 kVp photon beam. This was followed by the platinum NPs with DER value equal to 5.75, then silver NPs, iodine NPs, and iron oxide NPs with DER values equal to 5.06, 4.81, and 2.05, respectively. It is seen that the DER value increased with the increase of Z of the NPs. This is because the dose enhancement was due to the increased energy deposition at the lesion, resulting from the increased number of secondary electrons. These electrons are generally produced by photoelectric interaction, which is dominant in the kV energy range. The increase of compositional Z at the skin lesion enhanced the photoelectric effect, resulting in an increase of photoelectric electron yield [42]. As the cross-section of the photoelectric effect is proportional to Z^n (n varies between 4 and 5), it can be seen that the higher the Z, the higher the DER value of the lesion with the addition of NPs. Therefore, gold (Z = 79) had the highest DER value, followed by platinum (Z = 78), silver (Z = 53), iodine (Z = 47), and iron oxide (Z = 23).

In Figure 2, DER values of the NPs were found to increase with concentration. This is because higher concentrations of NPs contain more number of particles. These NPs generate more secondary electrons (e.g., photoelectric and Auger electrons) when interacting with the kV photons through the photoelectric and Auger effect [43]. These extra electrons deposit more energy in the lesion to enhance the dose. Moreover, such an increase of DER value is more sensitive for NPs with higher Z than lower. For example, considering the phantom with bone (Figure 1a) irradiated by the 105 kVp photon beam, gold NPs had their DER value increased at a rate of 0.12 $(mg/mL)^{-1}$. This was higher than that of the iron oxide NPs, at a rate of 0.026 $(mg/mL)^{-1}$.

4.2. Dependences of DER on the Presence of Bone and Photon Beam Energy

When bone is present underneath the skin lesion in photon beam irradiation, the radiation dose is reduced as the bone decreases the backscatter to the skin layer [24,38]. This effect is more significant when the NP concentration is high (e.g., 40 mg/mL). Moreover, this effect is more significant when a kV photon beam is used. Photoelectric effect is dominant in the kV energy range, and the photoelectric interaction increases with an increase of Z. Therefore, more photons are absorbed by the bone than the soft tissue, because bone has a higher Z. This results in a lower dose at the skin lesion when the presence of bone is considered [38]. However, in the calculation of DER using the bone phantom, the effect of reduction of skin dose was cancelled out in Equation (1) because both the numerator and denominator contained bone in the phantom.

When NPs were added to the skin lesion in this study, the dose enhancement with bone was higher than that without bone, as shown in Figure 2. For example, when the NP concentration was equal to 40 mg/mL using the 220 kVp photon beam, the DER value for the gold NPs was 3.90 with bone and 3.78 without bone. Similar trends of results were found with other NPs, NP concentrations, and beam energies. When NPs were added to the skin lesion, the number of photons arriving at the bone layer was decreased because the NP–skin lesion layer acted as a shield to reduce the photon fluence to the bone [44]. This caused a higher DER value as more NPs were added to the skin lesion with bone compared with that without bone underneath the skin. Therefore, by considering dose enhancement due to the addition of NPs, and the "shielding effect" on the bone due to the skin layer with added NPs, the DER value was found to be slightly increased when the bone's effect on dose enhancement due to the addition of gold NPs was considered in the calculation.

In Figure 2, the DER values for NPs using the 105 kVp photon beams were higher than those for 220 kVp. In addition, the higher the NP concentration, the larger was the difference between the DER values at the two beam energies. As the cross-section of the photoelectric effect is inversely proportional to the energy of the incident photon, the lower energy of 105 kVp resulted in a larger cross-section and hence a higher photoelectric electron yield compared with 220 kVp. This was reflected in the DER values of the corresponding photon beam energies in Figure 2.

4.3. Difference of DER with and without Presence of Bone

The effect of bone scatter on the variation in DER values is shown in Table 1, for different NPs, NP concentrations, and photon beam energies. The differences of DER were in the range 0.04% to 3.55%, and it was found that the value was lower for lower NP concentrations (e.g., 0.04–1.55% at 3 mg/mL), and higher for higher NP concentrations (e.g., 2.01–3.55% at 40 mg/mL). Since the uncertainty in the DER calculation was 2%, most differences of DER values (with or without bone scatter) were within the simulation uncertainty, except when the values were higher than 2%, which mostly occurred at higher NP concentrations (>18 mg/mL). In this event, the effect of bone scatter became significant enough to affect the dose enhancement at the skin lesion in radiotherapy. It was found that underestimation of the DER value for skin when neglecting the bone scatter would be more significant at higher NP concentrations.

5. Conclusions

Present trends in orthovoltage radiotherapy include enhancement of the effect of the therapy by adding NPs to the skin lesion. However, in absence of NPs the presence of bone tissue under the skin decreases the effective dose in the skin lesion. The present study addresses the question whether the presence of bone under the skin would increase or decrease the effective dose in the presence of NPs in the skin. By using Monte Carlo simulation methods with phantom models, it was found that in the presence of NPs the effective dose in the presence of bone was increased compared to the case without bone. The effect was better measurable for NP concentrations above 18 mg/mL. This threshold depends on the Z of the NP material: Z (26–79), and threshold (2.12–3.55%). This result should be taken into account in future clinical applications. It should be noted that the DER value for the bone phantom was independent of the reduction of skin dose due to the presence of bone, but the bone effect on the dose enhancement was due to the addition of gold NPs. Higher DER values were found when the bone scatter was considered in the simulation. Moreover, the DER values increased with higher Z of NPs, higher NP concentration, and lower photon beam energy. It is concluded that in NP-enhanced orthovoltage radiotherapy, dose enhancement may be slightly underestimated when bone scatter is neglected, particularly when the skin lesion has a high NP concentration. Considering dose enhancement with and without bone, the DER differences were found to vary between 0.04% and 3.55% for different NPs, NP concentrations, and beam energies. DER difference > 2% should be considered as unneglectable in clinical practice.

One limitation of this work is that variation of DER by NP size was not considered in this study. This is because it remains too complicated to create a realistic Monte Carlo model with billions of NPs in the simulation volume. Future work will include clinical results from real treatment of orthovoltage radiotherapy on real patients, where the material of the voxels inside the bone structure will be replaced by tissue material. The computed tomography image set used can verify the results from the Monte Carlo test, for effective dosimetry in orthovoltage radiotherapy.

Author Contributions: Conceptualization, J.C.L.C.; methodology, J.C.L.C.; software, J.C.L.C. and A.S.; validation, J.C.L.C. and A.S.; formal analysis, A.S.; investigation, A.S.; resources, J.C.L.C. and A.S.; data curation, A.S.; writing—original draft preparation, J.C.L.C. and A.S.; writing—review and editing, J.C.L.C.; visualization, J.C.L.C. and A.S.; supervision, J.C.L.C.; project administration, J.C.L.C. All authors have read and agreed to the published version of the manuscript.

Funding: This research received no external funding.

Acknowledgments: The authors would like to thank Xiao Zheng from Toronto Metropolitan University, Canada for her assistance in Monte Carlo simulation using the NP–soft-tissue mixture method.

Conflicts of Interest: The authors declare no conflict of interest.

References

1. Siddique, S.; Chow, J.C.L. Application of Nanomaterials in Biomedical Imaging and Cancer Therapy. *Nanomaterials* **2020**, *10*, 1700. [CrossRef]
2. Chithrani, D.B.; Jelveh, S.; Jalali, F.; Van Prooijen, M.; Allen, C.; Bristow, R.G.; Hill, R.P.; Jaffray, D.A. Gold nanoparticles as radiation sensitizers in cancer therapy. *Radiat. Res.* **2010**, *173*, 719–728. [CrossRef]
3. Abdulle, A.; Chow, J.C.L. Contrast enhancement for portal imaging in nanoparticle-enhanced radiotherapy: A Monte Carlo phantom evaluation using flattening-filter-free photon beams. *Nanomaterials* **2019**, *9*, 920. [CrossRef]
4. Albayedh, F.; Chow, J.C.L. Monte Carlo simulation on the imaging contrast enhancement in nanoparticle-enhanced radiotherapy. *J. Med. Phys.* **2018**, *43*, 195–199.
5. Chow, J.C.L. Application of Nanoparticle Materials in Radiation Therapy. In *Handbook of Ecomaterials*; Torres Martinez, L.M., Vasilievna Kharissova, O., Ildusovich Kharisov, B., Eds.; Springer Nature: Cham, Switzerland, 2017; Chapter 150; pp. 3661–3681.
6. Retif, P.; Pinel, S.; Toussaint, M.; Frochot, C.; Chouikrat, R.; Bastogne, T.; Barberi-Heyob, M. Nanoparticles for radiation therapy enhancement: The key parameters. *Theranostics* **2015**, *5*, 1030. [CrossRef]

7. Regulla, D.F.; Hieber, L.B.; Seidenbusch, M. Physical and biological interface dose effects in tissue due to X-ray-induced release of secondary radiation from metallic gold surfaces. *Radiat. Res.* **1998**, *150*, 92–100. [CrossRef]
8. Hainfeld, J.F.; Slatkin, D.N.; Smilowitz, H.M. The use of gold nanoparticles to enhance radiotherapy in mice. *Phys. Med. Biol.* **2004**, *49*, N309. [CrossRef]
9. Moore, J.; Chow, J.C.L. Recent progress and applications of gold nanotechnology in medical biophysics using artificial intelligence and mathematical modeling. *Nano Express* **2021**, *2*, 022001. [CrossRef]
10. Siddique, S.; Chow, J.C.L. Gold nanoparticles for drug delivery and cancer therapy. *Appl. Sci.* **2020**, *10*, 3824. [CrossRef]
11. Karathanasis, E.; Suryanarayanan, S.; Balusu, S.R.; McNeeley, K.; Sechopoulos, I.; Karellas, A.; Annapragada, A.V.; Bellamkonda, R.V. Imaging nanoprobe for prediction of outcome of nanoparticle chemotherapy by using mammography. *Radiology* **2009**, *250*, 398–406. [CrossRef]
12. Oh, N.; Park, J.H. Endocytosis and exocytosis of nanoparticles in mammalian cells. *Int. J. Nanomed.* **2014**, *9* (Suppl. 1), 51.
13. Hainfeld, J.F.; Dilmanian, F.A.; Zhong, Z.; Slatkin, D.N.; Kalef-Ezra, J.A.; Smilowitz, H.M. Gold nanoparticles enhance the radiation therapy of a murine squamous cell carcinoma. *Phys. Med. Biol.* **2010**, *55*, 3045. [CrossRef] [PubMed]
14. Cho, S.H. Estimation of tumour dose enhancement due to gold nanoparticles during typical radiation treatments: A preliminary Monte Carlo study. *Phys. Med. Biol.* **2005**, *50*, N163. [CrossRef]
15. Huynh, N.H.; Chow, J.C.L. DNA dosimetry with gold nanoparticle irradiated by proton beams: A Monte Carlo study on dose enhancement. *Appl. Sci.* **2021**, *11*, 10856. [CrossRef]
16. Jabeen, M.; Chow, J.C.L. Gold Nanoparticle DNA Damage by Photon Beam in a Magnetic Field: A Monte Carlo Study. *Nanomaterials* **2021**, *11*, 1751. [CrossRef]
17. Haume, K.; Rosa, S.; Grellet, S.; Śmiałek, M.A.; Butterworth, K.T.; Solov'yov, A.V.; Prise, K.M.; Golding, J.; Mason, N.J. Gold nanoparticles for cancer radiotherapy: A review. *Cancer Nanotechnol.* **2016**, *7*, 8. [CrossRef]
18. Peukert, D.; Kempson, I.; Douglass, M.; Bezak, E. Metallic nanoparticle radiosensitisation of ion radiotherapy: A review. *Phys. Med.* **2018**, *47*, 121–128. [CrossRef]
19. Zheng, X.J.; Chow, J.C.L. Radiation dose enhancement in skin therapy with nanoparticle addition: A Monte Carlo study on kilovoltage photon and megavoltage electron beams. *World J. Radiol.* **2017**, *9*, 63–71. [CrossRef]
20. Radiation: Ultraviolet (UV) Radiation and Skin Cancer. Available online: https://www.who.int/news-room/questions-and-answers/item/radiation-ultraviolet-(uv)-radiation-and-skin-cancer (accessed on 1 June 2022).
21. Fischbach, A.J.; Sause, W.T.; Plenk, H.P. Radiation therapy for skin cancer. *West. J. Med.* **1980**, *133*, 379.
22. Chen, Z.; Chow, J.C.L.; Sun, A.; Nagar, H.; Stevens, K.R.; Knisely, J.P.S. Cancers of the Skin, Including Mycosis Fungoides. In *Khan's Treatment Planning in Radiation Oncology*; Khan, F.M., Sperduto, P.W., Gibbons, J.P., Eds.; Wolters Kluwer Health: Philadelphia, PA, USA, 2022; Chapter 13; pp. 284–309.
23. Pearse, J.; Chow, J.C.L. An Internet of Things App for Monitor Unit Calculation in Superficial and Orthovoltage Skin Therapy. *IOP SciNotes* **2020**, *1*, 014002. [CrossRef]
24. Butson, M.J.; Cheung, T.; Peter, K.N. Measurement of dose reductions for superficial x-rays backscattered from bone interfaces. *Phys. Med. Biol.* **2008**, *53*, N329. [CrossRef] [PubMed]
25. Chow, J.C.L. Recent progress in Monte Carlo simulation on gold nanoparticle radiosensitization. *AIMS Biophys.* **2018**, *5*, 231–244. [CrossRef]
26. Sheeraz, Z.; Chow, J.C.L. Evaluation of dose enhancement with gold nanoparticles in kilovoltage radiotherapy using the new EGS geometry library in Monte Carlo simulation. *AIMS Biophys.* **2021**, *8*, 337–345. [CrossRef]
27. Sakata, D.; Kyriakou, I.; Tran, H.N.; Bordage, M.C.; Rosenfeld, A.; Ivanchenko, V.; Incerti, S.; Emfietzoglou, D.; Guatelli, S. Electron track structure simulations in a gold nanoparticle using Geant4-DNA. *Phys. Med.* **2019**, *63*, 98–104. [CrossRef]
28. Chun, H.; Chow, J.C.L. Gold nanoparticle DNA damage in radiotherapy: A Monte Carlo study. *AIMS Bioeng.* **2016**, *3*, 352–361.
29. Sharma, M.; Chow, J.C.L. Skin dose enhancement from the application of skin-care creams using FF and FFF photon beams in radiotherapy: A Monte Carlo phantom evaluation. *AIMS Bioeng.* **2020**, *7*, 82–90. [CrossRef]
30. Sotiropoulos, M.; Henthorn, N.T.; Warmenhoven, J.W.; Mackay, R.I.; Kirkby, K.J.; Merchant, M.J. Modelling direct DNA damage for gold nanoparticle enhanced proton therapy. *Nanoscale* **2017**, *9*, 18413–18422. [CrossRef]
31. Chow, J.C.L. A performance evaluation on Monte Carlo simulation for radiation dosimetry using cell processor. *J. Comp. Meth. Sci. Eng.* **2011**, *11*, 1–12. [CrossRef]
32. McMahon, S.J.; Hyland, W.B.; Muir, M.F.; Coulter, J.A.; Jain, S.; Butterworth, K.T.; Schettino, G.; Dickson, G.R.; Hounsell, A.R.; O'sullivan, J.M.; et al. Biological consequences of nanoscale energy deposition near irradiated heavy atom nanoparticles. *Sci. Rep.* **2011**, *1*, 18. [CrossRef]
33. Sung, W.; Ye, S.J.; McNamara, A.L.; McMahon, S.J.; Hainfeld, J.; Shin, J.; Smilowitz, H.M.; Paganetti, H.; Schuemann, J. Dependence of gold nanoparticle radiosensitization on cell geometry. *Nanoscale* **2017**, *9*, 5843–5853. [CrossRef]
34. Rogers, D.W.; Kawrakow, I.; Seuntjens, J.P.; Walters, B.R.; Mainegra-Hing, E. *NRC User Codes for EGSnrc*; NRCC Report PIRS-702 (Rev. B); NRCC: Ottawa, ON, Canada, 2003.
35. Rogers, D.W. Fifty years of Monte Carlo simulations for medical physics. *Phys. Med. Biol.* **2006**, *51*, R287. [CrossRef] [PubMed]
36. Kim, J.H.; Hill, R.; Kuncic, Z. An evaluation of calculation parameters in the EGSnrc/BEAMnrc Monte Carlo codes and their effect on surface dose calculation. *Phys. Med. Biol.* **2012**, *57*, N267. [CrossRef] [PubMed]

37. Moradi, F.; Saraee, K.R.; Sani, S.A.; Bradley, D.A. Metallic nanoparticle radiosensitization: The role of Monte Carlo simulations towards progress. *Rad. Phys. Chem.* **2021**, *180*, 109294. [CrossRef]
38. Chow, J.C.L.; Owrangi, A.M. Surface dose reduction from bone interface in kilovoltage x-ray radiation therapy: A Monte Carlo study of photon spectra. *J. Appl. Clin. Med. Phys.* **2012**, *13*, 215–222. [CrossRef]
39. Rogers, D.W.; Walters, B.; Kawrakow, I. *BEAMnrc Users Manual*; NRC Report Pirs.; NRCC: Ottawa, ON, Canada, 2009; Volume 509, p. 12.
40. Walters, B.R.; Kawrakow, I.; Rogers, D.W. *DOSXYZnrc Users Manual*; NRC Report Pirs.; NRCC: Ottawa, ON, Canada, 2005; Volume 794, pp. 57–58.
41. Chow, J.C.L. Dose Enhancement Effect in Radiotherapy: Adding Gold Nanoparticle to Tumour in Cancer Treatment. In *Nanostructures for Cancer Therapy*; Ficai, A., Grumezescu, A.M., Eds.; Elsevier: Amsterdam, The Netherlands, 2017; Chapter 15; pp. 383–400.
42. Cooper, D.R.; Bekah, D.; Nadeau, J.L. Gold nanoparticles and their alternatives for radiation therapy enhancement. *Front. Chem.* **2014**, *2*, 86. [CrossRef]
43. Leung, M.K.; Chow, J.C.L.; Chithrani, B.D.; Lee, M.J.; Oms, B.; Jaffray, D.A. Irradiation of gold nanoparticles by x-rays: Monte Carlo simulation of dose enhancements and the spatial properties of the secondary electrons production. *Med. Phys.* **2011**, *38*, 624–631. [CrossRef]
44. Chow, J.C.L. Depth dose enhancement on flattening-filter-free photon beam: A Monte Carlo study in nanoparticle-enhanced radiotherapy. *Appl. Sci.* **2020**, *10*, 7052. [CrossRef]

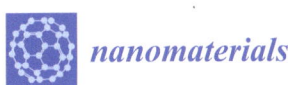

Review

Recent Advances in Functionalized Nanoparticles in Cancer Theranostics

Sarkar Siddique [1] and James C. L. Chow [2,3,*]

1. Department of Physics, Toronto Metropolitan University, Toronto, ON M5B 2K3, Canada
2. Radiation Medicine Program, Princess Margaret Cancer Centre, University Health Network, Toronto, ON M5G 1X6, Canada
3. Department of Radiation Oncology, University of Toronto, Toronto, ON M5T 1P5, Canada
* Correspondence: james.chow@rmp.uhn.ca; Tel.: +1-416-946-4501

Abstract: Cancer theranostics is the combination of diagnosis and therapeutic approaches for cancer, which is essential in personalized cancer treatment. The aims of the theranostics application of nanoparticles in cancer detection and therapy are to reduce delays in treatment and hence improve patient care. Recently, it has been found that the functionalization of nanoparticles can improve the efficiency, performance, specificity and sensitivity of the structure, and increase stability in the body and acidic environment. Moreover, functionalized nanoparticles have been found to possess a remarkable theranostic ability and have revolutionized cancer treatment. Each cancer treatment modality, such as MRI-guided gene therapy, MRI-guided thermal therapy, magnetic hyperthermia treatment, MRI-guided chemotherapy, immunotherapy, photothermal and photodynamic therapy, has its strengths and weaknesses, and combining modalities allows for a better platform for improved cancer control. This is why cancer theranostics have been investigated thoroughly in recent years and enabled by functionalized nanoparticles. In this topical review, we look at the recent advances in cancer theranostics using functionalized nanoparticles. Through understanding and updating the development of nanoparticle-based cancer theranostics, we find out the future challenges and perspectives in this novel type of cancer treatment.

Keywords: functionalized nanoparticles; MRI-guided therapy; molecular imaging; biomedical imaging; cancer therapy; cancer theranostics

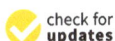

Citation: Siddique, S.; Chow, J.C.L. Recent Advances in Functionalized Nanoparticles in Cancer Theranostics. *Nanomaterials* **2022**, *12*, 2826. https://doi.org/10.3390/nano12162826

Academic Editors: Igor Nabiev and Pablo Botella

Received: 5 July 2022
Accepted: 16 August 2022
Published: 17 August 2022

Publisher's Note: MDPI stays neutral with regard to jurisdictional claims in published maps and institutional affiliations.

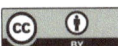

Copyright: © 2022 by the authors. Licensee MDPI, Basel, Switzerland. This article is an open access article distributed under the terms and conditions of the Creative Commons Attribution (CC BY) license (https:// creativecommons.org/licenses/by/ 4.0/).

1. Introduction

Cancer treatment has gained considerable attention in biomedical research over the past few decades due to the serious threat it poses to human health. The mortality rate of cancer increases every year, which leads to the need for the development of more efficient cancer therapeutic strategies [1]. Even though there is a major advance in cancer therapy, it continues to be a significant challenge due to tolerability and adherence [2]. Theranostics is a term first used by John Funkhouser at the beginning of the 1990s. It is defined as a combination of diagnostic tools that are the most suitable for specific diseases [3]. Theranostics portrays a close connection between diagnostics and the consequent therapy, and the theranostic principle has attracted huge attention in personalized medicine, in particular oncology. This allowed tumours at the advanced stage to be treated accurately with fewer side effects. For decades theranostics have been used for the therapy of benign and malignant thyroid diseases; however, recently, theranostics have been applied to other malignancies [4]. Theranostics agents such as radioisotopes, liposomes, quantum dots and plasmonic nanobubbles can be attached to anticancer drugs, imaging agents and cancer cell markers with the support of imaging techniques, providing the potential to facilitate the diagnosis, treatment and management of cancer patients [5]. The development of highly sensitive imaging modalities such as SPECT and PET with the synthesis of novel radio-labelled molecules specific for different biochemical targets promoted nuclear medicine into a new era [6]. These molecular imaging modalities have been applied in cardiology, neuroscience, oncology, gene therapy and theranostics. Nanoparticles (NPs) have been used as therapeutic or imaging agents that enhance the efficacy and control biodistribution and reduce the toxicity of drugs. In 2014–2015, there were 51 FDA-approved nanomedicines that met the definition of nanomedicines as therapeutic or imaging agents, and 77 products in clinical trial [7]. One of the crucial characteristics of nanomaterials is their small size. Their high affinity, high specificity, high thermal stability, low off-target accumulation and good solubility are among many adventurous characteristics they possess in cancer therapy. They can penetrate dense tissues of the tumour very well [8]. Nanotechnology in medicine is currently developed for drug delivery, and many substances are under study for cancer therapy. Solid NPs can be used for drug targeting when they reach the intended diseased site in the body, and the toxicology of the drug nanocarriers has been evaluated [9]. Active targeting is accomplished by conjugating tumour-specific ligands to the NPs' surface. It complements the enhanced permeability and retention effect (EPR). EPR is a universal pathophysiological phenomenon and mechanism where macromolecules with certain sizes above 40 kDa can progressively accumulate in the tumour vascularized area and achieve targeted delivery and retention of the anticancer compound into the solid tumour [10]. Some of the particles that are used to functionalize NPs are antibodies or antibody fragments, human transferrin protein, peptides, carbohydrates and vitamins. These biomarkers are recognized by their representative targeting ligands such as epidermal growth factor, human epidermal growth factor 2, Mucin-1, nucleolin, epithelial cell adhesion molecule and platelet-derived growth factor receptor 2. For anticancer drug delivery, Fu et al. [11] proposed to use aptamer-functionalized nanoparticles. This is because aptamers have favourable features such as a small size, very low immunogenicity, low cost of production and high affinity and specificity. The advantage of NPs as a theranostics agent is shown below in Figure 1 [12].

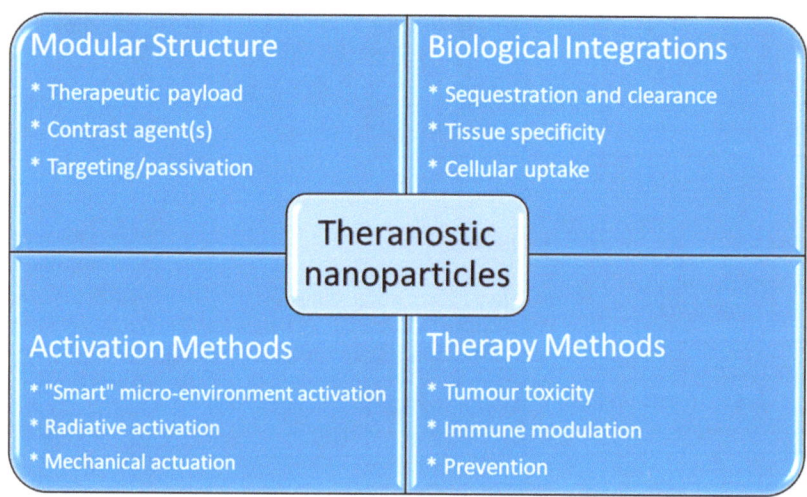

Figure 1. Advantages using nanoparticles in cancer theranostics.

A study of the functionalized NPs by wrapping them in the cancer cell membrane showed that the resulting particle possesses an antigenic exterior closely resembling that of the source cancer cells. These NPs allowed immunological adjuvant and membrane-bound tumour-associated antigens to be efficiently delivered to the cancer cell and promote an anticancer immune response [13]. Mesoporous silica NPs have a high potential in theranostic applications. They have a wide array of formulations and have significant in vivo efficacy for treating myriad malignant diseases in preclinical models [14]. The treatment of oral cancer is difficult and has a poor survival rate. Studies show that the proper inhibition of GST by NPs is promising in reversing pingyangmycin and carboplatin drug resistance in oral cancer, which improves the treatment outcome significantly [15]. One of the issues to keep in mind when using NPs is the formation of oxidative stress, which can have life-threatening consequences [16].

As there are many advantages of using functionalized nanoparticles in cancer theranostics, and there are various studies that have been carried out and are in progress, organizing and reviewing the recent works are necessary to see the big picture. From the current contributions in different aspects, we will be able to find out the future trends of work.

2. Magnetic Resonance Imaging (MRI)

MRI is one of the most powerful means of clinical detection and prognosis observation [17]. MRI is an imaging modality that is non-invasive, and it provides comprehensive multi-parametric information generally used for brain imaging [18]. MRI benefits from the contrast agent that provides a more improved depiction of large and medium-sized vassals and can provide dynamic vascular/perfusional properties of tissues. Gadolinium (Gd)-based contrast agents are widely used in MRI [19,20]. MRI can be coupled with other therapy to provide image-guided therapy for better treatment outcomes and tumour-targeting ability [21]. A study synthesized a multifunctional Gd-DTPA-ONB lipid by adding the Gd-DTPA contrast agent to an o-nitro-benzyl ester lipid. It combines the MRI tracking ability with dual trigger release capabilities, which allow maximum sensitivity without reducing the drug encapsulation rate. It can be activated by both PH-trigger hydrolysis and photo treatment [22]. Another Gd nanocomposite was synthesized by decorating Gd NPs onto the graphene oxide, and then functionalized with polyethylene glycol and folic acid. It was used to load doxorubicin to accomplish targeted image-guided drug delivery with MRI [23]. Liposomes are a useful class of NPs due to their tunable properties and multiple liposomal drug formulation. They have been clinically approved for cancer treatment. A vast number of Gd-based liposomal MRI contrast agents have been developed that can be used for targeted image-guided drug delivery [24]. Chemical exchange saturation transfer MRI has important advantages such as its ability to detect diamagnetic compounds that are not detectable using conventional MRI. It makes a broad spectrum of bioorganic agents, nanocarriers and natural compounds directly MRI detectable with a high resolution. It is advantageous for image-guided drug delivery [25]. An in vivo study looked at amphiphilic polymer-coated magnetic iron oxide NPs that were conjugated with near-infrared (NIR) dye-labelled HER2 affibody and chemotherapy drugs. Cisplatin was the drug used as the chemotherapy drug. MRI-guided therapy and the optical imaging detection of the therapy-resistant tumour were examined in an orthotopic human ovarian cancer xenograft model with a high level of HER2 expression. The result shows it significant inhibited the primary tumour and peritoneal and lung metastases in the ovarian cancer model in mice [26]. Another study looked at the NP with a unique morphology, which consists of a superparamagnetic iron oxide core and star-shaped plasmonic shell with high aspect ratio branches. Its strong near-infrared responsive plasmonic properties and magnetic properties allow it to be used in multimodal quantitative imaging, which combines the advantageous functions of MRI, magnetic particle imaging (MPI) and photoacoustic imaging. It can be used for image-guided drug delivery with tunable drug release capacity [27]. Drug resistance in chemotherapy has been a challenge for a long time in pancreatic cancer due to the stomal barrier making it difficult to reach the tumour microenvironment. A study developed IGF1 receptor-directed multifunctional theragnostic NPs for the targeted delivery of Dos into IGF1R-expressing drug-resistant tumour cells and tumour-associated stromal cells. NPs were prepared by combining IGF1 with magnetic iron oxide NPs carrying dox. They provided an excellent theranostics platform and showed good tumour control in an in vivo study [28]. Superparamagnetic iron oxide NPs have also been widely used in MRI and nanotheranostics. They can be coated with a biocompatible polymer such as polyethylene glycol or dextran, which allows chemical conjugation. They have a very high potential in MRI-guided drug delivery [29]. Figure 2 shows superparamagnetic iron oxide NPs being used in liver imaging and lymph node imaging [30].

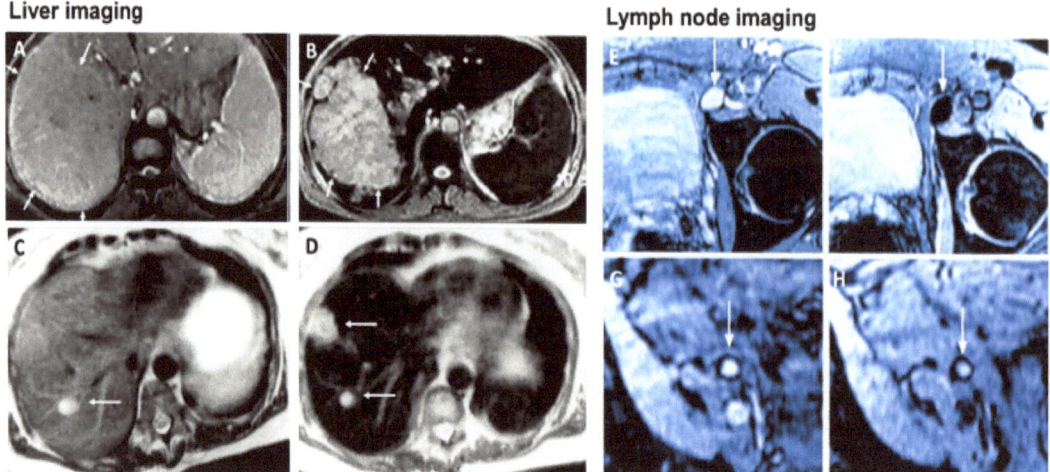

Figure 2. Superparamagnetic iron oxide NPs being used in liver imaging and lymph node imaging. (**A,B**): T2-weighted MR image of a liver with a large hepatocellular carcinoma before (**A**) and after (**B**) the administration of SPION. The lesion is demarcated with arrows. (**C,D**): Standard (**C**) and SPION-based contrast-enhanced (**D**) MR imaging of liver metastasis in a patient with colorectal cancer. After administration of ferumoxide SPION, a second metastasis becomes visible on T2-weighted MR image. (**E,H**): Lymph node in left iliac region (arrow), with and without metastatic infiltration. T2-weighted images before (**E,G**) and 24 h after (**F,H**) administration of ferumoxtran. Lymph node (arrow) appears bright before injection of UPIO (**E,G**). One day after injection, a signal loss in the lymph node (arrow) due to high UPIO macrophage uptake can be observed, thus indicating functionality and no metastasis (**F**). Conversely, in the lower panel, the lymph node (arrow) stays bright, indicating no trafficking of USPIO and thus metastatic colonization (**H**). Reprinted with permission from Ref. [30]. Copyright 2020 Elsevier.

2.1. MRI-Guided NPs for Gene Therapy

Gene therapy has gained considerable attention over the years and the health community has gained much more new information and knowledge regarding gene therapy [31]. Gene therapy is a form of engineered viruses carrying a therapeutic agent or containing genetically modified cells such as when chimeric antigen receptors are introduced to the T lymphocytes for cancer therapy such as for leukemia [32]. New gene therapy has shown its potential to significantly improve the survival rate of cancer patients [33]. For cancer gene therapy, the therapeutic agent generally requires a carrier such as an NP. MRI allows the tracking of that carrier and allows image-guided therapy, which can significantly improve the outcome [34]. A study looked at low molecular weight poly (ethylenimine)-poly (ethylene glycol) nanogels loaded with transforming growth factor -β1 siRNA and ultra-small iron oxide NPs for gene therapy and a T1-weighted MRI of tumour and tumour metastasis in a mouse sarcoma model. The study result shows it enhances the MRI image and effectively delivers the siRNA and inhibits tumour growth in the subcutaneous sarcoma tumour model and lung metastasis by silencing the TGF-β1 gene [35]. Another study investigated shaped, controlled magnetic mesoporous silica NPs and their performances in magnetic resonance image-guided targeted hyperthermia-enhanced suicide gene therapy of hepatocellular carcinoma. They had a higher loading capacity and better magnetic hyperthermia properties. They also had decreased cytotoxicity [36]. A bowl-shaped Fe_3O_4

NP with a self-assembly concept and appropriately surface-functionalized was studied with the aim for it to be used as a multifunctional carrier in combination therapy and gene therapy. The in vivo result shows promising results in the mouse breast cancer model [37]. The catalytic deoxy ribozyme has great potential in gene therapy via gene regulation but requires the carrier to reach the tumour target. A study showed polydopamine-Mn^{2+} NPs to be effective carriers and together they can be used as a photothermal agent and contrast agent for photoacoustic and magnetic resonance imaging [38]. Another study developed Fe_3O_4@PDA NPs to transport siRNA for gene therapy. The NPs were coated with mesenchymal stem cells to form a membrane. The overall complex showed good transport ability and photothermal functionality, and enhanced MRI capability [39].

2.2. MRI-Guided NPs for Thermal Therapy

Light-activated therapies have been introduced for cancer treatment for numerous cancers. Two of the main methods are localizing chemical exchange on the tumour known as photodynamic therapy (PDT) and localized thermal damage to the tumour, also known as photothermal therapy (PTT) [40]. Inorganic NPs have gained significant attention in image-guided thermal therapy in recent years, and the applications of inorganic NPs in tumour imaging and therapy are shown in Figure 3. The NPs contain metal, a semiconductor, metal oxide, nanocrystal and lanthanide-doped up conversion NPs. They can generate heat and reactive oxygen species, so they are ideal for image-guided PTT [41]. The thermal energy also promotes the gasification of perfluoropentane to enable the visualization of cancer tissue in ultrasound imaging, as well as enhances MRI imaging, and makes it ideal for dual MRI ultrasound imaging [42]. Core/shell nanoparticles were investigated for MRI imaging, magnetic hyperthermia and PTT due to their surface being coated with a porous shell. It can entrap large quantities of water around the nanoparticles and allows enhanced and efficient water exchange, which provides an improved magnetic resonance contrast signal. It also helps with NIR absorbance of the core and can have an enhanced thermal effect via synergistic PTT and magnetic hyperthermia. The nanoparticles investigated for this purpose were $MnFe_2O_4$/PB [43]. Another study developed temperature-activated engineered neutrophils by combining indocyanine green-loaded magnetic silica NIR sensitive nanoparticles. It provides a platform for dual-targeted PTT. The combination of magnetic targeting and neutrophil targeting provides an enhanced accumulation of the photothermal agent at the tumour site [44]. A study wrapped together gadolinium-DTPA, indocyanine green and perfluoropentane in a poly (lactic-co-glycolic) acid shell membrane by a double emulsion approach. Under NIR the indocyanine green converts the optic energy into thermal energy and converts oxygen to singlet oxygen, which destroys cancer cells through PTT and PDT. Another nanotheranostics agent was prepared via the participation of hydrophilic CuS nanoparticles, styrene, methacrylic acid, N-isopropylacrylamide and a polymerizable rare earth complex. It had good biocompatibility with a high loading capacity for DOX-HCl. Drug release can be activated via PH or high temperature. All these properties make it ideal for PTT and chemotherapy. MRI can also be used on it for image-guided drug delivery [45]. CuS material shows poor MRI ability but excellent photo absorption ability, whereas Fe-based materials have good MRI ability. A study combined the two and made a $Cu_xFe_yS_z$ sample that includes $CuFeS_2$, FeS_2 and Cu_5FeS_4 nanomaterials. The study result shows it to have high potential in MRI-guided photothermal enhanced chemo dynamic therapy [46].

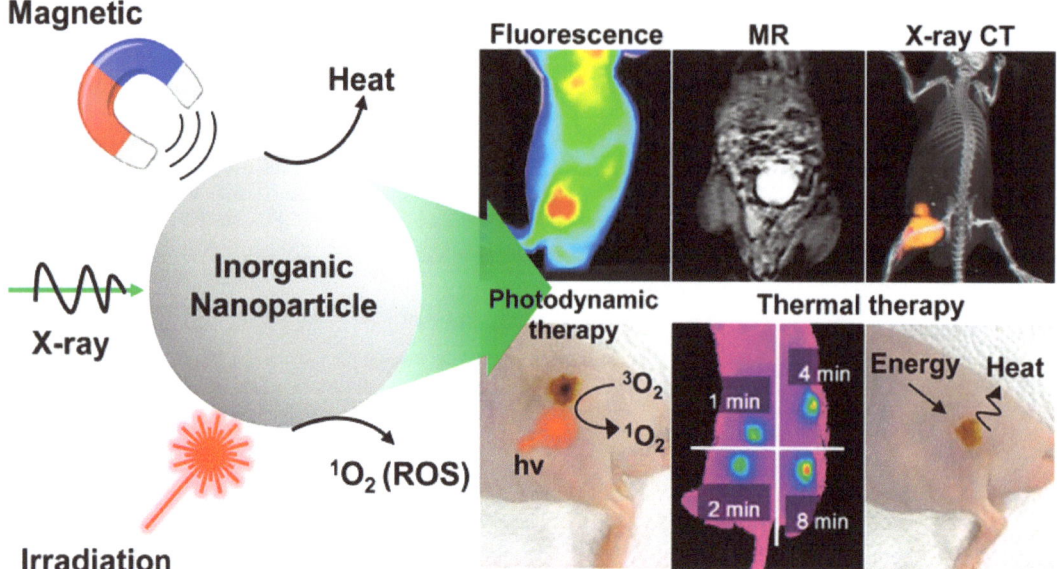

Figure 3. Applications of inorganic NPs for cancer therapy and imaging. Reproduced with permission from [40]. Copyright 2017 ACS Publications.

2.3. Magnetic Hyperthermia Treatment (MHT)

In cancer treatment, the use of a magnetic implant as a thermal seed exposed to the alternating magnetic field is the primary principle behind magnetic hypothermia. Magnetic hypothermia has been used for cancer treatment since the 1950s [47]. Traditionally, deep tumour treatment via magnetic fluid hyperthermia was not possible due to the very low-frequency excitation field being no longer than 100 m in vivo. Now it is possible due to NPs and magnetic particle imaging [48]. In magnetic hyperthermia, the tumour is heated to a moderate temperature of 40–30 °C to destroy cancer cells without the side effects associated with conventional treatment. It can also be co-administered with conventional treatment for better outcomes [49]. Iron oxide NPs have been employed as intra-tumour MTH agents in brain and prostate tumour clinical trials [50]. A study looked at encapsulating produced magnetic iron oxide nanocomposites due to their excellent magnetic saturation and superior magnetic to thermal conversion efficiency with a specific absorption range. It shows the good potential for magnetic hyperthermia therapy [51]. A side effect of magnetic hypothermia is heating of the tumour's surrounding tissue, which is aimed to be minimized as much as possible [52]. Using NPs can localize the heat and minimizes the damage to the tissue. One example is the release of heat due to the transfer of magnetic field energy into heat by adding magnetic NPs to the tumour in a time-varying magnetic field. This heats the cancer cells, whereas surrounding non-malignant tissues can be spared [53].

2.4. MRI-Guided Chemotherapy

NPs with magnetite composition and polymer encapsulation are used in many applications as theranostic agents for drug delivery and MRI [54]. MRI provides a high-resolution image of structures in the body, and when combined with other imaging modalities, together they can provide complementary diagnostic information for more accurate tumour characteristics identification and the precise guidance of anticancer therapy [55]. The applications of functionalized magnetic NPs in cancer nanotheranostics are shown in Figure 4. Magnetic NPs can be functionalized and guided by a magnetic field. They allow advanced MRI-guided gene and drug delivery, magnetic hyperthermia cancer therapy, cell tracking and bioseparation and tissue engineering [56]. Iron oxide NPs can be used in the diagnosis of liver, inflammation and liver and vascular imaging via MRI. They are also used for therapeutic applications such as iron supplementation in anaemia, macrophage polarization, magnetic drug targeting and magnetic fluid hyperthermia. Due to these properties, they are very useful in theranostic applications [30]. A multifunctional theranostic platform was developed based on amphiphilic hyaluronan/poly-(N-ε-Carbobenzyloxy-L-lysine) derivative (HA-g-PZLL) superparamagnetic iron oxide and aggregation-induced emission (AIR) NPs for magnetic resonance and fluorescence dual-modal image-guided PDT [57]. Gadolinium-based NPs have high relaxivity, passive uptake in the tumour due to an enhanced permeability and retention effect, and adapted biodistribution. These properties make them ideal contrast agents for positive MRI imaging. They can also act as an effective radiosensitizer in radiotherapy, neutron therapy and hadron therapy [58]. Ultra-small gold NPs have low toxicity, and they are non-immunogenic by nature. They have fast kidney clearance and can be used in NIR resonant biomedical imaging modalities. They can be used as an enhancer in MRI, photoacoustic imaging, X-ray and fluorescence imaging. They can also be used to generate heat and local hyperthermia of cancer tissue in PTT. They can also be functionalized to deliver the drug to the cancer cells. All these properties make them ideal for theranostic applications [59]. Another study synthesized a polydopamine-coated manganese oxide NP (FA-Mn$_3$O$_4$@PDA@PEG) conjugate for MRI-guided chemo (PTT). It has a relaxivity of 14.47 mM^{-1} s^{-1}, which makes it an excellent contrast agent for MRI [60].

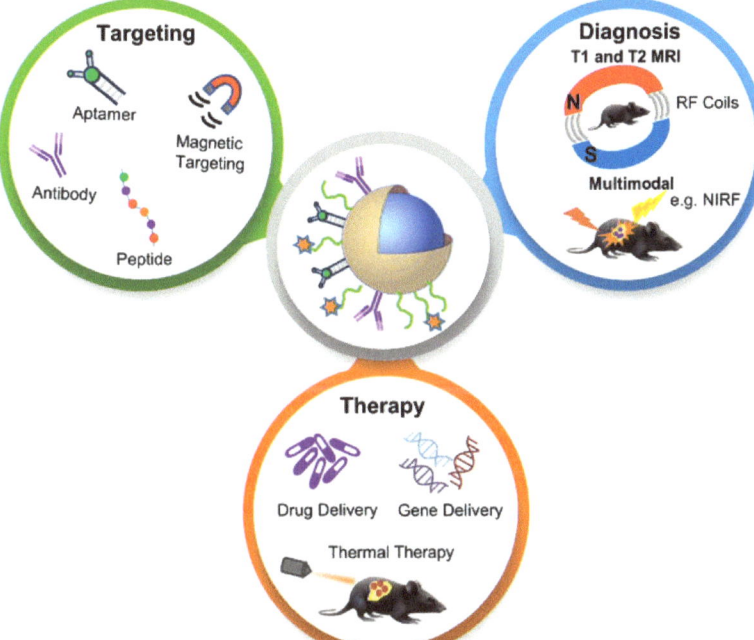

Figure 4. Schematic diagram showing applications of functionalized magnetic NPs in MRI-based diagnosis and anticancer therapy. Reproduced with permission from [55]. Copyright Anani et al. 2020.

3. Immunotherapy

Cancer immunotherapy aims to improve the antitumour immune response, which has advantages over chemotherapy such as fewer off-target effects [61]. T-cell checkpoint inhibitors are crucial in the management of advanced cancers such as melanoma and non-small cell lung cancer [62]. Immunotherapy needs to be personalized because of the variance in the immune response from patient to patient. Cancer immunotherapy includes pharmaceuticals such as monoclonal antibodies, immune checkpoints, cell therapy and vaccines. Programmed cell death is achieved in a combination of program cell death protein 1 and programmed cell death protein ligand 1 drugs and other immune therapy drugs such as antibody–drug conjugates, and other therapies such as chemotherapy and radiation therapy [63]. Immunotherapy can also be conjugated with positron emission tomography and single-photon emission computed tomography to evaluate the response to immune checkpoint therapy [64]. Nano immunotherapy has three different mechanisms, targeting cancer cells, targeting the peripheral immune system and targeting the tumour microenvironment. When it is targeting the cancer cells, it aims to promote immunogenic cell death by releasing the tumour antigens. When it is targeting the microenvironment, it inhibits immunosuppressive cells such as M2-like tumour-associated macrophages. It also reduces the expression of immunosuppressive molecules, e.g., changing growth factor beta. When it is targeting the peripheral immune system, it aims to promote T cell production in secondary lymphoid organs, and also engineer and strengthen the peripheral effector immune cell population, which ultimately promotes anticancer immunity [65]. Liposomal NPs have a very high potential to deliver immune modulators and act as theranostic agents [66]. NPs of different types such as graphene oxide, black phosphorous, silver, gold, copper, tellurium, iron oxide, zinc oxide and magnesium oxide, prepared using the aerosol method, have many advantages and show high potential in cancer theranostics [67]. Wrapping the NPs with a cellular membrane shows a high potential for cancer theranostics. They are generally isolated from immune cells, stem cells, blood cells and cancer cells and allow for superior tumour targeting through self-recognition, homotypic targeting and prolonged systemic circulation [68]. Magnetic NPs as novel agents for cancer theranostic purposes play a big role in treating malignant melanomas and significantly improves the treatment outcome [69].

4. Photothermal Therapy (PTT) and Photodynamic Therapy (PDT)

Research on gold NPs has increased significantly in recent years due to their property advantages and theragnostic compatibilities. They have been widely used in cancer theragnostics including photo imaging and PTT due to their stability, enhanced solubility, bifunctionality, biocompatibility and cancer-targeting ability [70]. A study functionalized AuNP with hyaluronic acid, polyethylene glycol and adipic dihydrazide. The antitumour drug was loaded into the NPs via the chemical method. The result shows the NPs had very low toxicity toward cells in high doses with a significant enhancement of the antitumour properties [71]. PTT therapy has high compatibility to be combined with other therapies to yield better treatment outcomes. One of the limitations of PPT is its light penetration depth that can cause the incomplete elimination of cancer cells, which could lead to tumour recurrence and metastases in distant organs. This shortcoming can be eliminated by combining PTT with other therapies [72]. Glioblastoma multiforme therapeutic efficacy is often limited due to the poor penetration of therapeutics through the blood–brain barrier. Functionalized up conversion of an NP-based delivery system can target brain tumours and convert deep tissue penetrating NIR light into visible light for PPT and PDT [73]. In PPT and PDT, the heat generation and the activation of photosensitizer drugs occurs in response to exogenously applied light of a specific wavelength. The NPs allow the generation of cytotoxic photothermal heating via a surface plasmon resonance phenomenon and reactive oxygen species. This cytotoxic heat promotes apoptotic and necrotic cancer cell death. Gold NPs can be used both as photothermal agents and photosensitize carriers due to their surface plasmon resonance effect that has a very high efficiency of light to hear conversion and simple thiolation chemistry for functionalization, which allows targeting [74]. The mechanism of the photothermal and photodynamic therapy using gold NPs can be seen in Figure 5 using near-infrared light. A study also looked at conjugating curcumin to the gold NPs to be used in PTT. Curcumin is a polyphenol with an anticancer and antimicrobial ability, and gold NPs allow it to be transported to the target site [75]. Gold NPs have proved themselves to be an excellent theranostic agent for carrier and synergistic PTT and PDT due to their properties [74]. PEGylated bovine serum albumin-coated silver core/shell NPs were proposed for PPT due to their advantageous properties and ability to transport indocyanine green, a clinically-approved NIR dye. The study shows it is an effective carrier and an efficient agent in PPT [76]. A study used magnetite (Fe_3O_4) NPs that were functionalized with chlorin e6 and folic acid as a theragnostic agent in PDT and showed that it can be used as a versatile therapeutic tool that can be used in diagnostic imaging [77]. A study synthesized novel carbon dots/hemin NPs. The fluorescence resonance energy transfer effect enhances their photothermal ability and synergises with PDT [78]. Another study synthesized selenide molybdenum nanoflower that is capable of delivering NIR-mediated synergetic PTT and PDT [79]. A cost-effective modified zinc oxide NP was also introduced that has NIR absorbance, which can be used in PTT and PDT for synergistic therapy [80]. A study also looked at gold doped hollow mesoporous organosilica NPs for PDT and PTT with multimodal imaging for gastric cancer [81]. These functionalized NPs have been suggested for non-invasive cancer treatment because the near-infrared-induced PTT and PDT effect can increase the cancer cell kills.

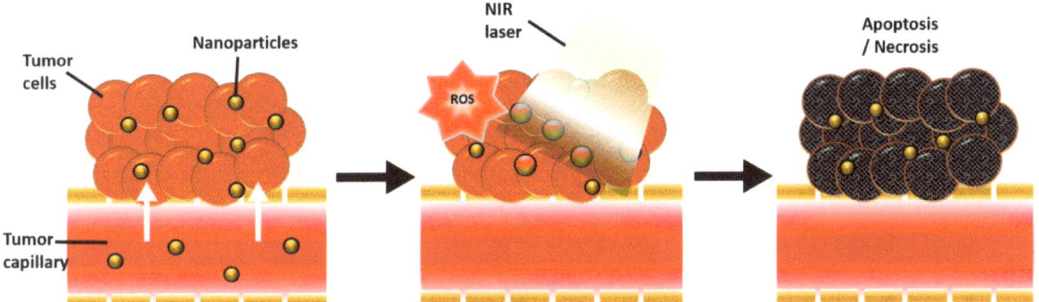

Figure 5. Schematic diagram showing the physiological and biological effects of gold nanoparticle-mediated photothermal therapy (PTT) and photodynamic therapy (PDT). A large amount of gold nanoparticles accumulate due to the leaky vasculature of the tumour, resulting in a photothermal effect in response to near-infrared (NIR) light and reactive oxygen species (ROS) generated by secondary delivered photosensitizer (PS), ultimately inducing apoptosis and necrosis of tumour tissue. Reproduced with permission from [74]. Copyright Kim et al. 2018.

5. Molecular Imaging

A nanoscaled material's size, shape surface chemistry and structure allow their functionalization and utilization in theranostic applications [82]. Molecular imaging shows their high potential in the identification of inflammatory cellular and molecular processes in cardiovascular disease. NPs have been studied as contrast agents in molecular imaging in the detection of vascular inflammation [83]. Quantum dot has also shown very good results in an in vivo study of molecular imaging as a contrast agent [84]. A preclinical study showed that molecular ultrasound imaging has high sensitivity and specificity in disease detection, classification and therapy response monitoring. The use of microbubbles may have high potential in cancer detection [85]. Perfluorocarbon NPs have a high potential to be used in combination with imaging modalities for targeted drug delivery. Their intravascular constraint from their particle size provides a unique advantage for angiogenesis imaging and antiangiogenesis therapy [86]. Gold NPs have been extensively used as a contrast agent in molecular imaging and as a theranostics platform [87]. Silica NPs have also been used in molecular imaging and as a theranostic platform due to their having different sizes in nanometer ranges, and this allows surface modification. It also allows conjugation of different biomolecules such as nucleic acid and proteins [88].

6. Chemotherapy

Some of the common issues with old therapeutic agents are their poor water solubility, non-specific distribution and lack of targeting capabilities. Now, functionalized NPs overcome those shortcomings and can also act as a contrast agent for diagnosis in therapeutic applications [89]. Therapeutic NPs can efficiently deliver chemotherapeutic drugs to the pathological site. This avoids accumulation in healthy organs and tissue and is based on an enhanced permeability and retention effect [90]. NPs offer several advantages in that they are drug-like, their capability to carry high payloads of a drug with reduced toxicity of the drug and prolonged half-life, and, most importantly, their increased targeting efficiency. All of these capabilities make them excellent theranostic agents and allow theranostic applications to flourish [91]. NPs are captured and eliminated by the natural immune system and this is an inconvenience for drug delivery. Camouflaging NPs with cell membrane provides a solution to this obstacle. A novel class of NPs such as biomimetic NPs was developed, which can inherit specific biological functions of the source cell-like immune cells, cancer cells or erythrocytes. This allows them to evade the immune system, and even in some cases, allows homing capabilities for cancer cell targeting [92]. A study conjugated gold NPs with folate and methotrexate in breast cancer cell lines due to the high expression of folate receptors. Low-level laser therapy had a proliferative effect on the breast cancer cell line. The combination of chemo and PTT with the functionalized NPs shows a significantly higher appetitive effect due to their targeting ability [93]. Table 1 below shows the gold NPs that have been investigated for drug delivery [94].

Table 1. Application of gold NPs in drug delivery. Reproduced with permission from [94].

Nanoparticle	Nanoparticle Size (nm)	Outcome	Cell Lines
MTX-AuNP	8–80	Higher cytotoxicity towards numerous cell lines as compared to free MTX. Suppression of tumour growth with MTX-AuNP but not with free MTX.	Lewis lung carcinoma (LL2) cells
DOX-Hyd@AuNP	30	Enhanced toxicity against multi drug-resistant cancer cells.	MCF-7/ADR cancer cells
(Pt(R,R-dach))-AuNP	26.7	Platinum-tethering exhibited higher cytotoxicity as compared to free oxaliplatin that could enter the nucleus.	A549 lung epithelial cancer cell line, HCT116, HCT15, HT29 and RKO colon cancer cell lines
Tfpep-AuNP conjugated with photodynamic pro-drug Pc 4	5.1	Cellular uptake of targeted particles was significantly higher than that of the non-targeted ones.	LN229 and U87 human glioma cancer lines
CPP-DOX-AuNP	25	Higher cell death as compared to previously tested 41 nm AuNP.	HeLa cells and A549 cells
FA-Au-SMCC-DOX		Enhanced drug accumulation and retention as compared to free DOX in multi drug-resistant cancer cells.	HepG2-R, C0045C and HDF
FA-BHC-AuNP	20–60	Increased efficacy of BHC against cancer cells.	Vero and HeLa
Au-P(LA-DOX)-b-PEG-OH/FA NP	34	Enhanced cellular uptake and cytotoxicity against cancer cells.	4T1 mouse mammary carcinoma cell line
DOX@PVP-AuNP	12	Induction of early and late apoptosis in lung cancer cells and upregulation of tumour suppression genes.	A549, H460 and H520 human lung cancer cells
DOX-BLM-PEG-AuNP	10	Enhanced half-maximal effective drug concentration, providing rationale for chemotherapy using two drugs.	HeLa cells
EpCam-RPAuN	48	The biomimetic nanoparticle loaded with PTX was used in combination treatment (PTT and chemotherapy).	4T1 mouse mammary carcinoma cell line

AuNP: gold nanoparticle, AuN: gold nanocage, BHC: berberine hydrochloride, BLM: bleomycin, CPP: cell penetrating peptides, DOX: doxorubicin, EpCam: epithelial cell adhesion molecule, FA: folic acid, Hyd: hydrazone, MTX: methotrexate, PEG: poly ethylene glycol, PLA: poly L-aspartate, (Pt (R,R-dach)): active ingredient of oxaliplatin, PTT: photothermal therapy, PTX: paclitaxel, PVP: polyvinylpyrrolidone, SMCC: succinimidyl 4-(N-maleimidomethyl) cyclohexane-1-carboxylate, Tfpep: transferrin peptide.

Breast cancer is often diagnosed with molecular imaging, and an NP conjugate with targeting moiety significantly enhances the output of optical imaging and can be used as a carrier in chemotherapy [95]. A polydopamine-coated magnetite NP and sphere with PAMAM dendrimers that were functionalized with NHS-PEG-Mal(N-hydroxysuccinimide-polyethylene glycol-maleimide) linker was developed to be able to functionalize with a folic acid derivative, which is a targeting moiety that can effectively kill cancer cells in dual chemo and PTT in liver cancer [96]. Microbubbles, when stabilized by a coating of magnetic or drug-containing NPs, have useful usages in theranostic applications. These microbubbles allow the transport of more efficient NP-mediated drug delivery [97]. Graphene-based NPs show good potential in photo chemotherapy. A study synthesized reduced graphene-based NPs with excellent biocompatibility capable of loading anticancer drugs for photo chemotherapy [98]. A study synthesized the polymerization of 3-caprolactone, 1,4,8-trioxa [4.6]spiro-9-undecanone and poly NPs for bladder cancer to be used as a chemotherapeutic agent with loaded DOX and zinc phthalocyanine, which enables synergistic PDT [99]. The potential risk of using NPs has yet to be fully explored. They pose a risk that is beyond the scope of chemical drug delivery. They can cross barriers that are not accessible to many other particles such as crossing the blood–brain barrier [9].

7. Clinical Research

Functionalized nanocarriers based on nanoparticles have been developed to improve the therapeutic efficiency of chemotherapy combined with other treatment options. The advantages of functionalized nanocarriers, namely, passive targeting capacity by the enhanced permeation and retention, ability to load drugs for targeting modification and the large surface-to-volume ratio, made various clinical research studies focusing on combined therapy possible [100]. For example, Katragadda et al. [101] demonstrated a safe and efficacious nanosized formulation for the delivery of paclitaxel and 17-AAG combination therapy, which has shown meagre responses in phase 1 clinical trials. Liu et al. [102] developed novel nanoparticles based on polymeric microspheres loaded with two anticancer drugs for pulmonary delivery. The in vivo pharmacokinetic and biodistribution studies showed that the microspheres demonstrated a prolonged circulation time and could accumulate in the lung. Araujo et al. [103] summarized the tyrosine kinase inhibitors in clinical practice for solid tumour treatment (Table 2). As SRC is a tyrosine kinase important in the oncogenic and bone-metastatic processes, it is a potential therapeutic agent to treat solid tumours. Dasatinib is one of the SRC inhibitors now being developed and is the most studied inhibitor. The current results provide valuable information to investigate if targeting SRC exhibits a viable therapeutic strategy. To date, various carrier-free prodrug NPs based on dasatinib have been designed. In vivo and in vitro experiments showed that the NPs had excellent antitumour activity and reduced toxicities [104].

Table 2. Some tyrosine kinase inhibitors used in clinical practice. Reproduced with permission from [103]. Copyright 2010 Elsevier.

Tyrosine Kinase Inhibitor	Kinase Target(s)	FDA-Approved Indications
Dasatinib (Sprycel)	SRC, SFKs, BCR-ABL, c-KIT, PDGFR, c-FMS, EPHA2	CML (2nd-line), Ph + ALL
Erlotinib (Tarceva)	EGFR	NSCLC
Gefitinib (Iressa)	EGFR	NSCLC
Imatinib (Gleevec/Glivec)	BCR-ABL, c-KIT, PDGFR	CML, Ph + ALL, GIST
Lapatinib (Tykerb)	EGFR, HER2/neu	Advanced breast cancer
Nilotinib (Tasigna)	BCR-ABL, c-KIT, PDGFR	CML (2nd-line)
Sorafenib (Nexavar)	VEGFR, PDGFR	Renal cell carcinoma, hepatocellular carcinoma
Sunitinib (Sutent)	VEGFR2, PDGFR, c-KIT, FLT3	GIST, renal cell carcinoma

CML, chronic myeloid leukemia; EGFR, epidermal growth factor receptor; EPHA, ephrin A; FLT3, FMS-like tyrosine kinase 3; GIST, gastrointestinal stromal tumours; NSCLC, non-small cell lung carcinoma; PDGFR, platelet-derived growth factor receptor; Ph + ALL, Philadelphia chromosome–positive acute lymphoblastic leukemia; VEGFR2, vascular endothelial growth factor receptor-2.

8. Future Prospects

In this topical review, though cancer nanotheranostics is quite a novel field within these last 10 years, it has high potential to be applied extensively for cancer therapy in personalized medicine oncology. From the current works and results, it can be seen that more efforts should be taken to study the microbiological environment of the disease, and investigate the stimuli-responsive nanomedicines and co-delivery of drugs using nanocarriers. Moreover, further work should focus on the development of a novel preclinical model resulting in the potential for more accurate clinical predictability. This should lead to more clinical trials on nanotheranostics. Regarding nanomaterials, future work should focus on the design and synthesis of functionalized nanoparticles in active delivery systems, and in targeted tumour and cancer marker detection in the human body serum.

9. Conclusions

Cancer treatment has advanced significantly over the last 10 years and it continues to advance. The development of more functionalized nanoparticles allows cancer therapy to be more precise and imaging modalities to provide more enhances images. The combination of imaging modalities and therapeutic application allows for more accurate patient-specific treatment and it is complemented by a new theranostic nanoagent, which can serve multiple purposes in combination modalities. This review is particularly important for researchers in either cancer diagnosis or therapy to see the big picture of the recent advances in nanotheranostics. Through understanding the current development and progress of functionalized nanoparticle application in theranostics, they can find out the most promising study directions in the future.

Author Contributions: Methodology, J.C.L.C. and S.S.; writing—original draft preparation, S.S.; writing—review and editing, J.C.L.C.; supervision, J.C.L.C. All authors have read and agreed to the published version of the manuscript.

Funding: This research received no external funding.

Institutional Review Board Statement: Not applicable.

Informed Consent Statement: Not applicable.

Data Availability Statement: No new data were created or analyzed in this study. Data sharing is not applicable to this article.

Conflicts of Interest: The authors declare no conflict of interest.

References

1. Xin, J.; Deng, C.; Aras, O.; Zhou, M.; Wu, C.; An, F. Chemodynamic nanomaterials for cancer theranostics. *J. Nanobiotechnol.* **2021**, *19*, 192. [CrossRef] [PubMed]
2. Mun, E.J.; Babiker, H.M.; Weinberg, U.; Kirson, E.D.; Von Hoff, D.D. Tumor-Treating Fields: A Fourth Modality in Cancer Treatment. *Clin. Cancer Res. Off. J. Am. Assoc. Cancer Res.* **2018**, *24*, 266–275. [CrossRef] [PubMed]
3. Choudhury, P.S.; Gupta, M. Theranostics and precision medicine special feature: Review Article Differentiated thyroid cancer theranostics: Radioiodine and beyond. *Br. J. Radiol.* **2018**, *91*, 20189004. [CrossRef]
4. Langbein, T.; Weber, W.A.; Eiber, M. Future of Theranostics: An Outlook on Precision Oncology in Nuclear Medicine. *J. Nucl. Med.* **2019**, *60*, 13S–19S. [CrossRef] [PubMed]
5. Jeyamogan, S.; Khan, N.A.; Siddiqui, R. Application and Importance of Theranostics in the Diagnosis and Treatment of Cancer. *Arch. Med. Res.* **2021**, *52*, 131–142. [CrossRef]
6. James, M.L.; Gambhir, S.S. A Molecular Imaging Primer: Modalities, Imaging Agents, and Applications. *Physiol. Rev.* **2012**, *92*, 897–965. [CrossRef]
7. Bobo, D.; Robinson, K.J.; Islam, J.; Thurecht, K.J.; Corrie, S.R. Nanoparticle-Based Medicines: A Review of FDA-Approved Materials and Clinical Trials to Date. *Pharm. Res.* **2016**, *33*, 2373–2387. [CrossRef]
8. Lecocq, Q.; De Vlaeminck, Y.; Hanssens, H.; D'Huyvetter, M.; Raes, G.; Goyvaerts, C.; Keyaerts, M.; Devoogdt, N.; Breckpot, K. Theranostics in immuno-oncology using nanobody derivatives. *Theranostics* **2019**, *9*, 7772–7791. [CrossRef]
9. Jong, W.H.; Borm, P.J.A. Drug delivery and nanoparticles: Applications and hazards. *Int. J. Nanomed.* **2008**, *3*, 133–149. [CrossRef]
10. Wu, J. The Enhanced Permeability and Retention (EPR) Effect: The Significance of the Concept and Methods to Enhance Its Application. *J. Pers. Med.* **2021**, *11*, 771. [CrossRef]

11. Fu, Z.; Xiang, J. Aptamer-Functionalized Nanoparticles in Targeted Delivery and Cancer Therapy. *Int. J. Mol. Sci.* **2020**, *21*, 9123. [CrossRef] [PubMed]
12. Andreou, C.; Pal, S.; Rotter, L.; Yang, J.; Kircher, M.F. Molecular Imaging in Nanotechnology and Theranostics. *Mol. Imaging Biol.* **2017**, *19*, 363–372. [CrossRef] [PubMed]
13. Fang, R.H.; Hu, C.-M.J.; Luk, B.T.; Gao, W.; Copp, J.A.; Tai, Y.; O'Connor, D.E.; Zhang, L. Cancer Cell Membrane-Coated Nanoparticles for Anticancer Vaccination and Drug Delivery. *Nano Lett.* **2014**, *14*, 2181–2188. [CrossRef]
14. Frickenstein, A.; Hagood, J.; Britten, C.; Abbott, B.; McNally, M.; Vopat, C.; Patterson, E.; MacCuaig, W.; Jain, A.; Walters, K.; et al. Mesoporous Silica Nanoparticles: Properties and Strategies for Enhancing Clinical Effect. *Pharmaceutics* **2021**, *13*, 570. [CrossRef] [PubMed]
15. Huang, G.; Pan, S.-T. ROS-Mediated Therapeutic Strategy in Chemo-/Radiotherapy of Head and Neck Cancer. *Oxidative Med. Cell. Longev.* **2020**, *2020*, 5047987. [CrossRef] [PubMed]
16. Balkrishna, A.; Kumar, A.; Arya, V.; Rohela, A.; Verma, R.; Nepovimova, E.; Krejcar, O.; Kumar, D.; Thakur, N.; Kuca, K. Phytoantioxidant Functionalized Nanoparticles: A Green Approach to Combat Nanoparticle-Induced Oxidative Stress. *Oxidative Med. Cell. Longev.* **2021**, *2021*, 3155962. [CrossRef] [PubMed]
17. Cai, X.; Zhu, Q.; Zeng, Y.; Zeng, Q.; Chen, X.; Zhan, Y. Manganese Oxide Nanoparticles As MRI Contrast Agents In Tumor Multimodal Imaging And Therapy. *Int. J. Nanomed.* **2019**, *14*, 8321–8344. [CrossRef]
18. Yousaf, T.; Dervenoulas, G.; Politis, M. Advances in MRI Methodology. *Int. Rev. Neurobiol.* **2018**, *141*, 31–76. [CrossRef]
19. Bashir, M.R.; Bhatti, L.; Marin, D.; Nelson, R.C. Emerging applications for ferumoxytol as a contrast agent in MRI. *J. Magn. Reson. Imaging* **2014**, *41*, 884–898. [CrossRef]
20. Lux, J.; Sherry, A.D. Advances in gadolinium-based MRI contrast agent designs for monitoring biological processes in vivo. *Curr. Opin. Chem. Biol.* **2018**, *45*, 121–130. [CrossRef]
21. Yang, X.; Atalar, E. MRI-guided gene therapy. *FEBS Lett.* **2006**, *580*, 2958–2961. [CrossRef] [PubMed]
22. Liu, C.; Ewert, K.K.; Wang, N.; Li, Y.; Safinya, C.R.; Qiao, W. A multifunctional lipid that forms contrast-agent liposomes with dual-control release capabilities for precise MRI-guided drug delivery. *Biomaterials* **2019**, *221*, 119412. [CrossRef] [PubMed]
23. Shi, J.; Wang, B.; Chen, Z.; Liu, W.; Pan, J.; Hou, L.; Zhang, Z. A Multi-Functional Tumor Theranostic Nanoplatform for MRI Guided Photothermal-Chemotherapy. *Pharm. Res.* **2016**, *33*, 1472–1485. [CrossRef] [PubMed]
24. Langereis, S.; Geelen, T.; Grüll, H.; Strijkers, G.; Nicolay, K. Paramagnetic liposomes for molecular MRI and MRI-guided drug delivery. *NMR Biomed.* **2013**, *26*, 728–744. [CrossRef]
25. Han, Z.; Liu, G. CEST MRI trackable nanoparticle drug delivery systems. *Biomed. Mater.* **2021**, *16*, 024103. [CrossRef]
26. Satpathy, M.; Wang, L.; Zielinski, R.J.; Qian, W.; Wang, Y.A.; Mohs, A.; Kairdolf, B.A.; Ji, X.; Capala, J.; Lipowska, M.; et al. Targeted Drug Delivery and Image-Guided Therapy of Heterogeneous Ovarian Cancer Using HER2-Targeted Theranostic Nanoparticles. *Theranostics* **2019**, *9*, 778–795. [CrossRef]
27. Tomitaka, A.; Arami, H.; Ahmadivand, A.; Pala, N.; McGoron, A.J.; Takemura, Y.; Febo, M.; Nair, M. Magneto-plasmonic nanostars for image-guided and NIR-triggered drug delivery. *Sci. Rep.* **2020**, *10*, 10115. [CrossRef]
28. Zhou, H.; Qian, W.; Uckun, F.M.; Wang, L.; Wang, Y.A.; Chen, H.; Kooby, D.; Yu, Q.; Lipowska, M.; Staley, C.A.; et al. IGF1 receptor targeted theranostic nanoparticles for targeted and image-guided therapy of pancreatic cancer. *ACS Nano* **2015**, *9*, 7976–7991. [CrossRef]
29. Wahajuddin; Arora, S. Superparamagnetic iron oxide nanoparticles: Magnetic nanoplatforms as drug carriers. *Int. J. Nanomed.* **2012**, *7*, 3445–3471. [CrossRef]
30. Dadfar, S.M.; Roemhild, K.; Drude, N.I.; Von, S. Europe PMC Funders Group Iron Oxide Nanoparticles: Diagnostic, Therapeutic and Theranostic Applications. *Gene* **2020**, *138*, 302–325. [CrossRef]
31. Wirth, T.; Parker, N.; Ylä-Herttuala, S. History of gene therapy. *Gene* **2013**, *525*, 162–169. [CrossRef] [PubMed]
32. Smith, E.; Blomberg, P. Gene therapy—From idea to reality. *Lakartidningen* **2017**, *114*, EWYL. (In Swedish) [PubMed]
33. Sun, W.; Shi, Q.; Zhang, H.; Yang, K.; Ke, Y.; Wang, Y.; Qiao, L. Advances in the techniques and methodologies of cancer gene therapy. *Discov. Med.* **2019**, *27*, 45–55. [PubMed]
34. Mohammadinejad, R.; Dadashzadeh, A.; Moghassemi, S.; Ashrafizadeh, M.; Dehshahri, A.; Pardakhty, A.; Sassan, H.; Sohrevardi, S.-M.; Mandegary, A. Shedding light on gene therapy: Carbon dots for the minimally invasive image-guided delivery of plasmids and noncoding RNAs—A review. *J. Adv. Res.* **2019**, *18*, 81–93. [CrossRef] [PubMed]
35. Peng, Y.; Gao, Y.; Yang, C.; Guo, R.; Shi, X.; Cao, X. Low-Molecular-Weight Poly(ethylenimine) Nanogels Loaded with Ultrasmall Iron Oxide Nanoparticles for T_1-Weighted MR Imaging-Guided Gene Therapy of Sarcoma. *ACS Appl. Mater. Interfaces* **2021**, *13*, 27806–27813. [CrossRef]
36. Wang, Z.; Chang, Z.; Lu, M.; Shao, D.; Yue, J.; Yang, D.; Zheng, X.; Li, M.; He, K.; Zhang, M.; et al. Shape-controlled magnetic mesoporous silica nanoparticles for magnetically-mediated suicide gene therapy of hepatocellular carcinoma. *Biomaterials* **2017**, *154*, 147–157. [CrossRef]
37. Wang, R.; Dai, X.; Duan, S.; Zhao, N.; Xu, F.-J. A flexible bowl-shaped magnetic assembly for multifunctional gene delivery systems. *Nanoscale* **2019**, *11*, 16463–16475. [CrossRef]
38. Feng, J.; Xu, Z.; Liu, F.; Zhao, Y.; Yu, W.; Pan, M.; Wang, F.; Liu, X. Versatile Catalytic Deoxyribozyme Vehicles for Multimodal Imaging-Guided Efficient Gene Regulation and Photothermal Therapy. *ACS Nano* **2018**, *12*, 12888–12901. [CrossRef]

39. Mu, X.; Li, J.; Yan, S.; Zhang, H.; Zhang, W.; Zhang, F.; Jiang, J. siRNA Delivery with Stem Cell Membrane-Coated Magnetic Nanoparticles for Imaging-Guided Photothermal Therapy and Gene Therapy. *ACS Biomater. Sci. Eng.* **2018**, *4*, 3895–3905. [CrossRef]
40. Li, X.; Lovell, J.F.; Yoon, J.; Chen, X. Clinical development and potential of photothermal and photodynamic therapies for cancer. *Nat. Rev. Clin. Oncol.* **2020**, *17*, 657–674. [CrossRef]
41. Yoon, H.Y.; Jeon, S.; You, D.G.; Park, J.H.; Kwon, I.C.; Koo, H.; Kim, K. Inorganic Nanoparticles for Image-Guided Therapy. *Bioconjug. Chem.* **2017**, *28*, 124–134. [CrossRef] [PubMed]
42. Shi, M.; Zuo, F.; Taoa, Y.; Liua, Y.; Lua, J.; Zhenga, S.; Lub, J.; Houcd, P.; Liab, J.; Xuab, K. Near-infrared laser-induced phase-shifted nanoparticles for US/MRI-guided therapy for breast cancer. *Colloids Surf. B Biointerfaces* **2020**, *196*, 111278. [CrossRef] [PubMed]
43. Zhou, X.; Lv, X.; Zhao, W.; Zhou, T.; Zhang, S.; Shi, Z.; Ye, S.; Ren, L.; Chen, Z. Porous MnFe$_2$O$_4$-decorated PB nanocomposites: A new theranostic agent for boosted T_1/T_2 MRI-guided synergistic photothermal/magnetic hyperthermia. *RSC Adv.* **2018**, *8*, 18647–18655. [CrossRef] [PubMed]
44. Wang, J.; Mei, T.; Liu, Y.; Zhang, Y.; Zhang, Z.; Hu, Y.; Wang, Y.; Wu, M.; Yang, C.; Zhong, X.; et al. Dual-targeted and MRI-guided photothermal therapy via iron-based nanoparticles-incorporated neutrophils. *Biomater. Sci.* **2021**, *9*, 3968–3978. [CrossRef] [PubMed]
45. Zhang, L.; Yang, Z.; Zhu, W.; Ye, Z.; Yu, Y.; Xu, Z.; Ren, J.; Li, P. Dual-Stimuli-Responsive, Polymer-Microsphere-Encapsulated CuS Nanoparticles for Magnetic Resonance Imaging Guided Synergistic Chemo-Photothermal Therapy. *ACS Biomater. Sci. Eng.* **2017**, *3*, 1690–1701. [CrossRef]
46. Wang, J.; Wang, Y.; Guo, H.; Yu, N.; Ren, Q.; Jiang, Q.; Xia, J.; Peng, C.; Zhang, H.; Chen, Z. Synthesis of one-for-all type Cu5FeS4 nanocrystals with improved near infrared photothermal and Fenton effects for simultaneous imaging and therapy of tumor. *J. Colloid Interface Sci.* **2021**, *592*, 116–126. [CrossRef]
47. Vilas-Boas, V.; Carvalho, F.; Espiña, B. Magnetic Hyperthermia for Cancer Treatment: Main Parameters Affecting the Outcome of In Vitro and In Vivo Studies. *Molecules* **2020**, *25*, 2874. [CrossRef]
48. Lu, Y.; Rivera-Rodriguez, A.; Tay, Z.W.; Hensley, D.; Fung, K.B.; Colson, C.; Saayujya, C.; Huynh, Q.; Kabuli, L.; Fellows, B.; et al. Combining magnetic particle imaging and magnetic fluid hyperthermia for localized and image-guided treatment. *Int. J. Hyperth.* **2020**, *37*, 141–154. [CrossRef]
49. Jose, J.; Kumar, R.; Harilal, S.; Mathew, G.E.; Parambi, D.G.T.; Prabhu, A.; Uddin, S.; Aleya, L.; Kim, H.; Mathew, B. Magnetic nanoparticles for hyperthermia in cancer treatment: An emerging tool. *Environ. Sci. Pollut. Res.* **2019**, *27*, 19214–19225. [CrossRef]
50. Gavilán, H.; Avugadda, S.K.; Fernández-Cabada, T.; Soni, N.; Cassani, M.; Mai, B.T.; Chantrell, R.; Pellegrino, T. Magnetic nanoparticles and clusters for magnetic hyperthermia: Optimizing their heat performance and developing combinatorial therapies to tackle cancer. *Chem. Soc. Rev.* **2021**, *50*, 11614–11667. [CrossRef]
51. Zhang, Y.; Wang, X.; Chu, C.; Zhou, Z.; Chen, B.; Pang, X.; Lin, G.; Lin, H.; Guo, Y.; Ren, E.; et al. Genetically engineered magnetic nanocages for cancer magneto-catalytic theranostics. *Nat. Commun.* **2020**, *11*, 5421. [CrossRef] [PubMed]
52. Tsiapla, A.-R.; Kalimeri, A.-A.; Maniotis, N.; Myrovali, E.; Samaras, T.; Angelakeris, M.; Kalogirou, O. Mitigation of magnetic particle hyperthermia side effects by magnetic field controls. *Int. J. Hyperth.* **2021**, *38*, 511–522. [CrossRef] [PubMed]
53. Tishin, A.M.; Shtil, A.A.; Pyatakov, A.P.; Zverev, V.I. Developing Antitumor Magnetic Hyperthermia: Principles, Materials and Devices. *Recent Pat. Anti-Cancer Drug Discov.* **2016**, *11*, 360–375. [CrossRef] [PubMed]
54. Perecin, C.J.; Gratens, X.P.M.; Chitta, V.A.; Leo, P.; de Oliveira, A.M.; Yoshioka, S.A.; Cerize, N.N.P. Synthesis and Characterization of Magnetic Composite Theranostics by Nano Spray Drying. *Materials* **2022**, *15*, 1755. [CrossRef] [PubMed]
55. Anani, T.; Rahmati, S.; Sultana, N.; David, A.E. MRI-traceable theranostic nanoparticles for targeted cancer treatment. *Theranostics* **2021**, *11*, 579–601. [CrossRef]
56. Morris, B.J.; Willcox, D.C.; Donlon, T.A.; Willcox, B.J. FOXO3: A major gene for human longevity-a mini-review. *Gerontology* **2015**, *61*, 515–525. [CrossRef]
57. Yang, H.; He, Y.; Wang, Y.; Yang, R.; Wang, N.; Zhang, L.-M.; Gao, M.; Jiang, X. Theranostic Nanoparticles with Aggregation-Induced Emission and MRI Contrast Enhancement Characteristics as a Dual-Modal Imaging Platform for Image-Guided Tumor Photodynamic Therapy. *Int. J. Nanomed.* **2020**, *15*, 3023–3038. [CrossRef]
58. Lux, F.; Sancey, L.; Bianchi, A.; Crémillieux, Y.; Roux, S.; Tillement, O. Gadolinium-based nanoparticles for theranostic MRI-radiosensitization. *Nanomedicine* **2015**, *10*, 1801–1815. [CrossRef]
59. Fan, M.; Han, Y.; Gao, S.; Yan, H.; Cao, L.; Li, Z.; Liang, X.-J.; Zhang, J. Ultrasmall gold nanoparticles in cancer diagnosis and therapy. *Theranostics* **2020**, *10*, 4944–4957. [CrossRef]
60. Ding, X.; Liu, J.; Li, J.; Wang, F.; Wang, Y.; Song, S.; Zhang, H. Polydopamine coated manganese oxide nanoparticles with ultrahigh relaxivity as nanotheranostic agents for magnetic resonance imaging guided synergetic chemo-/photothermal therapy. *Chem. Sci.* **2016**, *7*, 6695–6700. [CrossRef]
61. Riley, R.S.; June, C.H.; Langer, R.; Mitchell, M.J. Delivery technologies for cancer immunotherapy. *Nat. Rev. Drug Discov.* **2019**, *18*, 175–196. [CrossRef] [PubMed]
62. Caster, J.M.; Callaghan, C.; Seyedin, S.N.; Henderson, K.; Sun, B.; Wang, A.Z. Optimizing Advances in Nanoparticle Delivery for Cancer Immunotherapy. *Adv. Drug Deliv. Rev.* **2019**, *144*, 3–15. [CrossRef] [PubMed]
63. Jain, K.K. Personalized Immuno-Oncology. *Med Princ. Pract.* **2020**, *30*, 479–508. [CrossRef]
64. Chen, X.; Chen, M. Critical reviews of immunotheranostics. *Theranostics* **2020**, *10*, 7403–7405. [CrossRef]

65. Shi, Y.; Lammers, T. Combining Nanomedicine and Immunotherapy. *Acc. Chem. Res.* **2019**, *52*, 1543–1554. [CrossRef]
66. Gao, A.; Hu, X.-L.; Saeed, M.; Chen, B.-F.; Li, Y.-P.; Yu, H.-J. Overview of recent advances in liposomal nanoparticle-based cancer immunotherapy. *Acta Pharmacol. Sin.* **2019**, *40*, 1129–1137. [CrossRef]
67. Gautam, M.; Kim, J.O.; Yong, C.S. Fabrication of aerosol-based nanoparticles and their applications in biomedical fields. *J. Pharm. Investig.* **2021**, *51*, 361–375. [CrossRef]
68. Vijayan, V.; Uthaman, S.; Park, I.-K. Cell Membrane-Camouflaged Nanoparticles: A Promising Biomimetic Strategy for Cancer Theragnostics. *Polymers* **2018**, *10*, 983. [CrossRef]
69. Shevtsov, M.; Kaesler, S.; Posch, C.; Multhoff, G.; Biedermann, T. Magnetic nanoparticles in theranostics of malignant melanoma. *EJNMMI Res.* **2021**, *11*, 127. [CrossRef]
70. Kang, M.S.; Lee, S.Y.; Kim, K.S.; Han, D.-W. State of the Art Biocompatible Gold Nanoparticles for Cancer Theragnosis. *Pharmaceutics* **2020**, *12*, 701. [CrossRef]
71. Li, L.-S.; Ren, B.; Yang, X.; Cai, Z.-C.; Zhao, X.-J.; Zhao, M.-X. Hyaluronic Acid-Modified and Doxorubicin-Loaded Gold Nanoparticles and Evaluation of Their Bioactivity. *Pharmaceuticals* **2021**, *14*, 101. [CrossRef] [PubMed]
72. Tong, B.C.-K. Photothermal Therapy and Photoacoustic Imaging via Nanotheranostics in Fighting Cancer. *Physiol. Behav.* **2017**, *176*, 139–148. [CrossRef]
73. Tsai, Y.-C.; Vijayaraghavan, P.; Chiang, W.-H.; Chen, H.-H.; Liu, T.-I.; Shen, M.-Y.; Omoto, A.; Kamimura, M.; Soga, K.; Chiu, H.-C. Targeted Delivery of Functionalized Upconversion Nanoparticles for Externally Triggered Photothermal/Photodynamic Therapies of Brain Glioblastoma. *Theranostics* **2018**, *8*, 1435–1448. [CrossRef]
74. Kim, H.S.; Lee, D.Y. Near-Infrared-Responsive Cancer Photothermal and Photodynamic Therapy Using Gold Nanoparticles. *Polymers* **2018**, *10*, 961. [CrossRef] [PubMed]
75. Rahimi-Moghaddam, F.; Sattarahmady, N.; Azarpira, N. Gold-Curcumin Nanostructure in Photothermal Therapy on Breast Cancer Cell Line: 650 and 808 nm Diode Lasers as Light Sources. *J. Biomed. Phys. Eng.* **2018**, *9*, 473–482. [CrossRef] [PubMed]
76. Park, T.; Lee, S.; Amatya, R.; Cheong, H.; Moon, C.; Kwak, H.D.; Min, K.A.; Shin, M.C. ICG-Loaded PEGylated BSA-Silver Nanoparticles for Effective Photothermal Cancer Therapy. *Int. J. Nanomed.* **2020**, *15*, 5459–5471. [CrossRef]
77. Nam, K.C.; Han, Y.S.; Lee, J.-M.; Kim, S.C.; Cho, G.; Park, B.J. Photo-Functionalized Magnetic Nanoparticles as a Nanocarrier of Photodynamic Anticancer Agent for Biomedical Theragnostics. *Cancers* **2020**, *12*, 571. [CrossRef]
78. Yang, W.; Wei, B.; Yang, Z.; Sheng, L. Facile synthesis of novel carbon-dots/hemin nanoplatforms for synergistic photo-thermal and photo-dynamic therapies. *J. Inorg. Biochem.* **2019**, *193*, 166–172. [CrossRef]
79. Wang, Y.; Zhang, F.; Wang, Q.; Yang, P.; Lin, H.; Qu, F. Hierarchical $MoSe_2$ nanoflowers as novel nanocarriers for NIR-light-mediated synergistic photo-thermal/dynamic and chemo-therapy. *Nanoscale* **2018**, *10*, 14534–14545. [CrossRef]
80. Vasuki, K.; Manimekalai, R. NIR light active ternary modified ZnO nanocomposites for combined cancer therapy. *Heliyon* **2019**, *5*, e02729. [CrossRef]
81. Guo, W.; Chen, Z.; Chen, J.; Feng, X.; Yang, Y.; Huang, H.; Liang, Y.; Shen, G.; Liang, Y.; Peng, C.; et al. Biodegradable hollow mesoporous organosilica nanotheranostics (HMON) for multi-mode imaging and mild photo-therapeutic-induced mitochondrial damage on gastric cancer. *J. Nanobiotechnol.* **2020**, *18*, 99. [CrossRef] [PubMed]
82. Hoshyar, N.; Gray, S.; Han, H.; Bao, G. The effect of nanoparticle size on in vivo pharmacokinetics and cellular interaction. *Nanomedicine* **2016**, *11*, 673–692. [CrossRef] [PubMed]
83. McAteer, M.A.; Choudhury, R.P. Targeted molecular imaging of vascular inflammation in cardiovascular disease using nano- and micro-sized agents. *Vasc. Pharmacol.* **2013**, *58*, 31–38. [CrossRef] [PubMed]
84. Rosenblum, L.T.; Kosaka, N.; Mitsunaga, M.; Choyke, P.L.; Kobayashi, H. In vivo molecular imaging using nanomaterials: General in vivo characteristics of nano-sized reagents and applications for cancer diagnosis. *Mol. Membr. Biol.* **2010**, *27*, 274–285. [CrossRef]
85. Köse, G.; Darguzyte, M.; Kiessling, F. Molecular Ultrasound Imaging. *Nanomaterials* **2020**, *10*, 1935. [CrossRef]
86. Pauff, S.M.; Miller, S.C. Theragnostics for tumor and plaque angiogenesis with perfluorocarbon nanoemulsions. *Bone* **2012**, *78*, 711–716. [CrossRef]
87. Rashighi, M.; Harris, J.E. Recent advances in molecular imaging with gold nanoparticles. *Physiol. Behav.* **2017**, *176*, 139–148. [CrossRef]
88. Shirshahi, V.; Soltani, M. Solid silica nanoparticles: Applications in molecular imaging. *Contrast Media Mol. Imaging* **2014**, *10*, 1–17. [CrossRef]
89. Sun, T.; Zhang, Y.S.; Pang, B.; Hyun, D.C.; Yang, M.; Xia, Y. Engineered Nanoparticles for Drug Delivery in Cancer Therapy. *Angew. Chem. Int. Ed.* **2014**, *53*, 12320–12364. [CrossRef]
90. Baetke, S.C.; Lammers, T.; Kiessling, F. Applications of nanoparticles for diagnosis and therapy of cancer. *Br. J. Radiol.* **2015**, *88*, 20150207. [CrossRef]
91. Banerjee, D.; Sengupta, S. Nanoparticles in Cancer Chemotherapy. *Prog. Mol. Biol. Transl. Sci.* **2011**, *104*, 489–507. [CrossRef] [PubMed]
92. Wang, H.; Liu, Y.; He, R.; Xu, D.; Zang, J.; Weeranoppanant, N.; Dong, H.; Li, Y. Cell membrane biomimetic nanoparticles for inflammation and cancer targeting in drug delivery. *Biomater. Sci.* **2019**, *8*, 552–568. [CrossRef] [PubMed]

93. Agabeigi, R.; Rasta, S.H.; Rahmati-Yamchi, M.; Salehi, R.; Alizadeh, E. Novel Chemo-Photothermal Therapy in Breast Cancer Using Methotrexate-Loaded Folic Acid Conjugated Au@SiO$_2$ Nanoparticles. *Nanoscale Res. Lett.* **2020**, *15*, 62. [CrossRef] [PubMed]
94. Singh, P.; Pandit, S.; Mokkapati, V.; Garg, A.; Ravikumar, V.; Mijakovic, I. Gold Nanoparticles in Diagnostics and Therapeutics for Human Cancer. *Int. J. Mol. Sci.* **2018**, *19*, 1979. [CrossRef]
95. Shamsi, M.; Islamian, J.P. Breast cancer: Early diagnosis and effective treatment by drug delivery tracing. *Nucl. Med. Rev.* **2017**, *20*, 45–48. [CrossRef]
96. Jędrzak, A.; Grześkowiak, B.F.; Golba, K.; Coy, E.; Synoradzki, K.; Jurga, S.; Jesionowski, T.; Mrówczyński, R. Magnetite Nanoparticles and Spheres for Chemo- and Photothermal Therapy of Hepatocellular Carcinoma in vitro. *Int. J. Nanomed.* **2020**, *15*, 7923–7936. [CrossRef]
97. Jamburidze, A.; Huerre, A.; Baresch, D.; Poulichet, V.; De Corato, M.; Garbin, V. Nanoparticle-Coated Microbubbles for Combined Ultrasound Imaging and Drug Delivery. *Langmuir* **2019**, *35*, 10087–10096. [CrossRef]
98. Hu, Y.; He, L.; Ding, J.; Sun, D.; Chen, L.; Chen, X. One-pot synthesis of dextran decorated reduced graphene oxide nanoparticles for targeted photo-chemotherapy. *Carbohydr. Polym.* **2016**, *144*, 223–229. [CrossRef]
99. Huang, Z.; Xiao, H.; Lu, X.; Yan, W.; Ji, Z. Enhanced photo/chemo combination efficiency against bladder tumor by encapsulation of DOX and ZnPC into in situ-formed thermosensitive polymer hydrogel. *Int. J. Nanomed.* **2018**, *13*, 7623. [CrossRef]
100. Zhao, C.-Y.; Cheng, R.; Yang, Z.; Tian, Z.-M. Nanotechnology for Cancer Therapy Based on Chemotherapy. *Molecules* **2018**, *23*, 826. [CrossRef]
101. Katragadda, U.; Fan, W.; Wang, Y.; Teng, Q.; Tan, C. Combined Delivery of Paclitaxel and Tanespimycin via Micellar Nanocarriers: Pharmacokinetics, Efficacy and Metabolomic Analysis. *PLoS ONE* **2013**, *8*, e58619. [CrossRef] [PubMed]
102. Liu, K.; Chen, W.; Yang, T.; Wen, B.; Ding, D.; Keidar, M.; Tang, J.; Zhang, W. Paclitaxel and quercetin nanoparticles co-loaded in microspheres to prolong retention time for pulmonary drug delivery. *Int. J. Nanomed.* **2017**, *12*, 8239–8255. [CrossRef] [PubMed]
103. Araujo, J.; Logothetis, C. Dasatinib: A potent SRC inhibitor in clinical development for the treatment of solid tumors. *Cancer Treat. Rev.* **2010**, *36*, 492–500. [CrossRef]
104. Yang, L.; Xu, J.; Xie, Z.; Song, F.; Wang, X.; Tang, R. Carrier-free prodrug nanoparticles based on dasatinib and cisplatin for efficient antitumor in vivo. *Asian J. Pharm. Sci.* **2021**, *16*, 762–771. [CrossRef] [PubMed]

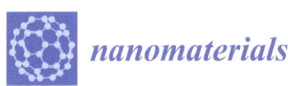

Review

Nanoparticle-Based Therapeutics to Overcome Obstacles in the Tumor Microenvironment of Hepatocellular Carcinoma

Yuanfei Lu [1], Na Feng [1], Yongzhong Du [2,*] and Risheng Yu [1,*]

1. Department of Radiology, Second Affiliated Hospital, School of Medicine, Zhejiang University, 88 Jiefang Road, Hangzhou 310009, China
2. Institute of Pharmaceutics, College of Pharmaceutical Sciences, Zhejiang University, 866 Yuhangtang Road, Hangzhou 310058, China
* Correspondence: duyongzhong@zju.edu.cn (Y.D.); risheng-yu@zju.edu.cn (R.Y.); Tel.: +86-571-88208435 (Y.D.); +86-571-87783925 (R.Y.)

Abstract: Hepatocellular carcinoma (HCC) is still a main health concern around the world, with a rising incidence and high mortality rate. The tumor-promoting components of the tumor microenvironment (TME) play a vital role in the development and metastasis of HCC. TME-targeted therapies have recently drawn increasing interest in the treatment of HCC. However, the short medication retention time in TME limits the efficiency of TME modulating strategies. The nanoparticles can be elaborately designed as needed to specifically target the tumor-promoting components in TME. In this regard, the use of nanomedicine to modulate TME components by delivering drugs with protection and prolonged circulation time in a spatiotemporal manner has shown promising potential. In this review, we briefly introduce the obstacles of TME and highlight the updated information on nanoparticles that modulate these obstacles. Furthermore, the present challenges and future prospects of TME modulating nanomedicines will be briefly discussed.

Keywords: hepatocellular carcinoma; tumor microenvironment; immunosuppression; nanoparticles

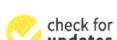

Citation: Lu, Y.; Feng, N.; Du, Y.; Yu, R. Nanoparticle-Based Therapeutics to Overcome Obstacles in the Tumor Microenvironment of Hepatocellular Carcinoma. *Nanomaterials* 2022, 12, 2832. https://doi.org/10.3390/nano12162832

Academic Editor: James C L Chow

Received: 7 July 2022
Accepted: 16 August 2022
Published: 17 August 2022

Publisher's Note: MDPI stays neutral with regard to jurisdictional claims in published maps and institutional affiliations.

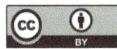

Copyright: © 2022 by the authors. Licensee MDPI, Basel, Switzerland. This article is an open access article distributed under the terms and conditions of the Creative Commons Attribution (CC BY) license (https://creativecommons.org/licenses/by/4.0/).

1. Introduction

Hepatocellular carcinoma (HCC) remains the most commonly diagnosed type of primary liver cancer [1]. According to the global cancer statistics 2020, HCC ranks sixth in terms of incidence and third in terms of mortality rates [1]. HCC accounts for ~80–90% of patients diagnosed with cirrhosis [2]. Therefore, the high prevalence of liver dysfunction in HCC patients limits the application of different treatments [2,3]. For HCC patients in early-stage and with well-preserved liver function, surgical approaches, including resection, ablation, and liver transplantation, are the possible curative options. However, high recurrence rates after resection locally continue to be a major obstacle [4]. Only a small subgroup (~15%) of patients are eligible for surgery, with a 5-year survival rate of 33–50% [5]. For the majority of patients found in the advanced stage, loco-regional and systemic therapies are the treatments of choice [6]. Sorafenib and Lenvatinib are the first Food and Drug Administration (FDA)-approved first-line therapies for advanced and unresectable HCC [7]. Unfortunately, because of overexpression of the multidrug resistance genes, HCC is inherently a chemotherapy-resistant tumor [8,9].

The management of cancer has changed dramatically since the rapid development of systemic treatments with immune therapies [10]. Immunotherapy, which employs immune cells to boost natural defenses to assault cancer cells, has achieved significant advances over the decades [11]. Nivolumab, the anti-PD-1 monoclonal antibody, has been approved by FDA for HCC immunotherapy [12]. In the CheckMate 040 study, nivolumab treatment showed durable responses and hopeful long-term survival in sorafenib-experienced patients with advanced HCC [13]. Though several major types of immunotherapies, including immune checkpoint inhibitors, cancer vaccines, adoptive cell transfer, etc., show durable anti-tumor effects, the limited response rate is one of the major obstacles in application [14,15], which may attribute to "immunological ignorance" and immune escape in the tumor microenvironment (TME) [16]. The overall objective response rate of nivolumab was approximately 15–20% [17]. Therefore, for better stimulating anti-tumor immunity, it is vital to comprehend and modify the microenvironment of HCC.

Until recently, pharmacological efforts to find new medications have primarily focused on oncogenic signaling networks, but the TME, where cancers originate, has just recently emerged as a prominent target for anti-cancer therapies. When cancer cells invade and alter homeostasis, the TME is formed. The cells of the immune system (e.g., T lymphocytes, dendritic cells (DCs), macrophages and neutrophils, and non-immune components (e.g., extracellular matrix (ECM), fibroblasts, and endothelial cells of vessels) form the TME, which immediately surrounds cancer cells. The TME not only provides a protective "ecological niche" for tumor cells to thrive, progress, and metastasize but also affects the responses to therapy [18,19]. Previous studies have demonstrated that immunosuppressive TME facilitates cancer evasion from immunosurveillance [20–22]. With the improved understanding of TME, modulation of TME from an immunosuppressive one toward an immune-promoting one provides a new direction in cancer immunotherapy. Reprogramming or re-educating tumor-promoting and suppressive TME may increase anti-tumor immunity by recognizing antigens by the reawakened immune system.

The TME plays an important role in the efficiency of HCC immunotherapy, which attracts increasing attention and drives TME-based research. Due to the impact of renal clearance and biological barriers, the majority of drugs cannot successfully reach the tumor site [23]. Therefore, nanoparticles are utilized as potential vehicles for medicine delivery for their function of prolonging retention time and targeting agents [24]. On the one hand, the enhanced permeability and retention (EPR) effect facilitates tumor accumulation of nanomedicines [25]. Besides passive medication delivery via nanoparticles, nanoparticles can also be modified to further increase their compatibility and efficacy. For instance, mannose-modified nanoparticles can actively target the mannose receptors on tumor-associated macrophages (TAM) which "re-educated" the TME, thus improving therapeutic efficacy [26]. Various innovative nanoparticle-based drugs targeting components of TME of HCC have emerged, with significant advances in both lab and clinic experiments [27–30]. This review mainly focuses on applications of different nanoparticles to modulate and reprogram components in TME that are major obstacles to HCC therapy. We first introduce the tumor-promoting components of TME and then discuss the recent achievements of TME modulating nanomedicines, which offer a critical perspective on the future development of TME modulating nanomedicines in HCC.

2. Major Constituents of the Tumor Microenvironment

The TME of HCC is a dynamic system, which consists of various types of cells (including cancer cells, immune cells, stromal cells, etc.), ECM, vasculature, and other secreted molecules [31,32]. Below, we describe the major components that are major obstacles to HCC therapy.

2.1. Abnormal Vasculature of TME

Like other solid tumors, the growth and progression of HCC will induce tumor angiogenesis in order to supply oxygen and nutrients during this period. Unlike normal vessels, tumor vessels are aberrant in structure and function, which impair blood perfusion in tumors, spatially and temporally [33]. The resulting hypoxia not only promotes tumor progression and metastasis by changing the gene expression of tumor cells but confers resistance to therapy [34,35], thereby creating a vicious cycle. The enhanced interstitial fluid pressure and inadequate perfusion caused by these leaky blood vessels increase the number of immunosuppressive cell types and decrease the delivery of therapeutic medications to the tumor [36]. HCC treatment can involve angiogenesis as a target. Major pro-angiogenic factors include but are not limited to vascular endothelial growth factor

(VEGF)-A, basic fibroblast growth factor (bFGF), and interleukin-8 (IL-8) [37]. Accumulating evidence indicates that increased VEGF levels in HCC are related to tumor angiogenesis and progression [38].

2.2. Cancer-Associated Fibroblasts and ECM

Cancer-associated fibroblasts (CAFs) constitute a dominant cellular component of the TME, which act as key players in the development of tumors and cancer cell evasion of therapies [39]. CAFs release a variety of ECM proteins (such as type I-V collagen and fibronectin), paracrine factors, cytokines, and vasculogenic mimicry, all of which aid in the start of HCC with a malignant character [40]. CAFs secrete angiogenic factors, including VEGF, bFGF, angiopoietin-1(ANG-1), and ANG-2, which induce neovascularization [41]. ECM is mainly produced by CAFs, which act as a scaffold in the tumor [42]. ECM undergoes extensive remodeling during cancer progression with characteristics of stiffness and degradation [43]. ECM stiffness is a physical barrier to the efficient absorption or transport of drugs to deeper regions of the tumor [44].

2.3. Immunosuppressive Immune Cells in TME

Tumor-associated immune cells can both assist and impede therapeutic efficacy, and their activation status and location within the TME can vary. Representative immunosuppressive immune cells are the focus of this essay.

2.3.1. Myeloid-Derived Suppressor Cells

Myeloid-derived suppressor cells (MDSCs) are immature myeloid cells with heterogeneity and immunosuppressive properties that are important components of the suppressive TME. MDSCs can be divided into two subsets: monocytic (M-MDSC) and polymorphonuclear (PMN-MDSC). M-MDSCs are more prevalent in tumors and have greater suppressive activity than PMN-MDSCs [45]. MDSCs induce immunosuppressive cells, regulatory T cells (Tregs), and M2-polarized TAM (M2-TAMs) or inhibited immune effector cells ($CD8^+$ T cells, DCs, NK cells, etc.) by a variety of methods [46]. Infection with the hepatitis B virus (HBV) is the most common risk factor for HCC, accounting for around 50–80% of all cases [47]. Importantly, MDSCs play a crucial role in maintaining immunotolerance to high levels of HBV replication [48]. Considerable evidence that has implicated the abundance of MDSCs could be employed as an independent prognostic and predictor in human HCC [49]. Infiltrated MDSCs in HCC overexpressed two enzymes: ARG1 and iNOS, which deplete the essential amino acid L-arginin for T cells [50,51]. Therefore, MDSCs could be a promising target for reversing the immunotolerant state in HCC.

2.3.2. Regulatory T Cells

A subgroup of $CD4^+$ T cells called Tregs is crucial for preserving immunological immune homeostasis and preventing excessive autoimmunity deleterious to the host [52]. In healthy conditions there is an equilibrium between Tregs and T helper 17 cells to keep peripheral tolerance [53]. However, this balance is disturbed in TME. The number of Tregs increases in TME of HCC patients, which links to compromised immune responses [54]. To mediate their suppressive functions, Tregs secrete inhibitory cytokines (such as transforming growth factor-β (TGF-β), IL-10, etc.), promote cytolysis, and "metabolic disruption" of the effector T cells, and inhibit the maturation of DCs [55].

2.3.3. M2-Polarized Macrophages

TAMs are another important component of immune cells in TME, which are broadly classified into M1-TAMs (tumor-suppressing subtype) and M2-TAMs (tumor-promoting subtype) [56]. As opposed to M1-TAMs, M2-TAMs, alternatively activated by TH2 cytokines IL-4/IL-13 [57], facilitate HCC progression by producing mediators that support tumor cell proliferation and immune escape [58,59]. According to several studies, HCC-derived exosomes can activate macrophages and exhibit the M2 phenotype, thereby promoting HCC development [60–62]. In theory, reprograming TAMs from M2 to M1 phenotype or eliminating present TAMs may be a considerable therapeutic approach to arouse their anti-tumor efficacy.

2.4. Crosstalk in the Dynamic TME

The TME of HCC is a dynamic network and complex connections affect the growth of HCC and hinder the immune system's ability to fight it by promoting the activation of immune cells with immunosuppressive qualities (Figure 1). For example, the hypoxia induced by abnormal vasculature drives tumor and stromal secretion of pro-angiogenic factors (hypoxia-inducible factor (HIF), VEGF, insulin-like growth factor-2 (IFG-2), etc.) [63]. Most immune cell types have their functions directly or indirectly modulated by hypoxia, which promotes the growth of tumors. IL-10 and interferon-γ (IFN-γ) produced by MDSDs affect Treg induction, while Tregs can, in turn, control the proliferation and function of MDSCs [64]. The CAFs can induce M2-TAMs via secretion of IL-6 and granulocyte-macrophage colony-stimulating factor (GM-CSF) [65]. Therefore, improvements in our knowledge of the local microenvironment of a growing tumor may present greater options for precise drug delivery.

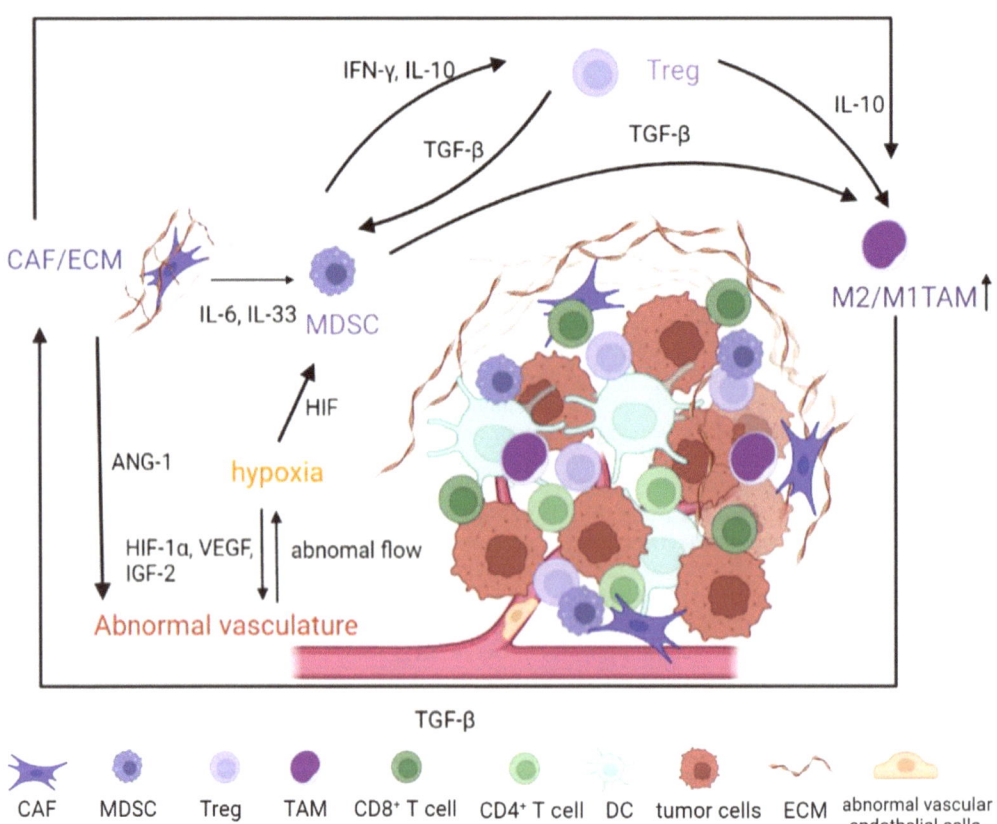

Figure 1. Schematic of the obstacles and their crosstalk in the dynamic TME of HCC. Complex connections affect the growth of HCC and hinder the immune system's ability to fight it by promoting the activation of immune cells with immunosuppressive qualities. The growth and progression of

HCC induce tumor abnormal vasculature and hypoxia, which negatively impacts the infiltration of immune cells and impairs host immunity. Immune suppressive cell types in the TME (MDSC, regulatory Tregs, and M2-TAM) secrete factors that establish immune tolerance to block cancer cell destruction. HCC: hepatocellular carcinoma; TME: tumor microenvironment; CAFs: cancer-associated fibroblasts; ECM: extracellular matrix; TAM: tumor-associated macrophages; MDSC: myeloid-derived suppressor cells; Tregs: regulatory T cells; GM-CSF: granulocyte-macrophage colony-stimulating factor; IL-6: interleukin-6; TGF-β: transforming growth factor-β; IFN-γ: Interferon-γ; HIF: hypoxia-inducible factor; VEGF: vascular endothelial growth factor; IFG-2: insulin-like growth factor-2; ANG-1: angiopoietin-1.

3. Nanomedicine-Based Strategies for TME Modulation

Nanotechnology offers a novel opportunity to deliver medicine to the site of the tumor via passive or active targeting ways. In passive targeting, the therapeutic substance is incorporated into a nanoparticle that passively travels to the target organ without a ligand. To increase the preferential accumulation of the drug at the targeted site, active targeting through the conjugation of receptor-specific ligands is a promising approach [66]. Compared with normal cells, some molecules and proteins are upregulated on the surface of HCC cells, such as asialoglycoprotein receptor, gycyrrhizin/glycyrrhetinic acid receptor [67], transferrin receptor [68], folate receptors [69], CD44 [70], and so on. Thus, their ligands can be used to decorate nanoparticles for active targeting. For example, folic acid (FA) can bind to folate receptors on cancer cells with high specificity. In vitro and in vivo data showed that the functional nanodroplets with FA enhance selective accumulation when targeting Hepa1–6 cells more than non-targeting nanodroplets [71]. Another study designed a type of FA-modified Fe_3O_4 nanoparticles to specifically co-deliver anti-tumor drugs to HCC [72].

A variety of nanomaterials, including polymeric nanoparticles, liposomes, and metal nanoparticles [73], have gained a lot of attention in potentiating cancer therapies, especially in cancer immunotherapy [74–76]. It is noteworthy that parameters such as shape, surface functionalization, and surface charge would have remarkable effects on drug delivery kinetics and biodistribution [77]. Pegylated liposomal formulation Doxil® showed promising activity and low cardiotoxicity compared with doxorubicin (DOX) in metastatic breast cancer [74]. Compared with free DOX, DOX-loaded liposomes significantly increased the uptake of DOX by HCC cells. DOX-loaded liposomes robustly enhanced mild ablation therapy in HCC and represented a viable nanoparticle-based therapeutic approach for HCC treatment [78]. Cubosomes, a type of lyotropic liquid crystalline lipid nanoparticles, are an emerging class of lipid-based nanoparticles. Recently, Pramanik, A. et al. developed Affimer-tagged cubosomes loaded with the anti-cancer drug copper acetylacetonate as a colorectal cancer therapeutic [75], which showed a higher survival rate than the control groups. A recent study revealed that compared with negatively charged PEG-stabilized polymeric nanoparticles, positive ones were better suited for HCC [76]. Furthermore, another study revealed the ability of metal-based ZnS@BSA nanoclusters to facilitate anti-tumor immunotherapy for HCC [79].

Cancer immunotherapy has undergone a revolution over the past decades. The application of nanomedicine has made significant progress in overcoming the constraints of immunological tolerance created by clinic-approved immunotherapies. With the advancement of nanotechnology, an increasing number of intelligent nanomaterials have been designed to re-mode the TME to improve the efficacy of anti-tumor therapies [80]. Since the first nano-drug was approved by the FDA in 1995 (Doxil®) [81], more researchers have an increasing interest in exploring novel nanomedicines targeting non-tumoral cells of TME [82], which held great promise in treating primary and metastatic tumors. Hence, in this section, we will review the nanomedicine-based strategies for TME modulation in HCC (Table 1).

3.1. Anti-Angiogenesis Nanotherapy

In response to the low level of oxygen, cancer cells promote the angiogenesis of tumors by an imbalance between pro-and anti-angiogenic factors [33]. Through neovascularization, more delivery of oxygen and nutrients promote tumor proliferation [63]. However, the rapid and uncontrolled growth of tumors causes more severe hypoxia thus creating a vicious cycle. Additionally, because of anatomical and functional vascular abnormalities, therapeutic drug delivery are strongly impaired [83]. So, modulating tumor vessels might be a viable approach to increase the effectiveness of tumor treatment.

Anti-angiogenic therapy is widely accepted and used in treating HCC [84]. In fact, most currently approved first- and second-line therapies for advanced HCC target angiogenic pathways, in which the VEGF/VEGF receptor (VEGFR) signaling pathway has been validated as a therapeutic target in HCC [85]. Though sorafenib and Lenvatinib exert anti-angiogenic and antiproliferative effects are the first-line treatment options, the drugs are rarely delivered at high concentrations to reach the cancerous tissues. Nanoparticles, as an effective platform for drug delivery, can overcome the adverse side effects of systemic chemotherapeutic administration by improving their pharmacokinetics and accumulation in tumor sites [86,87].

Nanomedicines can be delivered to tumor sites by active and/or passive targeting. In passive targeting, nanovectors are deposed within the TME due to the leaky vasculature and impaired lymphatic drainage [88]. Recently, a nanoassemblie based on biodegradable dendritic polymers poly(amidoamine)-poly(γ-benzyl-L-Glutamate)-b-D-α-tocopheryl polyethylene glycol 1000 succinate (PAM-PBLG-b-TPGS) to carry sorafenib have been developed. Under physiological conditions, the nanoassemblie releases a small portion of sorafenib, which indicates its characteristic stability [89]. Compared with the free sorafenib, the nanoassemblie induces higher therapy efficiency of HCC in both vitro and vivo, which may be attributed to the high accumulation of nanoparticles in HCC. In addition to anti-angiogenic drug delivery, down-regulating the production of VEGF is another nano-therapeutic strategy against angiogenesis in the HCC. Despite the great therapeutic potential of siRNA, the rapid degradation by nucleases and poor internalization by cancer cells restrict their application [90]. Thus, Han, L. et al. developed oral polymeric nanoparticles based on trimethyl chitosan-cysteine (GTC) conjugate to effectively deliver VEGF small interfering RNA (siVEGF) and survivin short hairpin RNA-expression pDNA (iSurpDNA) [91]. According to the ELISA assay, GTC nanoparticles can effectively silence VEGF with a reduction of 70.2%. Zheng, et al. have developed an ASGPR-targeting nanovector that delivers sorafenib and siVEGF simultaneously to enhance the targeting ability of the nanodrug delivery system and significantly induce cytotoxicity of three different HCC cell lines [92], which showed the high anti-tumor efficiency as a potential nanovector for targeted delivery to HCC (Figure 2).

Aside from VEGF inhibitors, vascular disruption agents (VDAs) are another type of medicine that can electively disrupt established tumor blood vessels causing necrosis in the center of HCC due to a lack of blood supply. As a representative VDA, combretastatin A4-phosphate (CA4P) has entered phase III clinical trials [93]. Wang, Y. et al. designed a pH-sensitive nanoparticle based on N-urocanyl pullulan (URPA) loaded with the anti-angiogenic drug combretastatin A4 (CA4) and cytotoxic drugs methotrexate (MTX) [94]. The experiments demonstrated that CA4/MTX-URPA exhibited significant inhibitory effects on tumor angiogenesis and growth. However, the use of CA4P frequently upregulates VEGF expression, which limits its application [95]. This disadvantage might be addressed when VDAs were combined with VEGF/VEGFR2 inhibitors which can inhibit the activity of VEGF in response to CA4P, momentarily normalizing the tumor vasculature. Bao, X. et al. designed poly (L-glutamic acid)-graft-methoxy poly (ethylene glycol) containing CA4 (CA4-NPs), and investigated the effectiveness of CA4-NPs together with VEGF/VEGFR2 inhibitor DC101 in improving anti-PD-1 therapy in an H22 tumor model [96]. Immunofluorescent images of the tumors showed that CA4-NP + DC101 co-treatment could normalize tumor vasculature, enhance tumor pericyte coverage, enhance tumor blood vessel perfusion, and overcome tumor hypoxia. Meanwhile, combining CA4-NP with DC101 raised the proportion of intra-tumoral CD8$^+$ T cells, which significantly improved the treatment efficacy of anti-PD-1 in HCC.

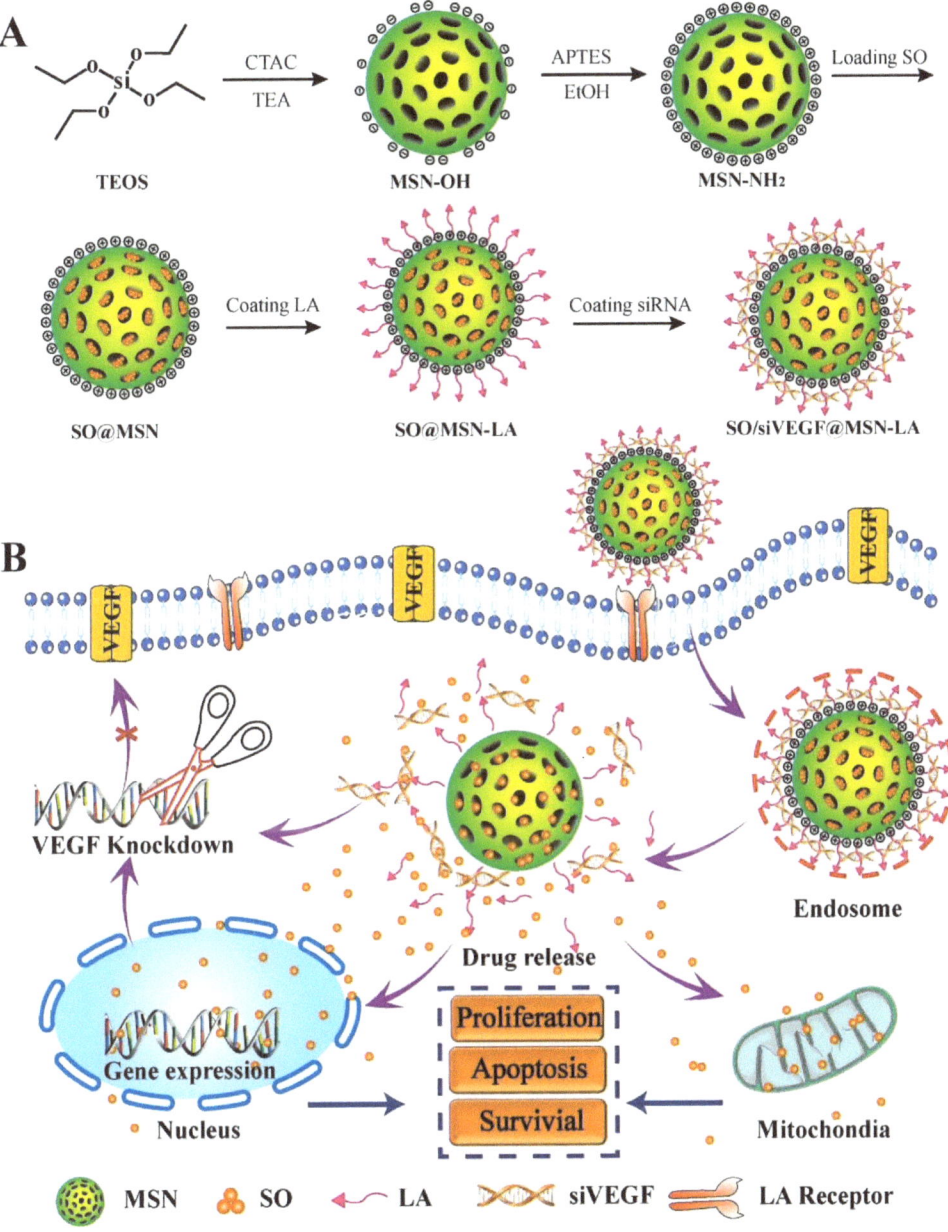

Figure 2. (A) Schematic illustration of synthesis procedure of SO/siVEGF@MSN-LA NPs and (B) inhibiting effect on the proliferation of cancer cells. MSN: mesoporous silica nanoparticles; SO: sorafenib; LA: lactobionic acid; siVEGF: vascular endothelial growth factor small interfering RNA. (Copyright © 2017 Elsevier B.V. All rights reserved, https://doi.org/10.1016/j.ejps.2017.10.036).

Moreover, nanoparticles can simultaneously deliver anti-angiogenic agents and other drugs to achieve their spatiotemporal cooperation in tumors, improving the efficacy of cancer treatment. Chang et al. developed a tumor-targeted multifunctional nanoparticle MnO_2 and a shell composed of lipids and poly(lactic-co-glycolic) acid (PLGA) loaded with sorafenib. These multifunctional nanoplatforms co-deliver sorafenib and MnO_2 for oxygen production to overcome hypoxia-induced drug resistance [97]. Since the favorable drug delivery system is expected to selectively deliver drug payloads in tumor sites and be time-release controlled, different stimulus-responsive nanoparticles, releasing drugs triggered by various external or internal stimuli, are tailored [98]. Zhang et al. designed a pH-sensitive nanoparticle for co-delivering the pro-apoptotic drug DOX and anti-angiogenic drug curcumin [99]. This nanoplatform promoted a spike in drug release in the acid TME. Curcumin inhibits the expression of VEGFR-1, VEGFR-2, VEGFR-3, and epidermal growth factor receptors [100]. Meanwhile, curcumin suppresses the main caspase pathway and activates the main caspase-independent pathway to reduce the adverse effects associated with doxorubicin [101]. Compared with chemotherapy alone, combining treatment with anti-angiogenic medications can enhance the therapeutic efficiency synergistically.

Anti-angiogenic therapy, on the other hand, must address a number of concerns. Firstly, new targets for anti-angiogenic therapy are needed. To date, the majority of anti-angiogenic drugs have targeted VEGF/VEGFR signaling pathways in tumor endothelial cells. However, tumor endothelial cells are heterogeneous [102]. Therefore, more investigation is necessary to explore new targets for anti-angiogenic therapy that increase angiogenesis capability. Moreover, achieving efficient and accurate delivery of nanocarrier to tumor sites remains a stumbling block in nanomedicine. For the application of nanomedicine in HCC, circulation, stability, degradability, and the balance between side effects and curative efficacy must all be carefully studied.

3.2. Nanomedicines Designed to Overcome Tumor Physiological Barrier

Current studies aim to regulate the ECM in two ways: degradation and stiffness. The disruption of the balance between degradation and stiffening is contributed to tumor growth and progression [103]. ECM stiffness can be targeted by reprogramming CAFs and blocking the TGF-β signal pathway [43]. Matrix metalloproteinase (MMP) inhibitors can be used to suppress ECM degradation [104]. For example, Liang, S. et al. constructed a stroma modulation nanosystem based on PEG–PLGA nanospheres [105]. The immunohistochemistry images showed that ECM formation collagen fibers were significantly reduced, via inhibiting TGF-β signaling. The regulation of the tumor ECM greatly enhanced the penetration of nanospheres and facilitated further tumor therapy. HCC is frequently accompanied by marked fibrosis [106]. Mycophenolic acid, the active metabolite of mycophenolate mofetil, exhibits a powerful antifibrotic activity [107]. Yang, Z. et al. designed nanoparticles loaded with mycophenolate mofetil based on 1, 2-distearoyl-sn-glycero-3-phosphoethanolamine-N-poly (ethylene glycol) (MMF-LA@DSPE-PEG) target CAFs [108] (Figure 3). It was shown that the number of CAFs accumulated in tumors was remarkably reduced, as the expression levels of proteins associated with CAF, such as α-smooth muscle actin (α-SMA), fibroblast activation protein (FAP), and collagen IV, were significantly decreased. In mouse models bearing HCC xenograft, mycophenolate mofetil-loaded nanoparticles significantly suppressed fibrotic as well as tumor progression.

In addition to regulating ECM stiffness, some researchers have focused on MMPs as a chemotherapy target in the HCC. MMPs are zinc-dependent endopeptidases that are responsible for degrading basement membrane and various proteins in EMC. According to unambiguous evidence, the release and activation of MMPs facilitate the migration and infiltration of the HCC cells through the damaged basement membrane [109,110]. Moreover, co-workers reported "two-in-one" nanofiber systems containing an anti-tumor drug (DOX) and an MMP inhibitor hexapeptide (KGFRWR) (DOX-KGFRWR) [111]. After administration, the initial liquid DOX-KGFRWR transitioned into nanofibers in the tumor sites, contributing to the inhibition of MPP and antiproliferative effect on HCC. As the results showed, DOX-KGFRWR enhanced the local concentration in the HCC and exerted a synergistic inhibiting effect on HCC cells (SMMC7721) migration. DOX-KGFRWR not only suppressed tumor growth in situ but decreased the number of metastatic nodules. On the other hand, Yeow et al. verified that specific ECM depletion is a viable strategy for boosting the accumulation and uptake of nanoparticles in poorly perfused malignancies such as HCC [112]. According to their results, the lectin-staining in HCC treated with ECM depletion was significantly higher than with PBS, which improved blood vessel function and perfusion in HCC. Notably, nanocarrier itself benefits from ECM depletion therapy. Decreasing the amount of ECM in advance induced significantly higher nanoparticle accumulation in HCC. So, the combination of nanoparticles and ECM depletion might be an ideal option. Based on the above hypothesis, Luo, J. et al. developed a chondroitin sulfate (CSN) modified lipid nanoparticles co-delivery, an ECM depletion drug (retinoic acid, RA), and a chemotherapy drug (DOX) (DOX + RA-CSNs) [113]. The nanoparticle delivery system DOX + RA-CSNs for the Golgi apparatus-specific delivery inhibited the production of type I collagen, which complements the anti-tumor effects of DOX loaded within the nanoparticles. Importantly, the collapse of the ECM barrier greatly boosted the accumulation of DOX + RA-CSNs in HCC and improved the uptake of DOX and RA in HCC cells.

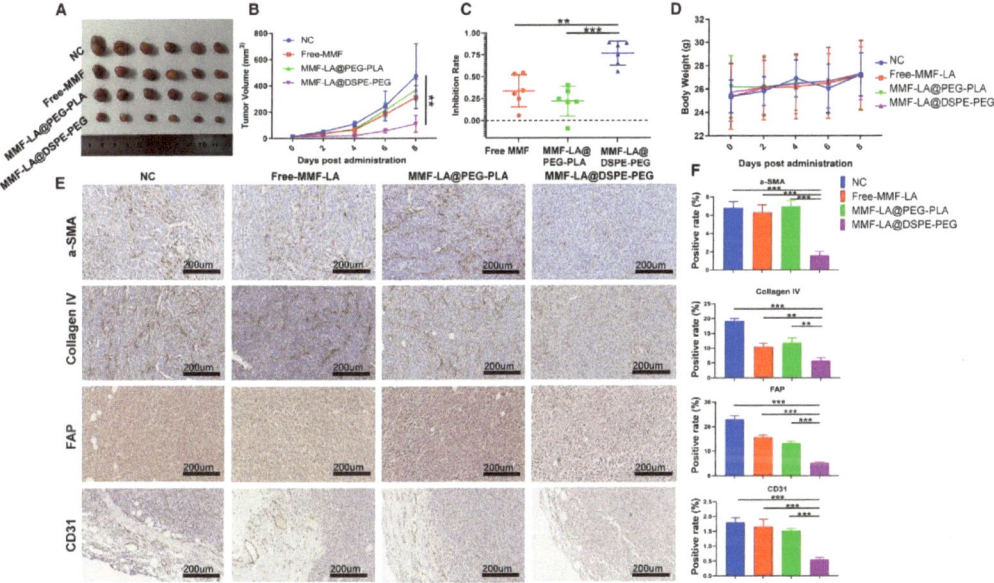

Figure 3. MMF-LA@DSPE-PEG inhibited HCC growth by depleting CAF. Mice were orally administrated with free MMF (20 mg/kg) or intravenously injected with MMF-LA NPs (at 20 mg/kg MMF-equivalent dose) every other day four times. (A), Tumor images of different groups, (n = 6). (B), Tumor growth curves of different groups, ** $p < 0.01$. (C), Tumor inhibition rates of different treatments. (n = 6), ** $p < 0.01$, *** $p < 0.001$. (D), Bodyweights (mean ± SD, n = 6) of mice in different groups. (E), Expression levels of α-SMA, FAP, collagen IV, and CD31 determined by Immunohistochemistry. The scale bars: 200 μm. (F), Quantitative analysis of panel E (Image J software), data are shown as the mean ± SD, (n = 3), ** $p < 0.01$, *** $p < 0.001$. MMF-LA: Mycophenolate mofetil-linoleic acid; DSPE-PEG: 1, 2-distearoyl-sn-glycero-3-phosphoethanolamine-N-poly (ethylene glycol); CAF: cancer-associated fibroblast; α-SMA: alpha-smooth muscle actin; FAP: fibroblast activation protein. (© 2021 The Authors. Journal of Cellular and Molecular Medicine published by Foundation for Cellular and Molecular Medicine and John Wiley & Sons Ltd. https://doi.org/10.1111/jcmm.16434).

3.3. Nanomedicine for Immunosuppressive Cells Inhibition

3.3.1. MDSCs Regulating Nanomedicine

The recruited MDSCs in TME act as a major obstacle for immunotherapy, which plays an important role in immune escape. The following steps have been proposed for therapeutic targeting of MDSCs: (1) interfering with their production by regulation of myelopoiesis, (2) promoting MDSCs differentiation into mature fully mature myeloid cells, (3) eliminating MDSCs, and (4) suppressing their immunosuppressive function.

The chemotherapeutic drug gemcitabine was able to selectively reduce the majority of s MDSCs in tumor-bearing animals while having no effect on macrophages, $CD4^+/CD8^+$ T cells, B cells, or NK cells [114]. To encapsulate Gem derivatives, Suzuki, E. et al. designed a lipid-coated calcium phosphate (LCP) nanocarrier which could effectively deplete MDSCs in the B16F10 mouse melanoma model. Plebanek, M.P. et al. designed high-density lipoprotein-like nanocarriers, with a strong affinity to scavenger receptor type B expressed by MDSCs, to suppress the function of MDSCs [115]. For instance, Lai, C. et al. designed folate (FA) modified chitosan nanoparticles loaded with mouse interferon-γ-inducible protein-10 (mIP-10) plasmid (FA-chitosan/mIP-10) which could efficiently attract and activate T cells, B cells and NK cells with an increase in the number of MDSCs [116] on HCC tumor models. Therefore, Hu, Z. et al. combined FA-chitosan/mIP-10 with DC/tumor fusion vaccine to improve the immunosuppressive TME and enhance anti-cancer efficiency [117]. The results showed that compared with the administration of FA-chitosan/mIP-10 alone, the growth of implanted HCC tumors was effectively inhibited upon the treatment with both FA-chitosan/mIP-10 and DC/tumor fusion vaccine. The results suggested that DC/tumor fusion vaccine, together with FA-chitosan/mIP-10, greatly increased anti-tumor immune responses which inhibited the recruitment of MDSCs. In comparison to other malignancies, however, a few researchers have looked at the regulatory influence of nanoparticles on MDSCs in HCC. At present, MDSCs were generally regulated by combining other immune cell therapy. Further studies targeting MDSCs specifically are necessary due to the importance of MDSCs in HCC progression.

3.3.2. T Cell-Modulating Nanoparticles

T cells are crucial components of the adaptive immune system that help to defend against pathogens like viruses, bacteria, and cancers. T cells are classified into three categories based on their functions: helper T lymphocytes (HTLs), Tregs, and cytotoxic T lymphocytes (CTLs). The presence of a large number of Treg cells in the TME, as well as a low $CD8^+$ T cells to Treg cells ratio, is linked to poor prognosis, suggesting that Treg cells block tumor antigen-specific T cell immune responses [118]. Treg cell elimination or modulation of its activities may provide potential immunotherapies. In view of the vital key of T cells in cancer immunotherapy, we look at nanoparticles that control T cell viability in the following section.

IL-2, which is recognized as a T cell growth factor to enhance memory T cell responses and regulate T cell maintenance, is the first FDA-approved immunotherapy for human cancer [119]. Treg cells that express the transcription factor Foxp3 play an important role in immune tolerance and autoimmunity prevention and a low dose of IL-2 has been proven to boost Tregs and improve their suppressive abilities [120]. Tregs consume IL-2 primarily through high-affinity IL-2 receptors (CD25), which limit the amount of IL-2 available for effector T cell proliferation and activation. Therefore, injection of a sufficient dose of IL-2 can neutralize Tregs suppressive abilities. In order to obtain sufficient exposure at tumor sites and induce tumor suppression with decreasing side effects, several investigations have focused on nanocarrier-based IL-2 application. Wu, J. et al. developed an N, N, N-trimethyl chitosan (TMC) based nanocarrier to realize co-delivery DOX and recombinant human IL-2 (FTCD/rhIL-2) which increased the anti-cancer therapeutic benefits with toxicity reduced [121]. These nanoparticles could suppress tumor progression through apoptosis induced by DOX and enhance anti-cancer immunity by rhIL-2. The nanocomplexes FTCD/rhIL-2 could promote humoral and cellular immunity by activating the vitality of T, B lymphocytes, and NK cells. The in vivo investigations in an HCC model have revealed that FTCD/rhIL-2 exhibited stronger anti-tumor efficacy than DOX or rhIL-2, respectively. In addition to administrating IL-2 protein directly, delivery of immunostimulatory IL-2–encoding plasmid DNA (Pdna) can also remodel the immunosuppressive TME of HCC. Huang, K.-W. et al. developed tumor-targeted lipid-dendrimer-calcium-phosphate nanoparticles (TT-LDCP) loaded with siRNA silencing immune checkpoint ligand PD-L1 gene and Pdna upregulating expression of the immunostimulating cytokine IL-2 [122] (Figure 4). Confocal microscopy detection of fluorescence intensity showed that TT-LDCP nanoparticles could efficiently deliver siRNA and Pdna into two HCC cell lines (murine HCA-1 and human Hep3B) with effective gene transfection. Experiments showed that TT-LDCP nanoparticles that co-delivered PD-L1 siRNA and IL-2 Pdna could reverse the immunosuppressive TME of HCC by increasing tumoral infiltration CD8$^+$ T cells and promote the maturation of tumor-infiltrating DCs.

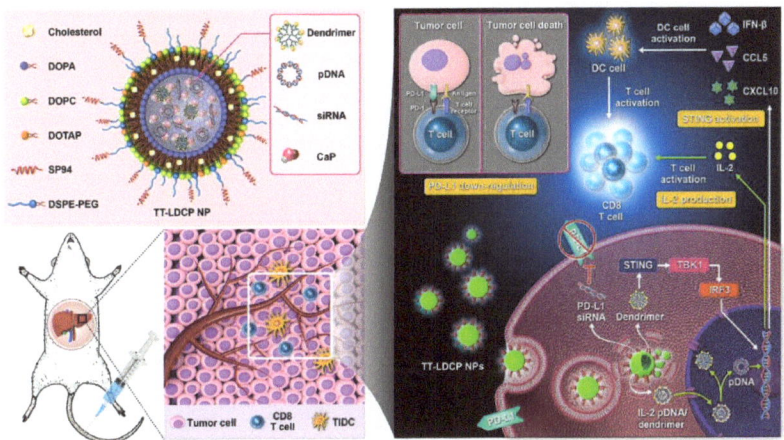

Figure 4. Schematic representation of the mechanism of immunogene therapy by TT-LDCP NPs containing siRNA against the immune checkpoint PD-L1 and Pdna encoding the immunostimulating cytokine IL-2. Active tumor targeting was achieved through the addition of the HCC-targeted SP94 peptide to the surface of the NPs.

The thymine-capped PAMAM dendrimer/CaP complexes achieved highly efficient gene transfection efficacy by enhancing the nuclear delivery of the Pdna. Furthermore, thymine-capped PAMAM dendrimers stimulate the STING pathway and serve as an adjuvant to promote the maturation of intra-tumoral DCs. Efficient tumor-targeted co-delivery of PD-L1 siRNA and IL-2 Pdna achieves tumor-specific expression of IL-2 and down-regulation of PD-L1, increases infiltration and activation of CD8+ T cells in HCC, and induces a strong tumor-suppressive effect in HCC in synergy with a vaccine. CaP, calcium phosphate; TIDC, tumor-infiltrating dendritic cell; TT-LDCP NPs, tumor-targeted lipid-dendrimer-calcium-phosphate NPs; IFN-γ, interferon-γ. (Copyright © 2020 The Authors, some rights reserved; exclusive licensee American Association for the Advancement of Science. http://dx.doi.org/10.1126/sciadv.aax5032).

IL-12 is another potent cytokine in provoking anti-tumor immune responses [123]. Li, J. et al. newly created CD8 and Glypican-3 antibodies modified PLGA nanoparticles loaded with IL-12 [123]. Cell counting revealed that compared with other groups, the proliferation of CD8$^+$ T cells was more effective in the group treated with the targeted immune nanoparticles (TINPs). TINPs are attached precisely to the two target cells (CD8$^+$ T cells and HepG-2 cells) to form T cell-HepG-2 cell clusters to induce robust immune responses. Moreover, compared to soluble IL-12, the expression of CD107a, which was a degranulation marker and a predictor of T lymphocytes' ability to lyse tumor cells, was 5-fold higher when treated with TINPs.

The metabolism in tumors differs from the normal tissues from which they develop, indicating that metabolic pathways may make effective targets for cancer therapy [124]. Accelerated glycolysis of a tumor, known as the "Warburg effect", leads to increased lactate production [125]. Lactate, which drives cancer cells, has been demonstrated to strongly inhibited the activation of T cells [126,127]. 2-Deoxy-D-glucose (2DG), a hexokinase inhibitor, can interrupt glycolysis [128]. Sasaki, K. et al. designed 2DG-encapsulated PLGA nanoparticles (2DG-PLGA-NPs) to improve the delivery efficiency of 2DG to HCC [129]. It was found that 2DG-PLGA-NPs may boost T-cell trafficking in the TME by reducing the generation of lactate by tumor cells and increase the production of IFN-γ and the uptake of glucose by $CD8^+$ T cells.

3.3.3. TAM Modulating Nanoparticles

In view of the key role of macrophages in cancer immunity, current therapies targeting TAMs utilize four strategies: (1) restricting macrophage recruitment, (2) depleting TAMs, (3) re-educating TAMs, and (4) blocking the CD47-signal regulatory protein alpha (SIRPα) pathway.

Several studies have proven that hypoxia induced by sorafenib could upregulate the expression of stromal-derived factor 1α (SDF-1α) and its receptor, C-X-C receptor type 4 (CXCR4) in HCC [130,131]. AMD3100, a CXCR4 inhibitor, could suppress cancer cell proliferation and M2-TAM polarization by blocking SDF1α/CXCR4 pathway [130]. Gao, D. et al. contrasted AMD3100 modified lipid-coated PLGA nanoparticles with sorafenib-containing (ADOPSor-NPs) [132]. These ADOPSor-NPs delivered sorafenib and AMD3100 into HCC, triggered tumor apoptosis, prevented the infiltration of TAMs, and overcame the acquired sorafenib resistance. In the orthotopic HCC mice model, ADOPSor-NPs effectively suppressed primary HCC development and metastasis and thus improved overall survival. Li, G. et al. prepared a nanoliposome loaded a sphingolipid metabolite C6-ceramide (LipC6). In liver tumor-bearing mice, LipC6 administration decreased the quantity of TAMs and their capacity to inhibit the anti-tumor immune response [133].

Apart from decreasing TAMs infiltration, another strategy is to re-educate TAMs. In response to changes in the TME during tumor progression, the TAMs go through a shift of polarized phenotypes from M1 to M2. The macrophage, on the other hand, retains the ability for plasticity, including the capacity to transition between M1/M2 status in response to microenvironmental signals. A number of studies have looked into the applications of nanoparticles to modulate TAM polarization from an immune-suppressive phenotype to an immune-promoting one [134]. Wang, T. et al. created twin-like core-shell nanoparticles: SF loaded cationic lipid-based nanoparticles (CLN) coated with O-Carboxymethyl-chitosan (CMCS) (CMCS/SF-CLN) and mannose-modified IMD-0354 (a TAM re-polarization agents) loaded CLN coated with CMCS (M-IMD-CLN) [135]. To improve tumor-localized chemoimmunotherapy, CMCS/SF-CLN and CMCS/M-IMD-CLN could simultaneously target cancer cells and TAM separately via SF and mannose on the surface of CLN. Flow cytometry assay showed that the M1/M2 ratio of CMCS/M-IMD-CLN was ~2.5-fold higher than the PBS group, which indicated enhanced polarization. Immunogenic cytokines IFN-γ and IL-12 secreted by M1-TAM were higher than those in CMCS/SF-CLN. Moreover, the administration of CMCS/M-IMD-CLN normalized abnormal tumor blood vessels induced by CMCS/SF-CLN. These findings revealed that CMCS/M-IMD-CLN considerably improved the immunosuppression caused by CMCS/SF-CLN via M2-TAM polarization. In order to deliver siRNA to M2-TAM selectively, Kaps, L. et al. prepared α-mannosyl modified cationic nanohydrogel particles (ManNP) loaded with siRNA [136]. ManNP specifically targeted M2-TAMs with no organ or cellular toxicity, indicting them as promising nanocarriers for macrophage repolarization in HCC.

Hypoxia is frequent in HCC, which leads to an inhibitory TME, such as macrophage recruitment and polarization. In other words, improving hypoxia contributes to a reduction in the amounts of TAMs as well as in transit pro-tumor M2-TAM into anti-tumor M1-TAM [137]. Dai, X. et al. synthesized oxygen microcapsules based on polydopamine nanoparticles to improve the hypoxia microenvironment in HCC [138]. The ratio of TAMs to total lymphocytes in the TME of radiation + oxygen microcapsules group showed a significant drop of 55.8% when compared with the PBS group, indicating the suppressed TAMs recruitment. Meanwhile, radiotherapy combined with oxygen microcapsules reprogramed M2-TAMs towards an M1-type phenotype. In detail, the ratio of M1/M2 in the radiotherapy + oxygen microcapsules group was 33-fold higher than in the PBS group.

The binding of the SPIRα on macrophages to CD47, a "don't eat me" signal on cancer cells, protects cancer cells from being phagocytosed. Thus, blocking the CD47-SIRPα pathway can enhance the phagocytosis of macrophages. Comparetti, E.J. et al. reported that plasma membrane-derived nanostructures (MNPs), co-delivery siRNA (inactivation of the proto-oncogene c-MYC), and the immune adjuvant monophosphoryl lipid A (MPLA) (MNPs-MPLA-siRNA) [139]. The prepared MNPs-MPLA-siRNA downregulated CD47 and PD-L1 expression on Hep-G2 cells and upregulated expression of classical activation markers on macrophages, such as CD64, CD80, CD83, and CD86 (Table 1).

Table 1. Nanomedicine-based strategies for TME modulation in HCC.

Target	NP	Size (nm)	Mechanism	Animal Model	Cell Lines	Ref
Anti-angiogenesis	encapsulating sorafenib with PAM-PBLG-b-TPGS	118.3 ± 5.1	release sorafenib target angiogenic pathways	Balb/C nude mice	HepG2 and LO2	[89]
	galactose modified GTC co-delivery iSur-Pdna and siVEGF	130–160	VEGF was depleted with siVEGF	female Balb/c nude mice and female Kunming mice	BEL-7402	[91]
	co-delivery of sorafenib and siVEGF based on mesoporous silica nanoparticles	148.5 ± 3.5	sustained release of sorafenib and siVEGF	NA	HepG2, Huh, HeLa and A549	[92]
	MTX and CA4 loaded N-urocanyl pullulan	187.1 ± 15.2	Release anti-tumor drug MTX and vascular disruption agents CA4	Balb/c and nude mice	HepG2, PLC/PRF/5 and A549	[94]
ECM/CAF	loaded MMF based on 1, 2-distearoyl-sn-glycero-3-phosphoethanolamine-N-poly	156.23 ± 60.38	MMF inhibited fibroblasts proliferation and tubulin expression; reduced CAF density	C57BL/6 mice, nude mice	Huh7, SUN 449, LM3, LX2, Hep1-6, NIH-3T3	[108]
	DOX-KGFRWR	long nanofibers with average widths of 10.51 nm	MMP inhibition and antiproliferative effects	male Sprague–Dawley rats; male Institute of Cancer Research mice	SMMC7721	[111]
	RA- and DOX-loaded lipid nanoparticles modified with chondroitin sulfate	smaller than 100	RA disrupted the ECM barrier by destroying the Golgi structure of hepatoma cells and HSCs, while DOX-induced cell death.	Male Kunming mice	SMMC-7721 and H22	[113]
MDSC	FA-chitosan/mIP-10 nanoparticles	315.5	sustained local IP-10 expression reduced the number of MDSCs, and attracted $CXCR^{3+}CD^{8+}$ T cells to the tumor	Female C57BL/6 mice	Hepa1-6	[117]

Table 1. Cont.

Target	NP	Size (nm)	Mechanism	Animal Model	Cell Lines	Ref
T cell	FA modified TMC co-delivery DOX and IL-2	198.1 ± 1.4	improve the amounts of infiltrated cytotoxic T lymphocytes cells.	Female Kunming mice	SMMC-7721 and A549	[121]
	poly(d,l-lactide-co-glycolide) nanoparticle, by loading IL-12 and modifying with CD8 and Glypican-3 antibodies o	145−172	target T cells and deliver IL-12 to T cells for effective activation and proliferation.	NA	HepG-2	[123]
	2DG-encapsulated PLGA nanoparticles	120	activated CD8+ T-cell chemotaxis in the tumor microenvironment via the decreased production of lactate in tumors, the increased IFN-γ production and glucose uptake in CD8+ T cells, and production of CXCL9/CXCL10/CXCL11 in both the tumors and CD8+ T cells	nude mice with xenograft tumors	The Huh7, HepG2, B16F10, BxPC3, OS-RC-2, and HT29 cells	[129]
TAM	AMD3100 modified lipid-coated PLGA nanoparticles with sorafenib-containing	150−200	suppressed the infiltration of TAMs	Male C3H/HeNCrNarl mice	HCA-1 and JHH-7	[132]
	a nanoliposome-loaded C6-ceramide	NA	reduces not only TAM frequency but also its suppressive function and increased the activity of CD8+ T cells	Male C57BL/6 mice	TAg-transformed B6/WT-19 cells	[133]
	mannose-modified IMD-0354 loaded cationic lipid-based nanoparticles coated with polymer O-carboxymethyl-chitosan	129.4 ± 6.8	TAM re-polarization	C57BL/6 mice	Hepa1-6	[135]
	MNPs-MPLA-siRNA	40−400	inhibiting the activity of c-MYC oncogene to reduce the pro-tumoral response from M2 macrophages	NA	Hep-G2	[139]

PAM-PBLG-b-TPGS: poly(amidoamine)-poly(γ-benzyl-L-Glutamate)-b-D-α-tocopheryl polyethylene glycol 1000 succinate; GTC: trimethyl chitosan-cysteine; VEGF: vascular endothelial growth factor; NA: not available; MTX: methotrexate; CA4: combretastatin A4; ECM: extracellular matrix; CAF: cancer-associated fibroblasts; MMF: mycophenolate mofetil; DOX-KGFRWR: doxorubicin-conjugated hexapeptide; MMP: matrix metalloproteinases; RA: retinoic acid; HSCs: Hepatic stellate cells; MDSC: Myeloid-derived suppressor cells; FA: folate; mIP-10: mouse interferon-induced protein-10 gene; TMC: N,N,N-trimethyl chitosan; IL-2: Interleukin-2; 2DG: 2-deoxy-D-glucose; PLGA: poly(lactic-co-glycolic acid); IFN-γ: Interferon-γ; TAM: tumor-associated macrophage; MNPs: Plasma membrane-derived nanoparticles co-delivery monophosphoryl lipid A and small interfering RNA.

4. Conclusions and Future Perspectives

HCC is one of the most prevalent malignancies in the world, with rising incidence and high mortality rates. Immunotherapy for HCC is both promising and challenging due to its unique characteristic of immunity and immune tolerance. As a protective "ecological niche" for tumor cells, the different components and complex crosstalk in TME promote HCC progression and impair therapeutic effects. Since the TME of HCC plays a key role in its initiation and progression, it is worth considering the regulation of TME to enhance anti-cancer immune responses. Given the rapid development of nanotechnology and the success of cancer immunotherapy in the clinic, the convergence of the two therapies will certainly achieve significant progress in cancer treatment. In this study, we review recent advancements in the treatment of HCC using nano-delivery technologies to regulate immunosuppressive TME. There is a plethora of studies to reprogram the components of TME, such as tumor cells, T lymphocytes, tumor endothelial cells, TAMs, and ECM. TME-modulating nanoparticles can contain various drugs and be modified by targeting ligands in order to highly and specifically accumulate in tumor sites while reducing side effects.

However, there exist a few obstacles to be faced and overcome when it comes to regulating the HCC microenvironment. For example, despite the fact that TME-modulating nanoparticles have demonstrated promising results in preclinical studies, several challenges remain in their clinical translation. First of all, the potential toxicity and immunogenicity of nanomaterials restrict their application in clinical experiments. Immune responses toward the nanomaterials may induce severe complications, such as allergic reactions, thrombogenesis, and so on [140]. Thus, future clinical translations of nanoparticles should concentrate on the low antigenicity with a carefully controlled dose. Secondly, considering the unique immunological landscape of HCC, which contains large amounts of immune cells and some of these, such as Kupffer cells, cannot be found in any other parts of the body, the components in the HCC microenvironment should be further investigated. The TME is a complex network and the impact of one component's depletion or suppression on the entire system is unknown. Inhibition of one or more components in HCC may be compensated by overexpression of other pathways. A better understanding of components in TME of HCC and the long-term effects of nanoparticles targeting these TME components is critical in future research. Thirdly, because of the existing individual differences in reactions to nanomedicines, it will also be important to develop biomarkers that are both reliable and predictive.

Altogether, modulation of the TME of HCC is seen to be promising as it can effectively improve anti-cancer immunity. Significant progress in the treatment of HCC is believed to be made in the near future.

Author Contributions: Conceptualization, Y.L. and N.F.; Formal Analysis, Y.D. and R.Y.; Investigation, Y.L. and N.F.; Visualization, Y.L.; Writing—Review and Editing, Y.D. and R.Y. All authors have read and agreed to the published version of the manuscript.

Funding: This study was supported in part by grants from the Natural Science Foundation of Zhejiang province (LZ22H180002), and the National Natural Science Foundation of China (General Program: 82171998).

Institutional Review Board Statement: Not applicable.

Informed Consent Statement: Not applicable.

Data Availability Statement: Not applicable.

Conflicts of Interest: The authors declare no conflict of interest.

Abbreviations

HCC: hepatocellular carcinoma; TME: tumor microenvironment; FDA: Food and Drug Administration; DC: dendritic cells; ECM: extracellular matrix; EPR: the enhanced permeability and retention; TAM: tumor-associated macrophages; MDSC: myeloid-derived suppressor cells; VEGF: vascular endothelial growth factor; bFGF: basic fibroblast growth factor; IL-8: interleukin-8; CAFs: cancer-associated fibroblasts; PMN-MDSC: polymorphonuclear-MDSC; M-MDSC: monocytic MDSC; HBV: hepatitis B virus; Tregs: regulatory T cells; TGFβ: transforming growth factor-β; VEGFR: VEGF receptor; PAM-PBLG-b-TPGS: poly(amidoamine)-poly(γ-benzyl-L-Glutamate)-b-D-α-tocopheryl polyethylene glycol 1000 succinate; GTC: trimethyl chitosan-cysteine; siVEGF: VEGF small interfering RNA; iSur-pDNA: survivin hort hairpin RNA-expression pDNA; ASGPR: asialoglycoprotein receptor; VDAs: vascular disruption agents; CA4P: combretastatin A4-phosphate; URPA: N-urocanyl pullulan; MTX: methotrexate; PLGA: poly(lactic-co-glycolic) acid; MMP: matrix metalloproteinase; DOX: doxorubicin; CSN: chondroitin sulfate; LCP: lipid-coated calcium phosphate; mIP-10: mouse interferon-γ-inducible protein-10; FA: folate; HTLs: helper T lymphocytes; CTLs: cytotoxic T lymphocytes; TMC: N, N, N-trimethyl chitosan; rhIL-2: recombinant human IL-2;pDNA: plasmid DNA; TT-LDCP: tumor-targeted lipid-dendrimer-calcium-phosphate; TINPs: targeted immune nanoparticles; SDF-1α: stromal-derived factor 1α; CXCR4: C-X-C receptor type 4; CLN: cationic lipid-based nanoparticles; CMCS: O-Carboxymethyl-chitosan; MNPs: plasma membrane-derived nanostructures; MPLA: monophosphoryl lipid A; MMF-LA: Mycophenolate mofetil-linoleic acid; DSPE-PEG: 1, 2-distearoyl-sn-glycero-3-phosphoethanolamine-N-poly (ethylene glycol); α-SMA: alpha-smooth muscle actin; FAP: fibroblast activation protein.

References

1. Sung, H.; Ferlay, J.; Siegel, R.L.; Laversanne, M.; Soerjomataram, I.; Jemal, A.; Bray, F. Global Cancer Statistics 2020: GLOBOCAN Estimates of Incidence and Mortality Worldwide for 36 Cancers in 185 Countries. *CA Cancer J. Clin.* **2021**, *71*, 209–249. [CrossRef] [PubMed]
2. Llovet, J.M.; Kelley, R.K.; Villanueva, A.; Singal, A.G.; Pikarsky, E.; Roayaie, S.; Lencioni, R.; Koike, K.; Zucman-Rossi, J.; Finn, R.S. Hepatocellular carcinoma. *Nat. Rev. Dis. Primers* **2021**, *7*, 6. [CrossRef] [PubMed]
3. Pinato, D.J.; Sharma, R.; Allara, E.; Yen, C.; Arizumi, T.; Kubota, K.; Bettinger, D.; Jang, J.W.; Smirne, C.; Kim, Y.W.; et al. The ALBI grade provides objective hepatic reserve estimation across each BCLC stage of hepatocellular carcinoma. *J. Hepatol.* **2017**, *66*, 338–346. [CrossRef] [PubMed]
4. Roayaie, S.; Obeidat, K.; Sposito, C.; Mariani, L.; Bhoori, S.; Pellegrinelli, A.; Labow, D.; Llovet, J.M.; Schwartz, M.; Mazzaferro, V. Resection of hepatocellular cancer ≤2 cm: Results from two Western centers. *Hepatology* **2013**, *57*, 1426–1435. [CrossRef]
5. Roxburgh, P.; Evans, T.R.J. Systemic therapy of hepatocellular carcinoma: Are we making progress? *Adv. Ther.* **2008**, *25*, 1089–1104. [CrossRef]
6. Jin, H.; Qin, S.; He, J.; Xiao, J.; Li, Q.; Mao, Y.; Zhao, L. New insights into checkpoint inhibitor immunotherapy and its combined therapies in hepatocellular carcinoma: From mechanisms to clinical trials. *Int. J. Biol. Sci.* **2022**, *18*, 2775–2794. [CrossRef]
7. Al-Salama, Z.T.; Syed, Y.Y.; Scott, L.J. Lenvatinib: A Review in Hepatocellular Carcinoma. *Drugs* **2019**, *79*, 665–674. [CrossRef]
8. Thomas, M. Molecular targeted therapy for hepatocellular carcinoma. *J. Gastroenterol.* **2009**, *44*, 136–141. [CrossRef]
9. Tang, W.; Chen, Z.; Zhang, W.; Cheng, Y.; Zhang, B.; Wu, F.; Wang, Q.; Wang, S.; Rong, D.; Reiter, F.P.; et al. The mechanisms of sorafenib resistance in hepatocellular carcinoma: Theoretical basis and therapeutic aspects. *Signal Transduct. Target. Ther.* **2020**, *5*, 87. [CrossRef]
10. Van den Bulk, J.; Verdegaal, E.M.; de Miranda, N.F. Cancer immunotherapy: Broadening the scope of targetable tumours. *Open Biol.* **2018**, *8*, 180037. [CrossRef]
11. Hoos, A.; Britten, C. The immuno-oncology framework: Enabling a new era of cancer therapy. *Oncoimmunology* **2012**, *1*, 334–339. [CrossRef]
12. Marrero, J.A.; Kulik, L.M.; Sirlin, C.B.; Zhu, A.X.; Finn, R.S.; Abecassis, M.M.; Roberts, L.R.; Heimbach, J.K. Diagnosis, Staging, and Management of Hepatocellular Carcinoma: 2018 Practice Guidance by the American Association for the Study of Liver Diseases. *Hepatology* **2018**, *68*, 723–750. [CrossRef]
13. Yau, T.; Hsu, C.; Kim, T.Y.; Choo, S.P.; Kang, Y.K.; Hou, M.M.; Numata, K.; Yeo, W.; Chopra, A.; Ikeda, M.; et al. Nivolumab in advanced hepatocellular carcinoma: Sorafenib-experienced Asian cohort analysis. *J. Hepatol.* **2019**, *71*, 543–552. [CrossRef]
14. Pan, C.; Liu, H.; Robins, E.; Song, W.; Liu, D.; Li, Z.; Zheng, L. Next-generation immuno-oncology agents: Current momentum shifts in cancer immunotherapy. *J. Hematol. Oncol.* **2020**, *13*, 29. [CrossRef]
15. Yan, Y.; Zheng, L.; Du, Q.; Yan, B.; Geller, D.A. Interferon regulatory factor 1 (IRF-1) and IRF-2 regulate PD-L1 expression in hepatocellular carcinoma (HCC) cells. *Cancer Immunol. Immunother. CII* **2020**, *69*, 1891–1903. [CrossRef]
16. Sharma, P.; Hu-Lieskovan, S.; Wargo, J.A.; Ribas, A. Primary, Adaptive, and Acquired Resistance to Cancer Immunotherapy. *Cell* **2017**, *168*, 707–723. [CrossRef]
17. El-Khoueiry, A.B.; Sangro, B.; Yau, T.; Crocenzi, T.S.; Kudo, M.; Hsu, C.; Kim, T.-Y.; Choo, S.-P.; Trojan, J.; Welling, T.H.R.; et al. Nivolumab in patients with advanced hepatocellular carcinoma (CheckMate 040): An open-label, non-comparative, phase 1/2 dose escalation and expansion trial. *Lancet* **2017**, *389*, 2492–2502. [CrossRef]
18. Sheng, H.; Huang, Y.; Xiao, Y.; Zhu, Z.; Shen, M.; Zhou, P.; Guo, Z.; Wang, J.; Wang, H.; Dai, W.; et al. ATR inhibitor AZD6738 enhances the antitumor activity of radiotherapy and immune checkpoint inhibitors by potentiating the tumor immune microenvironment in hepatocellular carcinoma. *J. Immunother. Cancer* **2020**, *8*, e000340. [CrossRef]
19. Wu, Y.; Kuang, D.M.; Pan, W.D.; Wan, Y.L.; Lao, X.M.; Wang, D.; Li, X.F.; Zheng, L. Monocyte/macrophage-elicited natural killer cell dysfunction in hepatocellular carcinoma is mediated by CD48/2B4 interactions. *Hepatology* **2013**, *57*, 1107–1116. [CrossRef]

20. Hato, T.; Goyal, L.; Greten, T.F.; Duda, D.G.; Zhu, A.X. Immune checkpoint blockade in hepatocellular carcinoma: Current progress and future directions. *Hepatology* **2014**, *60*, 1776–1782. [CrossRef]
21. Quail, D.F.; Joyce, J.A. Microenvironmental regulation of tumor progression and metastasis. *Nat. Med.* **2013**, *19*, 1423–1437. [CrossRef]
22. Eggert, T.; Greten, T.F. Tumor regulation of the tissue environment in the liver. *Pharm. Ther.* **2017**, *173*, 47–57. [CrossRef]
23. Sun, K.; Yu, J.; Hu, J.; Chen, J.; Song, J.; Chen, Z.; Cai, Z.; Lu, Z.; Zhang, L.; Wang, Z. Salicylic acid-based hypoxia-responsive chemodynamic nanomedicines boost antitumor immunotherapy by modulating immunosuppressive tumor microenvironment. *Acta Biomater.* **2022**, *148*, 230–243. [CrossRef]
24. Dai, Q.; Wilhelm, S.; Ding, D.; Syed, A.M.; Sindhwani, S.; Zhang, Y.; Chen, Y.Y.; MacMillan, P.; Chan, W.C.W. Quantifying the Ligand-Coated Nanoparticle Delivery to Cancer Cells in Solid Tumors. *ACS Nano* **2018**, *12*, 8423–8435. [CrossRef]
25. Golombek, S.K.; May, J.-N.; Theek, B.; Appold, L.; Drude, N.; Kiessling, F.; Lammers, T. Tumor targeting via EPR: Strategies to enhance patient responses. *Adv. Drug Deliv. Rev.* **2018**, *130*, 17–38. [CrossRef]
26. Zhao, P.; Wang, Y.; Kang, X.; Wu, A.; Yin, W.; Tang, Y.; Wang, J.; Zhang, M.; Duan, Y.; Huang, Y. Dual-targeting biomimetic delivery for anti-glioma activity via remodeling the tumor microenvironment and directing macrophage-mediated immunotherapy. *Chem. Sci.* **2018**, *9*, 2674–2689. [CrossRef]
27. Wan, J.L.; Wang, B.; Wu, M.L.; Li, J.; Gong, R.M.; Song, L.N.; Zhang, H.S.; Zhu, G.Q.; Chen, S.P.; Cai, J.L.; et al. MTDH antisense oligonucleotides reshape the immunosuppressive tumor microenvironment to sensitize Hepatocellular Carcinoma to immune checkpoint blockade therapy. *Cancer Lett.* **2022**, *541*, 215750. [CrossRef]
28. Wang, Y.; Wang, Z.; Jia, F.; Xu, Q.; Shu, Z.; Deng, J.; Li, A.; Yu, M.; Yu, Z. CXCR4-guided liposomes regulating hypoxic and immunosuppressive microenvironment for sorafenib-resistant tumor treatment. *Bioact. Mater.* **2022**, *17*, 147–161. [CrossRef]
29. Xiao, Y.; Chen, J.; Zhou, H.; Zeng, X.; Ruan, Z.; Pu, Z.; Jiang, X.; Matsui, A.; Zhu, L.; Amoozgar, Z.; et al. Combining p53 mRNA nanotherapy with immune checkpoint blockade reprograms the immune microenvironment for effective cancer therapy. *Nat. Commun.* **2022**, *13*, 758. [CrossRef]
30. Zhang, J.; Shan, W.F.; Jin, T.T.; Wu, G.Q.; Xiong, X.X.; Jin, H.Y.; Zhu, S.M. Propofol exerts anti-hepatocellular carcinoma by microvesicle-mediated transfer of miR-142-3p from macrophage to cancer cells. *J. Transl. Med.* **2014**, *12*, 279. [CrossRef]
31. Bejarano, L.; Jordāo, M.J.C.; Joyce, J.A. Therapeutic Targeting of the Tumor Microenvironment. *Cancer Discov.* **2021**, *11*, 933–959. [CrossRef] [PubMed]
32. Petitprez, F.; Meylan, M.; de Reyniès, A.; Sautès-Fridman, C.; Fridman, W.H. The Tumor Microenvironment in the Response to Immune Checkpoint Blockade Therapies. *Front. Immunol.* **2020**, *11*, 784. [CrossRef] [PubMed]
33. Jain, R.K. Normalizing tumor microenvironment to treat cancer: Bench to bedside to biomarkers. *J. Clin. Oncol.* **2013**, *31*, 2205–2218. [CrossRef] [PubMed]
34. Wilson, W.R.; Hay, M.P. Targeting hypoxia in cancer therapy. *Nat. Rev. Cancer* **2011**, *11*, 393–410. [CrossRef]
35. Facciabene, A.; Peng, X.; Hagemann, I.S.; Balint, K.; Barchetti, A.; Wang, L.-P.; Gimotty, P.A.; Gilks, C.B.; Lal, P.; Zhang, L.; et al. Tumour hypoxia promotes tolerance and angiogenesis via CCL28 and Treg cells. *Nature* **2011**, *475*, 226–230. [CrossRef]
36. Carmeliet, P.; Jain, R.K. Principles and mechanisms of vessel normalization for cancer and other angiogenic diseases. *Nat. Rev. Drug Discov.* **2011**, *10*, 417–427. [CrossRef]
37. Schaaf, M.B.; Garg, A.D.; Agostinis, P. Defining the role of the tumor vasculature in antitumor immunity and immunotherapy. *Cell Death Dis.* **2018**, *9*, 115. [CrossRef]
38. Poon, R.T.-P.; Fan, S.-T.; Wong, J. Clinical Implications of Circulating Angiogenic Factors in Cancer Patients. *J. Clin. Oncol.* **2001**, *19*, 1207–1225. [CrossRef]
39. Kalluri, R. The biology and function of fibroblasts in cancer. *Nat. Rev. Cancer* **2016**, *16*, 582–598. [CrossRef]
40. Yin, Z.; Dong, C.; Jiang, K.; Xu, Z.; Li, R.; Guo, K.; Shao, S.; Wang, L. Heterogeneity of cancer-associated fibroblasts and roles in the progression, prognosis, and therapy of hepatocellular carcinoma. *J. Hematol. Oncol.* **2019**, *12*, 101. [CrossRef]
41. Kubo, N.; Araki, K.; Kuwano, H.; Shirabe, K. Cancer-associated fibroblasts in hepatocellular carcinoma. *World J. Gastroenterol.* **2016**, *22*, 6841–6850. [CrossRef]
42. Fu, R.; Zhang, Y.-W.; Li, H.-M.; Lv, W.-C.; Zhao, L.; Guo, Q.-L.; Lu, T.; Weiss, S.J.; Li, Z.-Y.; Wu, Z.-Q. LW106, a novel indoleamine 2,3-dioxygenase 1 inhibitor, suppresses tumour progression by limiting stroma-immune crosstalk and cancer stem cell enrichment in tumour micro-environment. *Br. J. Pharm.* **2018**, *175*, 3034–3049. [CrossRef]
43. Najafi, M.; Farhood, B.; Mortezaee, K. Extracellular matrix (ECM) stiffness and degradation as cancer drivers. *J. Cell. Biochem.* **2019**, *120*, 2782–2790. [CrossRef]
44. Carloni, V.; Luong, T.V.; Rombouts, K. Hepatic stellate cells and extracellular matrix in hepatocellular carcinoma: More complicated than ever. *Liver Int.* **2014**, *34*, 834–843. [CrossRef]
45. Kumar, V.; Patel, S.; Tcyganov, E.; Gabrilovich, D.I. The Nature of Myeloid-Derived Suppressor Cells in the Tumor Microenvironment. *Trends Immunol.* **2016**, *37*, 208–220. [CrossRef]
46. Hao, X.; Sun, G.; Zhang, Y.; Kong, X.; Rong, D.; Song, J.; Tang, W.; Wang, X. Targeting Immune Cells in the Tumor Microenvironment of HCC: New Opportunities and Challenges. *Front. Cell Dev. Biol.* **2021**, *9*, 775462. [CrossRef]
47. Venook, A.P.; Papandreou, C.; Furuse, J.; de Guevara, L.L. The incidence and epidemiology of hepatocellular carcinoma: A global and regional perspective. *Oncologist* **2010**, *15* (Suppl. S4), 5–13. [CrossRef]

48. Pallett, L.J.; Gill, U.S.; Quaglia, A.; Sinclair, L.V.; Jover-Cobos, M.; Schurich, A.; Singh, K.P.; Thomas, N.; Das, A.; Chen, A.; et al. Metabolic regulation of hepatitis B immunopathology by myeloid-derived suppressor cells. *Nat. Med.* **2015**, *21*, 591–600. [CrossRef]
49. Zhang, X.; Fu, X.; Li, T.; Yan, H. The prognostic value of myeloid derived suppressor cell level in hepatocellular carcinoma: A systematic review and meta-analysis. *PLoS ONE* **2019**, *14*, e0225327. [CrossRef]
50. Rodríguez, P.C.; Ochoa, A.C. Arginine regulation by myeloid derived suppressor cells and tolerance in cancer: Mechanisms and therapeutic perspectives. *Immunol. Rev.* **2008**, *222*, 180–191. [CrossRef]
51. Wang, Y.; Zhang, T.; Sun, M.; Ji, X.; Xie, M.; Huang, W.; Xia, L. Therapeutic Values of Myeloid-Derived Suppressor Cells in Hepatocellular Carcinoma: Facts and Hopes. *Cancers* **2021**, *13*, 5127. [CrossRef] [PubMed]
52. Sakaguchi, S.; Yamaguchi, T.; Nomura, T.; Ono, M. Regulatory T Cells and Immune Tolerance. *Cell* **2008**, *133*, 775–787. [CrossRef] [PubMed]
53. Eisenstein, E.M.; Williams, C.B. The Treg/Th17 Cell Balance: A New Paradigm for Autoimmunity. *Pediatr. Res.* **2009**, *65*, 26–31. [CrossRef] [PubMed]
54. Fu, J.; Xu, D.; Liu, Z.; Shi, M.; Zhao, P.; Fu, B.; Zhang, Z.; Yang, H.; Zhang, H.; Zhou, C.; et al. Increased regulatory T cells correlate with CD8 T-cell impairment and poor survival in hepatocellular carcinoma patients. *Gastroenterology* **2007**, *132*, 2328–2339. [CrossRef]
55. Vignali, D.A.A.; Collison, L.W.; Workman, C.J. How regulatory T cells work. *Nat. Rev. Immunol.* **2008**, *8*, 523–532. [CrossRef]
56. Murray, P.J.; Allen, J.E.; Biswas, S.K.; Fisher, E.A.; Gilroy, D.W.; Goerdt, S.; Gordon, S.; Hamilton, J.A.; Ivashkiv, L.B.; Lawrence, T.; et al. Macrophage activation and polarization: Nomenclature and experimental guidelines. *Immunity* **2014**, *41*, 14–20. [CrossRef]
57. Cassetta, L.; Pollard, J.W. Tumor-associated macrophages. *Curr. Biol.* **2020**, *30*, R246–R248. [CrossRef]
58. Yang, J.; Zhang, J.-X.; Wang, H.; Wang, G.-L.; Hu, Q.-G.; Zheng, Q.-C. Hepatocellular carcinoma and macrophage interaction induced tumor immunosuppression via Treg requires TLR4 signaling. *World J. Gastroenterol.* **2012**, *18*, 2938–2947. [CrossRef]
59. Ju, C.; Tacke, F. Hepatic macrophages in homeostasis and liver diseases: From pathogenesis to novel therapeutic strategies. *Cell Mol. Immunol.* **2016**, *13*, 316–327. [CrossRef]
60. Yin, C.; Han, Q.; Xu, D.; Zheng, B.; Zhao, X.; Zhang, J. SALL4-mediated upregulation of exosomal miR-146a-5p drives T-cell exhaustion by M2 tumor-associated macrophages in HCC. *Oncoimmunology* **2019**, *8*, 1601479. [CrossRef]
61. Hou, P.-p.; Luo, L.-j.; Chen, H.-z.; Chen, Q.-t.; Bian, X.-l.; Wu, S.-f.; Zhou, J.-x.; Zhao, W.-x.; Liu, J.-m.; Wang, X.-m.; et al. Ectosomal PKM2 Promotes HCC by Inducing Macrophage Differentiation and Remodeling the Tumor Microenvironment. *Mol. Cell* **2020**, *78*, 1192–1206.e1110. [CrossRef]
62. Chen, J.; Lin, Z.; Liu, L.; Zhang, R.; Geng, Y.; Fan, M.; Zhu, W.; Lu, M.; Lu, L.; Jia, H.; et al. GOLM1 exacerbates CD8(+) T cell suppression in hepatocellular carcinoma by promoting exosomal PD-L1 transport into tumor-associated macrophages. *Signal Transduct. Target. Ther.* **2021**, *6*, 397. [CrossRef]
63. LaGory, E.L.; Giaccia, A.J. The ever-expanding role of HIF in tumour and stromal biology. *Nat. Cell Biol.* **2016**, *18*, 356–365. [CrossRef]
64. Dysthe, M.; Parihar, R. Myeloid-Derived Suppressor Cells in the Tumor Microenvironment. *Adv. Exp. Med. Biol.* **2020**, *1224*, 117–140. [CrossRef]
65. Cho, H.; Seo, Y.; Loke, K.M.; Kim, S.W.; Oh, S.M.; Kim, J.H.; Soh, J.; Kim, H.S.; Lee, H.; Kim, J.; et al. Cancer-Stimulated CAFs Enhance Monocyte Differentiation and Protumoral TAM Activation via IL6 and GM-CSF Secretion. *Clin. Cancer Res. Off. J. Am. Assoc. Cancer Res.* **2018**, *24*, 5407–5421. [CrossRef]
66. Ranganathan, R.; Madanmohan, S.; Kesavan, A.; Baskar, G.; Krishnamoorthy, Y.R.; Santosham, R.; Ponraju, D.; Rayala, S.K.; Venkatraman, G. Nanomedicine: Towards development of patient-friendly drug-delivery systems for oncological applications. *Int. J. Nanomed.* **2012**, *7*, 1043–1060. [CrossRef]
67. Turato, C.; Balasso, A.; Carloni, V.; Tiribelli, C.; Mastrotto, F.; Mazzocca, A.; Pontisso, P. New molecular targets for functionalized nanosized drug delivery systems in personalized therapy for hepatocellular carcinoma. *J. Control. Release Off. J. Control. Release Soc.* **2017**, *268*, 184–197. [CrossRef]
68. Martin, D.N.; Uprichard, S.L. Identification of transferrin receptor 1 as a hepatitis C virus entry factor. *Proc. Natl. Acad. Sci. USA* **2013**, *110*, 10777–10782. [CrossRef]
69. Pramanik, A.; Laha, D.; Pramanik, P.; Karmakar, P. A novel drug "copper acetylacetonate" loaded in folic acid-tagged chitosan nanoparticle for efficient cancer cell targeting. *J. Drug Target.* **2014**, *22*, 23–33. [CrossRef]
70. Wang, J.; Qian, Y.; Xu, L.; Shao, Y.; Zhang, H.; Shi, F.; Chen, J.; Cui, S.; Chen, X.; Zhu, D.; et al. Hyaluronic acid-shelled, peptide drug conjugate-cored nanomedicine for the treatment of hepatocellular carcinoma. *Mater. Sci. Eng. C* **2020**, *117*, 111261. [CrossRef]
71. Maghsoudinia, F.; Tavakoli, M.B.; Samani, R.K.; Hejazi, S.H.; Sobhani, T.; Mehradnia, F.; Mehrgardi, M.A. Folic acid-functionalized gadolinium-loaded phase transition nanodroplets for dual-modal ultrasound/magnetic resonance imaging of hepatocellular carcinoma. *Talanta* **2021**, *228*, 122245. [CrossRef] [PubMed]
72. Zhan, X.; Guan, Y.-Q. Design of magnetic nanoparticles for hepatocellular carcinoma treatment using the control mechanisms of the cell internal nucleus and external membrane. *J. Mater. Chem. B* **2015**, *3*, 4191–4204. [CrossRef] [PubMed]
73. Kumari, P.; Ghosh, B.; Biswas, S. Nanocarriers for cancer-targeted drug delivery. *J. Drug Target.* **2016**, *24*, 179–191. [CrossRef] [PubMed]

74. Shafei, A.; El-Bakly, W.; Sobhy, A.; Wagdy, O.; Reda, A.; Aboelenin, O.; Marzouk, A.; El Habak, K.; Mostafa, R.; Ali, M.A.; et al. A review on the efficacy and toxicity of different doxorubicin nanoparticles for targeted therapy in metastatic breast cancer. *Biomed. Pharmacother.* **2017**, *95*, 1209–1218. [CrossRef] [PubMed]
75. Pramanik, A.; Xu, Z.; Shamsuddin, S.H.; Khaled, Y.S.; Ingram, N.; Maisey, T.; Tomlinson, D.; Coletta, P.L.; Jayne, D.; Hughes, T.A.; et al. Affimer Tagged Cubosomes: Targeting of Carcinoembryonic Antigen Expressing Colorectal Cancer Cells Using In Vitro and In Vivo Models. *ACS Appl. Mater. Interfaces* **2022**, *14*, 11078–11091. [CrossRef] [PubMed]
76. Wang, Q.; Sun, Y.; Zhang, Z.; Duan, Y. Targeted polymeric therapeutic nanoparticles: Design and interactions with hepatocellular carcinoma. *Biomaterials* **2015**, *56*, 229–240. [CrossRef]
77. Lou, J.; Zhang, L.; Zheng, G. Advancing Cancer Immunotherapies with Nanotechnology. *Adv. Ther.* **2019**, *2*, 1800128. [CrossRef]
78. Wu, S.; Zhang, D.; Yu, J.; Dou, J.; Li, X.; Mu, M.; Liang, P. Chemotherapeutic Nanoparticle-Based Liposomes Enhance the Efficiency of Mild Microwave Ablation in Hepatocellular Carcinoma Therapy. *Front. Pharmacol.* **2020**, *11*, 85. [CrossRef]
79. Cen, D.; Ge, Q.; Xie, C.; Zheng, Q.; Guo, J.; Zhang, Y.; Wang, Y.; Li, X.; Gu, Z.; Cai, X. ZnS@BSA Nanoclusters Potentiate Efficacy of Cancer Immunotherapy. *Adv. Mater.* **2021**, *33*, 2104037. [CrossRef]
80. Liao, J.; Jia, Y.; Wu, Y.; Shi, K.; Yang, D.; Li, P.; Qian, Z. Physical-, chemical-, and biological-responsive nanomedicine for cancer therapy. *WIREs Nanomed. Nanobiotechnol.* **2020**, *12*, e1581. [CrossRef]
81. Barenholz, Y. Doxil®—The first FDA-approved nano-drug: Lessons learned. *J. Control. Release* **2012**, *160*, 117–134. [CrossRef]
82. Shi, J.; Kantoff, P.W.; Wooster, R.; Farokhzad, O.C. Cancer nanomedicine: Progress, challenges and opportunities. *Nat. Rev. Cancer* **2017**, *17*, 20–37. [CrossRef]
83. Azzi, S.; Hebda, J.K.; Gavard, J. Vascular permeability and drug delivery in cancers. *Front. Oncol.* **2013**, *3*, 211. [CrossRef]
84. Berretta, M.; Rinaldi, L.; Di Benedetto, F.; Lleshi, A.; De Re, V.; Facchini, G.; De Paoli, P.; Di Francia, R. Angiogenesis Inhibitors for the Treatment of Hepatocellular Carcinoma. *Front. Pharmacol.* **2016**, *7*, 428. [CrossRef]
85. Taketomi, A. Clinical trials of antiangiogenic therapy for hepatocellular carcinoma. *Int. J. Clin. Oncol.* **2016**, *21*, 213–218. [CrossRef]
86. Zhang, Y.N.; Poon, W.; Tavares, A.J.; McGilvray, I.D.; Chan, W.C.W. Nanoparticle-liver interactions: Cellular uptake and hepatobiliary elimination. *J. Control. Release Off. J. Control. Release Soc.* **2016**, *240*, 332–348. [CrossRef]
87. Hao, Q.; Wang, Z.; Zhao, W.; Wen, L.; Wang, W.; Lu, S.; Xing, D.; Zhan, M.; Hu, X. Dual-Responsive Polyprodrug Nanoparticles with Cascade-Enhanced Magnetic Resonance Signals for Deep-Penetration Drug Release in Tumor Therapy. *ACS Appl. Mater. Interfaces* **2020**, *12*, 49489–49501. [CrossRef]
88. Bazak, R.; Houri, M.; Achy, S.E.; Hussein, W.; Refaat, T. Passive targeting of nanoparticles to cancer: A comprehensive review of the literature. *Mol. Clin. Oncol.* **2014**, *2*, 904–908. [CrossRef]
89. Li, Z.; Ye, L.; Liu, J.; Lian, D.; Li, X. Sorafenib-Loaded Nanoparticles Based on Biodegradable Dendritic Polymers for Enhanced Therapy of Hepatocellular Carcinoma. *Int. J. Nanomed.* **2020**, *15*, 1469–1480. [CrossRef]
90. Kanasty, R.; Dorkin, J.R.; Vegas, A.; Anderson, D. Delivery materials for siRNA therapeutics. *Nat. Mater.* **2013**, *12*, 967–977. [CrossRef]
91. Han, L.; Tang, C.; Yin, C. Oral delivery of shRNA and siRNA via multifunctional polymeric nanoparticles for synergistic cancer therapy. *Biomaterials* **2014**, *35*, 4589–4600. [CrossRef]
92. Zheng, G.; Zhao, R.; Xu, A.; Shen, Z.; Chen, X.; Shao, J. Co-delivery of sorafenib and siVEGF based on mesoporous silica nanoparticles for ASGPR mediated targeted HCC therapy. *Eur. J. Pharm. Sci. Off. J. Eur. Fed. Pharm. Sci.* **2018**, *111*, 492–502. [CrossRef]
93. Chase, D.M.; Chaplin, D.J.; Monk, B.J. The development and use of vascular targeted therapy in ovarian cancer. *Gynecol. Oncol.* **2017**, *145*, 393–406. [CrossRef]
94. Wang, Y.; Chen, H.; Liu, Y.; Wu, J.; Zhou, P.; Wang, Y.; Li, R.; Yang, X.; Zhang, N. pH-sensitive pullulan-based nanoparticle carrier of methotrexate and combretastatin A4 for the combination therapy against hepatocellular carcinoma. *Biomaterials* **2013**, *34*, 7181–7190. [CrossRef] [PubMed]
95. Inglis, D.J.; Lavranos, T.C.; Beaumont, D.M.; Leske, A.F.; Brown, C.K.; Hall, A.J.; Kremmidiotis, G. The vascular disrupting agent BNC105 potentiates the efficacy of VEGF and mTOR inhibitors in renal and breast cancer. *Cancer Biol. Ther.* **2014**, *15*, 1552–1560. [CrossRef] [PubMed]
96. Bao, X.; Shen, N.; Lou, Y.; Yu, H.; Wang, Y.; Liu, L.; Tang, Z.; Chen, X. Enhanced anti-PD-1 therapy in hepatocellular carcinoma by tumor vascular disruption and normalization dependent on combretastatin A4 nanoparticles and DC101. *Theranostics* **2021**, *11*, 5955–5969. [CrossRef] [PubMed]
97. Chang, C.-C.; Dinh, T.K.; Lee, Y.-A.; Wang, F.-N.; Sung, Y.-C.; Yu, P.-L.; Chiu, S.-C.; Shih, Y.-C.; Wu, C.-Y.; Huang, Y.-D.; et al. Nanoparticle Delivery of MnO_2 and Antiangiogenic Therapy to Overcome Hypoxia-Driven Tumor Escape and Suppress Hepatocellular Carcinoma. *ACS Appl. Mater. Interfaces* **2020**, *12*, 44407–44419. [CrossRef] [PubMed]
98. Karimi, M.; Ghasemi, A.; Sahandi Zangabad, P.; Rahighi, R.; Moosavi Basri, S.M.; Mirshekari, H.; Amiri, M.; Shafaei Pishabad, Z.; Aslani, A.; Bozorgomid, M.; et al. Smart micro/nanoparticles in stimulus-responsive drug/gene delivery systems. *Chem. Soc. Rev.* **2016**, *45*, 1457–1501. [CrossRef]
99. Zhang, J.; Li, J.; Shi, Z.; Yang, Y.; Xie, X.; Lee, S.M.; Wang, Y.; Leong, K.W.; Chen, M. pH-sensitive polymeric nanoparticles for co-delivery of doxorubicin and curcumin to treat cancer via enhanced pro-apoptotic and anti-angiogenic activities. *Acta Biomater.* **2017**, *58*, 349–364. [CrossRef]

100. Arbiser, J.L.; Klauber, N.; Rohan, R.; van Leeuwen, R.; Huang, M.T.; Fisher, C.; Flynn, E.; Byers, H.R. Curcumin is an in vivo inhibitor of angiogenesis. *Mol. Med.* **1998**, *4*, 376–383. [CrossRef]
101. Sadzuka, Y.; Nagamine, M.; Toyooka, T.; Ibuki, Y.; Sonobe, T. Beneficial effects of curcumin on antitumor activity and adverse reactions of doxorubicin. *Int. J. Pharm.* **2012**, *432*, 42–49. [CrossRef]
102. Xiong, Y.-Q.; Sun, H.-C.; Zhang, W.; Zhu, X.-D.; Zhuang, P.-Y.; Zhang, J.-B.; Wang, L.; Wu, W.-z.; Qin, L.-X.; Tang, Z.-Y. Human Hepatocellular Carcinoma Tumor–derived Endothelial Cells Manifest Increased Angiogenesis Capability and Drug Resistance Compared with Normal Endothelial Cells. *Clin. Cancer Res.* **2009**, *15*, 4838–4846. [CrossRef]
103. Chaudhuri, O.; Koshy, S.T.; Branco da Cunha, C.; Shin, J.W.; Verbeke, C.S.; Allison, K.H.; Mooney, D.J. Extracellular matrix stiffness and composition jointly regulate the induction of malignant phenotypes in mammary epithelium. *Nat. Mater.* **2014**, *13*, 970–978. [CrossRef]
104. Bourboulia, D.; Stetler-Stevenson, W.G. Matrix metalloproteinases (MMPs) and tissue inhibitors of metalloproteinases (TIMPs): Positive and negative regulators in tumor cell adhesion. *Semin. Cancer Biol.* **2010**, *20*, 161–168. [CrossRef]
105. Liang, S.; Hu, J.; Xie, Y.; Zhou, Q.; Zhu, Y.; Yang, X. A polyethylenimine-modified carboxyl-poly(styrene/acrylamide) copolymer nanosphere for co-delivering of CpG and TGF-β receptor I inhibitor with remarkable additive tumor regression effect against liver cancer in mice. *Int. J. Nanomed.* **2016**, *11*, 6753–6762. [CrossRef]
106. Affo, S.; Yu, L.-X.; Schwabe, R.F. The Role of Cancer-Associated Fibroblasts and Fibrosis in Liver Cancer. *Annu. Rev. Pathol.* **2017**, *12*, 153–186. [CrossRef]
107. Greupink, R.; Bakker, H.I.; Reker-Smit, C.; van Loenen-Weemaes, A.M.; Kok, R.J.; Meijer, D.K.; Beljaars, L.; Poelstra, K. Studies on the targeted delivery of the antifibrogenic compound mycophenolic acid to the hepatic stellate cell. *J. Hepatol.* **2005**, *43*, 884–892. [CrossRef]
108. Yang, Z.; Zhang, L.; Zhu, H.; Zhou, K.; Wang, H.; Wang, Y.; Su, R.; Guo, D.; Zhou, L.; Xu, X.; et al. Nanoparticle formulation of mycophenolate mofetil achieves enhanced efficacy against hepatocellular carcinoma by targeting tumour-associated fibroblast. *J. Cell Mol. Med.* **2021**, *25*, 3511–3523. [CrossRef]
109. Arii, S.; Mise, M.; Harada, T.; Furutani, M.; Ishigami, S.; Niwano, M.; Mizumoto, M.; Fukumoto, M.; Imamura, M. Overexpression of matrix metalloproteinase 9 gene in hepatocellular carcinoma with invasive potential. *Hepatology* **1996**, *24*, 316–322. [CrossRef]
110. Cui, N.; Hu, M.; Khalil, R.A. Biochemical and Biological Attributes of Matrix Metalloproteinases. *Prog. Mol. Biol. Transl. Sci.* **2017**, *147*, 1–73. [CrossRef]
111. Ji, Y.; Xiao, Y.; Xu, L.; He, J.; Qian, C.; Li, W.; Wu, L.; Chen, R.; Wang, J.; Hu, R.; et al. Drug-Bearing Supramolecular MMP Inhibitor Nanofibers for Inhibition of Metastasis and Growth of Liver Cancer. *Adv. Sci.* **2018**, *5*, 1700867. [CrossRef]
112. Yeow, Y.L.; Wu, J.; Wang, X.; Winteringham, L.; Feindel, K.W.; Tirnitz-Parker, J.E.E.; Leedman, P.J.; Ganss, R.; Hamzah, J. ECM Depletion Is Required to Improve the Intratumoral Uptake of Iron Oxide Nanoparticles in Poorly Perfused Hepatocellular Carcinoma. *Front. Oncol.* **2022**, *12*, 837234. [CrossRef]
113. Luo, J.; Gong, T.; Ma, L. Chondroitin-modified lipid nanoparticles target the Golgi to degrade extracellular matrix for liver cancer management. *Carbohydr. Polym.* **2020**, *249*, 116887. [CrossRef]
114. Suzuki, E.; Kapoor, V.; Jassar, A.S.; Kaiser, L.R.; Albelda, S.M. Gemcitabine Selectively Eliminates Splenic Gr-1+/CD11b+ Myeloid Suppressor Cells in Tumor-Bearing Animals and Enhances Antitumor Immune Activity. *Clin. Cancer Res.* **2005**, *11*, 6713–6721. [CrossRef]
115. Plebanek, M.P.; Bhaumik, D.; Bryce, P.J.; Thaxton, C.S. Scavenger Receptor Type B1 and Lipoprotein Nanoparticle Inhibit Myeloid-Derived Suppressor Cells. *Mol. Cancer* **2018**, *17*, 686–697. [CrossRef]
116. Lai, C.; Yu, X.; Zhuo, H.; Zhou, N.; Xie, Y.; He, J.; Peng, Y.; Xie, X.; Luo, G.; Zhou, S.; et al. Anti-tumor immune response of folate-conjugated chitosan nanoparticles containing the IP-10 gene in mice with hepatocellular carcinoma. *J. Biomed. Nanotechnol.* **2014**, *10*, 3576–3589. [CrossRef]
117. Hu, Z.; Chen, J.; Zhou, S.; Yang, N.; Duan, S.; Zhang, Z.; Su, J.; He, J.; Zhang, Z.; Lu, X.; et al. Mouse IP-10 Gene Delivered by Folate-modified Chitosan Nanoparticles and Dendritic/tumor Cells Fusion Vaccine Effectively Inhibit the Growth of Hepatocellular Carcinoma in Mice. *Theranostics* **2017**, *7*, 1942–1952. [CrossRef]
118. Wang, Z.; He, L.; Li, W.; Xu, C.; Zhang, J.; Wang, D.; Dou, K.; Zhuang, R.; Jin, B.; Zhang, W.; et al. GDF15 induces immunosuppression via CD48 on regulatory T cells in hepatocellular carcinoma. *J. Immunother. Cancer* **2021**, *9*, e002787. [CrossRef]
119. Rosenberg, S.A. IL-2: The first effective immunotherapy for human cancer. *J. Immunol.* **2014**, *192*, 5451–5458. [CrossRef]
120. Tahvildari, M.; Dana, R. Low-Dose IL-2 Therapy in Transplantation, Autoimmunity, and Inflammatory Diseases. *J. Immunol.* **2019**, *203*, 2749–2755. [CrossRef]
121. Wu, J.; Tang, C.; Yin, C. Co-delivery of doxorubicin and interleukin-2 via chitosan based nanoparticles for enhanced antitumor efficacy. *Acta Biomater.* **2017**, *47*, 81–90. [CrossRef] [PubMed]
122. Huang, K.-W.; Hsu, F.-F.; Qiu, J.T.; Chern, G.-J.; Lee, Y.-A.; Chang, C.-C.; Huang, Y.-T.; Sung, Y.-C.; Chiang, C.-C.; Huang, R.-L.; et al. Highly efficient and tumor-selective nanoparticles for dual-targeted immunogene therapy against cancer. *Sci. Adv.* **2020**, *6*, eaax5032. [CrossRef] [PubMed]
123. Li, J.; Lin, W.; Chen, H.; Xu, Z.; Ye, Y.; Chen, M. Dual-target IL-12-containing nanoparticles enhance T cell functions for cancer immunotherapy. *Cell. Immunol.* **2020**, *349*, 104042. [CrossRef] [PubMed]
124. Tennant, D.A.; Durán, R.V.; Gottlieb, E. Targeting metabolic transformation for cancer therapy. *Nat. Rev. Cancer* **2010**, *10*, 267–277. [CrossRef]

125. Warburg, O. On the facultative anaerobiosis of cancer cells and its use in chemotherapy. *Munch. Med. Wochenschr. (1950)* **1961**, *103*, 2504–2506.
126. Dietl, K.; Renner, K.; Dettmer, K.; Timischl, B.; Eberhart, K.; Dorn, C.; Hellerbrand, C.; Kastenberger, M.; Kunz-Schughart, L.A.; Oefner, P.J.; et al. Lactic Acid and Acidification Inhibit TNF Secretion and Glycolysis of Human Monocytes. *J. Immunol.* **2010**, *184*, 1200. [CrossRef]
127. Brand, A.; Singer, K.; Koehl, G.E.; Kolitzus, M.; Schoenhammer, G.; Thiel, A.; Matos, C.; Bruss, C.; Klobuch, S.; Peter, K.; et al. LDHA-Associated Lactic Acid Production Blunts Tumor Immunosurveillance by T and NK Cells. *Cell Metab.* **2016**, *24*, 657–671. [CrossRef]
128. Raez, L.E.; Papadopoulos, K.; Ricart, A.D.; Chiorean, E.G.; Dipaola, R.S.; Stein, M.N.; Rocha Lima, C.M.; Schlesselman, J.J.; Tolba, K.; Langmuir, V.K.; et al. A phase I dose-escalation trial of 2-deoxy-D-glucose alone or combined with docetaxel in patients with advanced solid tumors. *Cancer Chemother. Pharmacol.* **2013**, *71*, 523–530. [CrossRef]
129. Sasaki, K.; Nishina, S.; Yamauchi, A.; Fukuda, K.; Hara, Y.; Yamamura, M.; Egashira, K.; Hino, K. Nanoparticle-Mediated Delivery of 2-Deoxy-D-Glucose Induces Antitumor Immunity and Cytotoxicity in Liver Tumors in Mice. *Cell. Mol. Gastroenterol. Hepatol.* **2021**, *11*, 739–762. [CrossRef]
130. Chen, Y.; Huang, Y.; Reiberger, T.; Duyverman, A.M.; Huang, P.; Samuel, R.; Hiddingh, L.; Roberge, S.; Koppel, C.; Lauwers, G.Y.; et al. Differential effects of sorafenib on liver versus tumor fibrosis mediated by stromal-derived factor 1 alpha/C-X-C receptor type 4 axis and myeloid differentiation antigen–positive myeloid cell infiltration in mice. *Hepatology* **2014**, *59*, 1435–1447. [CrossRef]
131. Duda, D.G.; Kozin, S.V.; Kirkpatrick, N.D.; Xu, L.; Fukumura, D.; Jain, R.K. CXCL12 (SDF1alpha)-CXCR4/CXCR7 pathway inhibition: An emerging sensitizer for anticancer therapies? *Clin. Cancer Res. Off. J. Am. Assoc. Cancer Res.* **2011**, *17*, 2074–2080. [CrossRef]
132. Gao, D.-Y.; Lin, T.-T.; Sung, Y.-C.; Liu, Y.C.; Chiang, W.-H.; Chang, C.-C.; Liu, J.-Y.; Chen, Y. CXCR4-targeted lipid-coated PLGA nanoparticles deliver sorafenib and overcome acquired drug resistance in liver cancer. *Biomaterials* **2015**, *67*, 194–203. [CrossRef]
133. Li, G.; Liu, D.; Kimchi, E.T.; Kaifi, J.T.; Qi, X.; Manjunath, Y.; Liu, X.; Deering, T.; Avella, D.M.; Fox, T.; et al. Nanoliposome C6-Ceramide Increases the Anti-tumor Immune Response and Slows Growth of Liver Tumors in Mice. *Gastroenterology* **2018**, *154*, 1024–1036.e1029. [CrossRef]
134. Ngambenjawong, C.; Gustafson, H.H.; Pun, S.H. Progress in tumor-associated macrophage (TAM)-targeted therapeutics. *Adv. Drug Deliv. Rev.* **2017**, *114*, 206–221. [CrossRef]
135. Wang, T.; Zhang, J.; Hou, T.; Yin, X.; Zhang, N. Selective targeting of tumor cells and tumor associated macrophages separately by twin-like core–shell nanoparticles for enhanced tumor-localized chemoimmunotherapy. *Nanoscale* **2019**, *11*, 13934–13946. [CrossRef]
136. Kaps, L.; Leber, N.; Klefenz, A.; Choteschovsky, N.; Zentel, R.; Nuhn, L.; Schuppan, D. In Vivo siRNA Delivery to Immunosuppressive Liver Macrophages by α-Mannosyl-Functionalized Cationic Nanohydrogel Particles. *Cells* **2020**, *9*, 1905. [CrossRef]
137. Boutilier, A.J.; Elsawa, S.F. Macrophage Polarization States in the Tumor Microenvironment. *Int. J. Mol. Sci.* **2021**, *22*, 6995. [CrossRef]
138. Dai, X.; Ruan, J.; Guo, Y.; Sun, Z.; Liu, J.; Bao, X.; Zhang, H.; Li, Q.; Ye, C.; Wang, X.; et al. Enhanced radiotherapy efficacy and induced anti-tumor immunity in HCC by improving hypoxia microenvironment using oxygen microcapsules. *Chem. Eng. J.* **2021**, *422*, 130109. [CrossRef]
139. Comparetti, E.J.; Lins, P.M.P.; Quitiba, J.; Zucolotto, V. Cancer cell membrane-derived nanoparticles block the expression of immune checkpoint proteins on cancer cells and coordinate modulatory activity on immunosuppressive macrophages. *J. Biomed. Mater. Res. Part A* **2022**, *110*, 1499–1511. [CrossRef]
140. Li, Y.; Ayala-Orozco, C.; Rauta, P.R.; Krishnan, S. The application of nanotechnology in enhancing immunotherapy for cancer treatment: Current effects and perspective. *Nanoscale* **2019**, *11*, 17157–17178. [CrossRef]

MDPI AG
Grosspeteranlage 5
4052 Basel
Switzerland
Tel.: +41 61 683 77 34

Nanomaterials Editorial Office
E-mail: nanomaterials@mdpi.com
www.mdpi.com/journal/nanomaterials

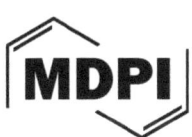

Disclaimer/Publisher's Note: The statements, opinions and data contained in all publications are solely those of the individual author(s) and contributor(s) and not of MDPI and/or the editor(s). MDPI and/or the editor(s) disclaim responsibility for any injury to people or property resulting from any ideas, methods, instructions or products referred to in the content.

www.ingramcontent.com/pod-product-compliance
Lightning Source LLC
LaVergne TN
LVHW072337090526
838202LV00019B/2437